Treating Complex Trauma

Tamara McClintock Greenberg

Treating Complex Trauma

Combined Theories and Methods

Springer

Tamara McClintock Greenberg
Clinical Psychologist, Private Practice
San Francisco, CA, USA

ISBN 978-3-030-45284-1 ISBN 978-3-030-45285-8 (eBook)
https://doi.org/10.1007/978-3-030-45285-8

This Springer imprint is published by the registered company Springer Nature Switzerland AG
The registered company address is: Gewerbestrasse 11, 6330 Cham, Switzerland

Preface

Despite significant increases in the numbers of therapeutic treatments offered to the public, people who have experienced complex trauma struggle to find relief from debilitating symptoms. Complex trauma or complex post-traumatic stress disorder (cPTSD) differs substantially from a diagnosis of PTSD. Complex PTSD impacts the identity of people afflicted and is thought to be more difficult to treat. Common symptoms of cPTSD include relationship difficulties, suicidality, physical symptoms, substance use, dissociation, difficulty regulating and modulating emotions, and a sense of meaninglessness. These latter three experiences (referred to in some literature as disturbances of self-regulation) often co-occur with what we think of as traditional PTSD symptoms, such as hypervigilance, re-experiencing traumatic events, psychic numbing, and avoidance. Though many people who have experienced trauma can appear to have lives that are well-adjusted, some are so impacted by symptoms they have not been able to develop careers or have meaningful relationships.

As I will argue throughout this book, complicated clients need multiple and flexible approaches to help them get better. I think we can help people who have been impacted by severe trauma, but it requires viewing them through a different lens. This starts with considering developmental adaptations required of trauma survivors and that some of the labels we have ascribed, especially ideas that they have personality disorders, no longer suit us or the people we care for.

I think the recent rise in interest of complex trauma is a healthy reaction to decades of pathologizing clients and worse, leading people to believe their conditions are beyond help. Current research and clinical observations support the idea that a trauma-informed approach to treatment provides hope for clients who may have not had the benefit of a more empathic and comprehensive understanding. It's not just minds that are impacted by trauma, bodies are too. Many of the symptoms we can find difficult and vexing often have neurobiological underpinnings, meaning clients who often want to have different kinds of lives feel forced into patterns they cannot help but repeat. Dissociation is common in people who have cPTSD, which means that clients have built-in defenses that can challenge our assessment and intervention skills. People who have survived repeated trauma need us to adapt and shift in order to accommodate where someone lives emotionally at a given point and time. This includes willingness to be flexible with and knowledgeable of different therapeutic techniques and methods.

This volume will focus on several aspects of therapeutic treatment for persons who have experienced complex childhood and adult trauma. It will focus on what we know, which is that empathy and the stability of the therapeutic relationship explain therapeutic outcome more than any other variable. However, while our relationships are vital, treatment with people who have cPTSD also requires clinicians who can think in a flexible and moment-to-moment way about what clients need. Some therapists emphasize one or two main approaches and then assume or hope that these approaches can apply to the many diverse clients that present for help. While advocates of different theories claim they have the right answer, therapeutic technique accounts for only roughly 15% of the variance of therapeutic outcome. Adding to the confusion, there is no one superior theory for treating trauma. All empirically validated approaches have roughly equal efficacy. Clinicians, who have become increasingly tribal in the wars on theory, have failed to utilize combined approaches, which I'll argue is a great tragedy for the people who need our help.

In this book, I will provide a framework for helping the most complicated and challenging people we face as clinicians. Despite a large number of therapeutic theories and modalities within our field, there is confusion among even very skilled clinicians about how to be helpful. However, what concerns me most is the trend among some to advocate one or two theories and accompanying techniques and then to apply these techniques to most or all clients that seek treatment. Such an approach is limited. There is no one-size-fits-all approach to the treatment of complex trauma.

There was a time when clinicians were taught multiple ways to help people and were encouraged to use all available "tools in the toolbox." A person needing help walked in the door and the clinician decided which approach would work best based on symptoms and presentation, including DSM diagnoses, values and beliefs, cognitive and learning style, coping skills, behaviors, character structure, current and past relational attachments, and family history. While many approaches may still be taught in graduate programs, the current climate of psychotherapy research and practice is akin to a horse race. Clinicians have a curious investment in proving that they have the best theory and technique, as opposed to thoughtfully considering which approaches work best for whom and, most importantly, what techniques the client can tolerate.

We are fortunate to have a number of options for helping people. In this book I will focus on my nearly 30 years of experience of helping clients, what I have learned from them, as well as supervising and teaching younger colleagues eager to learn about the variety of ways to alleviate human suffering. This book will be a guide for therapists who may not have had the benefit of learning multiple approaches. For people who are new to the field, I hope to provide examples of how to think in ways that move beyond just techniques and that my explanations of my missteps can be useful and informative. It may also be helpful to well-seasoned clinicians who are looking for additional ways to think about the multiple avenues we can use to help clients with cPTSD. I'll offer client examples, ideas for interventions, and explanations regarding what I say to clients and why. I'll introduce the concept and technique of clinical hypothesis testing and how constant evaluation of people in our care can lead us to choose or alter treatment approaches; often this is necessary in just one session. I'll discuss ways to provide ongoing assessment of clients and ideas for when specific therapies should be used or avoided.

It was as gratifying as it was challenging to weave in multiple theories and methods for treating complex trauma, many of which literally have different languages and typologies to describe the impact of the many terrifying experiences faced by the people we are trying to help. There are many important ideas about how to help people who have survived repetitive and multiple traumas. But no theory can do it all, and I learned as I talked with talented clinicians and researchers that we all can learn a lot from each other.

In this book I will offer a number of overarching themes about what seems to make therapy work for people who have endured trauma. These include the therapeutic relationship, clinical hypothesis testing, the use of several and flexible approaches, and the importance of mentalizing and the imagining of psychic experience as key aspects of facilitating therapeutic change. At times, I will express my preference for various CBT approaches; at others. I might imply my use of modern psychodynamic methods that focus on the present and current relational functioning. I assume the reader of this book already has ideas about how to help people with their own preferred methods. My disclosure of what techniques I use and when is not meant to be implemented in a rigid way. I trust the reader can determine for herself or himself what works best for whom and when. My main goal is just to implore us to think about how we need to use many techniques to help people. Flexibility is what I am advocating for here.

I will address the most challenging aspects of care. After describing the benefits and limitations of multiple empirically validated approaches, I will focus on how to help clients feel safe, including the important aspects of neurobiology and physiological responses that work together with psychological constructs to reinforce that the world is a dangerous place. I'll emphasize the importance and clinical utility of thinking about, imagining, and managing fear. I will address suicidality early on in this book as suicide and deaths of despair are at near-epidemic levels in the United States and elsewhere. Following that, I will describe the important phenomena of dissociation and how understanding this process is vital to clinical work. I will discuss substance use in detail and the variety of ways we can think about and help people who need to excessively numb themselves from their own thoughts and feelings. As trauma often lands in the body, an entire chapter is devoted to physical concerns among trauma survivors. Another problem that has both physical and psychological etiology is aggression and anger. I'll describe ways to provide support and safety among clients who simply cannot control more aggressive aspects of their behavior, as well as the devastating impact of anger when turned on the self. As we increasingly realize that cultural and systemic aspects of racism and other forms of discrimination are important contributors to mental health and can be traumatic, I will describe research and clinical experiences impacting people who have historically been negated and minimized. Finally, I will discuss the very real impact of vicarious trauma and self-care in the trauma therapist and ways we can consider how to take care of ourselves while taking care of others.

A few notes about how I describe clinical material and emotionally charged topics. A lot of trauma books go into details about specific kinds of abuse, victimization, and traumatic events. Since I am assuming that the reader is aware of the many kinds of traumas people experience, I am going to limit details of traumatic events. In my experience as a reader of books on trauma, I sometimes find detailed discussions of horrific events to be unnecessary. Additionally, since statistics suggest that a number of people reading this book might have histories of trauma, I'd like to keep the material from being too overstimulating. It's not that I don't discuss difficult material, but I do so with the least amount of information possible, so that I can still get my point across. This is also to protect confidentiality. And on that note, although cases are described in this book, they are heavily and judiciously composite. Any details have been additionally disguised to protect privacy.

San Francisco, CA, USA Tamara McClintock Greenberg

Acknowledgments

I am delighted to again be publishing a book with Springer Nature and am very thankful to Sofia Geck and Sharon Panulla who offered enthusiastic support when my ideas for this project were in their infancy.

I am so grateful to many colleagues who took time to comment on aspects of this book and to fill in gaps regarding my understanding of research and clinical developments. Laura Brown, Ph.D., helped me understand the history of trauma therapy and what was involved in the advocacy of treatment for trauma survivors. Thalia Robakis, M.D., Ph.D., fielded endless questions from me regarding how to understand and articulate the neurobiology of trauma. Bethany Brand, Ph.D., Constance Dalenberg, Ph.D., and Richard Chefetz, M.D., generously offered time to educate me on resources and controversies regarding dissociation. John Norcross, Ph.D., was similarly generous in sharing his work on the healing aspects of the therapeutic relationship as well as his writing on the importance of therapist self-care. Lisa Najavits, Ph.D., provided a great deal of context for working with people who have both complex PTSD and substance use problems. David Rudd, Ph.D., offered hope and inspiration as a clinician specializing in suicide and he helped me appreciate how so many theories are linked together by one common value, the reparative relationship we can offer as therapists.

I am especially grateful to Ghislaine Boulanger, Ph.D., Juli Fraga, Ph.D., Tom Rosbrow, Ph.D., and Lee Rather, Ph.D., who read chapters and offered valuable feedback. I am especially thankful to Andrew McClintock Greenberg, M.D., Ph.D. As my partner for 20 years, he's provided a foundation and an anchor for everything that I do. His clinical skills with people from a variety of backgrounds, especially those who have experienced discrimination and the insults a lack of privilege provides, inspires me every day. He's been through a few writing projects with me, but this particular book took more of my time and a lot more of his patience and understanding than previous works.

Finally, though, if it were not for my clients who entrusted me with their care, this book would not be possible. It is from them I have learned and continue to learn how to heal trauma. This book is because of them and for them. I hope it speaks to their experience and to the many lost voices and identities that trauma has attempted to take away.

Contents

Chapter 1
The Need for Utilizing Multiple Approaches for Complex PTSD: No Theory Has It All

Introduction: Complex Clients Need Multiple Approaches

Despite significant increases in the numbers of therapeutic treatments offered to the public, people who have experienced complex trauma struggle to find relief from debilitating symptoms. Complex trauma or complex post-traumatic stress disorder (cPTSD) differs substantially from a diagnosis of PTSD. Introduced by Herman (1992) and expanded upon most notably by Van der Kolk (e.g., 1994, 1996; Van der Kolk et al. 2012) and Courtois and Ford (2009, 2013), cPTSD impacts the identity of people afflicted and is difficult to treat. Common symptoms include relationship difficulties, suicidality, physical symptoms, substance use, dissociation, difficulty regulating and modulating emotions, and a sense of meaninglessness. These latter three experiences (referred to in some literature as disturbances of self-regulation, or DOS) often co-occur with what we think of as traditional PTSD symptoms, such as hypervigilance (that may co-occur or be misconstrued as hypomania; I'll speak to this more in subsequent chapters), re-experiencing traumatic events, psychic numbing, and avoidance. Though many people who have experienced trauma can appear to have lives that are well-adjusted, some are so impacted by symptoms they have not been able to develop careers or have meaningful relationships. Consider the following case example:

Melanie is a 30-year-old woman who came to therapy after a partial hospitalization program. She landed in San Francisco a few years ago after getting her "dream job" as a software engineer at a start-up. Though she was excited about moving from another part of the country, by the time we met, she had been fired from her third job. She could not tell me exactly why she was let go from her previous positions, though was able to say that she didn't like her most of her co-workers or bosses. After she lost her third position, Melanie became increasingly anxious, with frequent panic attacks. She thought in these moments she was dying. Her anxiety, however, was equally matched by severe episodes of depression, and she had days where she could not get out of bed. Eventually she thought a lot about suicide and

T. M. Greenberg, *Treating Complex Trauma*,
https://doi.org/10.1007/978-3-030-45285-8_1

on the eve of a visit from her family emailed her mother and told her she was going to kill herself. Her panicked mother called the police and Melanie was brought to a hospital for evaluation. She denied being suicidal and said she did not even remember sending the email. The psychiatrist assessing her was concerned but did not feel he had enough evidence for a mandatory psychiatric hold but convinced Melanie to enter into a partial hospitalization program, which she attended for 3 weeks.

When we met, Melanie appeared to be very astute psychologically. Though she initially told me this was her first time having difficulties, I eventually learned that she started therapy in college and had seen "six or eight" therapists before myself. She couldn't tell me much about her life, except that she knew she needed to find a job and she worried about what her parents might think if she remains unemployed. She had a boyfriend, but it was hard to get a sense of how serious the two were, as they had been dating roughly 3 months. Regarding her upbringing, she reported stoically that her parents were "good to her" with very vague details about their lives and careers, and she denied any difficulties growing up that might contribute to her current situation. She said she kept thinking if she could just find the right job, with people who understood her abilities, then everything would be okay. When asked if she had thoughts about starting therapy again, she looked at me blankly and said, "Well, if this helps, that would be good. I don't know if it will."

Compared with other clinical issues, we know relatively little about cPTSD. For example, the diagnosis was not included in the most recent edition of the *Diagnostic and Statistical Manual of Mental Disorders*, though it will be included in the ICD-11 (Brewin 2019). Part of the reason for the DSM omission and the relative lack of attention paid to this diagnosis may be because cPTSD symptoms overlap with other symptoms of mental illnesses. For example, researchers have noted overlap between cPTSD and borderline personality disorder (e.g., Ford and Courtois 2014). Among many clinicians, cPTSD is a euphemism for personality disorders. I was recently talking with a younger clinician finishing his fourth year of graduate school. When I told him I was writing a book about complex PTSD, he said, "Oh, so personality disorders." I'll discuss this issue in much more detail in the next chapter, but the complexity of treating people who have experienced severe, repetitive traumas, I think, has led to difficulties involving both inaccurate and compassionate diagnoses. Some people, especially those who have more symptoms of disturbances of self-regulation, may seem *personality disordered* to some clinicians. What is often meant by this moniker is that patients seem brittle in their defensive structure, they may have little external support due to social isolation (presumably because they have difficulty with relationships), they may be prone to suicidal thoughts and/or excessive use of substances, they may appear overly concrete or literal in their thinking (suggesting to some clinicians that they may not appreciate symbolic or abstract interpretations), and sometimes, we feel uncomfortable in their presence. Maybe they seem angry, or perhaps they are envious or hesitant to be dependent on us and trust our authority. Suspicious people often fall into the category of "difficult" and are certainly not sought after as patients. And yet, many of these symptoms are common among people with cPTSD.

Some people with cPTSD have been viewed as being too challenging to help, as their character styles are already baked in. Childhood trauma does impact how or if we develop a cohesive sense of self, as well as our personality style, the capacity to tolerate stress, the ability to form healthy relationships, etc. Adult trauma can shake the foundation of self-structure, at times causing it to collapse (Boulanger 2007).

No matter how we theorize it, these clients are often complex and vexing. Some of us also worry these clients will be aggressive and may be unable to form a good working relationship, and for those who use structured cognitive behavioral therapies, worries abound that the client will not be compliant. Yet despite the challenges, there's something just not quite right and a bit unfair regarding how some of these clients have been viewed. One problem with the ways we've focused on maladaptive personality traits is that if we begin treatment with the idea that someone is "characterologically disturbed," we tend to lack sympathy. Some may also worry that these clients cannot be helped, a hangover from the older teachings on the treatment of people with personality disorders. Conversely, if we think of someone as having survived trauma, we generally tend to not only have more empathy, but we may try harder to help. Additionally, we may rightly assume that it will take the client a long time to trust us, and our expectations regarding compliance and the development of therapeutic alliance could be more tempered. As we will see throughout the course of this book, we often have to be creative and flexible in order to help some of the clients who show up in our offices. My main point is that if we think of people through a trauma-focused lens, we are often more able to access empathy and our own motivation as helping professionals. Indeed, no matter what kind of therapy we practice, no matter what kind of techniques we prefer, we are often treating coping mechanisms that originate from something that worked at some point before they met us. If we start with that premise, we may be more inspired to find ways to help.

I think the recent rise in interest of complex trauma is a healthy reaction to decades of pathologizing clients and worse, leading people to believe their conditions are beyond help. Modern research and clinical observations support the idea that a trauma-informed approach to treatment provides hope for clients who may have not had the benefit of a more empathic and comprehensive understanding. It's not just minds that are impacted by trauma, bodies are too. Many of the symptoms we can find difficult and vexing often have neurobiological underpinnings, meaning clients who often want to have different kinds of lives feel forced into patterns they cannot help but repeat. Dissociation is common in people who have cPTSD, which means that clients have built-in defenses that can challenge our assessment and intervention skills. People who have survived repeated trauma need us to adapt and shift in order to accommodate where someone lives emotionally at a given point and time. This includes willingness to be flexible with and knowledgeable of different therapeutic techniques and methods.

This volume will focus on several aspects of therapeutic treatment for persons who have experienced complex childhood and adult trauma. It will focus on what we know, which is that empathy and the stability of the therapeutic relationship explain therapeutic outcome more than every other variable. However, more than a good relationship is needed for patients to get better. Our relationships are vital but also require clinicians who can think in a flexible and moment-to-moment way about what clients need. Some therapists emphasize one or two main approaches and then assume or hope that these approaches can apply to the many diverse clients that present for help. While advocates of different theories claim they have the right approach, therapeutic technique accounts for only roughly 15% of the variance of therapeutic outcome. Adding to the confusion, there is no one superior theory for treating trauma. All approaches have roughly equal efficacy. Clinicians, who have become increasingly tribal in the wars on theory, have failed to utilize combined approaches, which I'll argue is a great tragedy for the people who need our help.

In this book, I will provide a framework for helping the most complicated and challenging people we face as clinicians. Clients such as Melanie often bounce from one therapist to another looking for help. Despite a large number of therapeutic theories and modalities within our field, there is confusion among even very skilled clinicians about how to be helpful. However, what concerns me most is the trend in the field to advocate one or two theories and accompanying techniques and then to apply these techniques to most or all clients that seek treatment. Sometimes clients who see therapists who have only one or two tools in their toolbox can feel that they, as clients and trauma survivors, are broken and unfixable. This is often not true. There is no one-size-fits-all approach to the treatment of complex trauma. And the reality is that for people with cPTSD, during one session, a particular method may work. The next session, a whole new approach may need to be used. As one trauma expert described, "We need to be able to just sit in a room with clients before rushing in with our approach or technique." No matter which therapy we use, it's all about the relationship and relating to a client in a human and authentic way.

There was a time when clinicians who went to grad school were taught multiple ways to help people. A person needing help walked in the door and the clinician decided which approach would work best based on symptoms and presentation, including DSM diagnoses, values and beliefs, cognitive and learning style, coping skills, behaviors, character, and current and past relational attachments and family history. While many approaches may still be taught in graduate programs, the current climate of psychotherapy is akin to a horse race, in which clinicians have a curious investment in proving that they have the best theory and technique, as opposed to thoughtfully considering which approaches work best for whom and most importantly, what techniques the patient can tolerate. We are fortunate to have a number of options for helping people. In this book I will focus on my nearly 30 years of experience of helping clients, what I have learned from them, as well as supervising and teaching younger colleagues eager to learn about the variety of ways to alleviate human suffering. This book will be a guide for therapists who may not have had the benefit of learning multiple approaches. I'll offer client examples, ideas for interventions, and explanations regarding what I say to clients and why. I'll introduce the practice of clinical hypothesis testing and how constant evaluation of people in our care can lead us to choose or alter treatment approaches; often this is necessary in just one session. I'll discuss ways to provide ongoing assessment of clients and ideas for when specific therapies should be used or avoided.

The rest of this chapter will review the data on efficacy in psychotherapy and how overreliance on technique or theory neglects the most robust indicator of therapeutic success—the relationship between therapist and client. That being said, I will also briefly review the most common empirically validated therapies used to address PTSD and cPTSD. I'll discuss the controversies that exist in the field and challenges in the study of people with PTSD and cPTSD, and I'll introduce the notion of clinical hypothesis testing and how we can begin to apply that concept from the first meeting. First, let's think about trauma and what it actually means.

What Is Trauma and Who Gets to Define It?

Upon hearing about this project, a few colleagues urged me to define trauma with specific concerns that this term has been overused and overapplied. At first I was a little defensive about these comments. I assumed that trauma and traumatic events were obvious. Then one of my colleagues showed me a flyer for a conference entitled, "The Trauma of Falling in Love." I started to get the point. At that time I wasn't aware that there have been calls for people in the mental health field to limit the use of the term trauma. One author noted that it's problematic for us to interpret adversity as trauma and describes this in the context of suffering as being integral to the human condition (Haslam 2016). In an opinion piece in the *Chicago Tribune*, Haslam describes the problem as when people describe trauma in response to "microaggression, reading something offensive without a trigger warning or even watching upsetting news unfold on television." He even refers to someone describing a "hair trauma" because she did not like the texture of her hair. I appreciate the point that Haslam and others have made about the overuse of the term trauma. I am also cognizant of the debates on college campuses, for example, regarding the request for "trigger warnings" when students are exposed to something that might be unpleasant. I can understand where it could go too far, the idea that people should be protected from certain facts because they make them uncomfortable. However, it also occurs to me that what may be described as traumatic by some has meaning that could be explored in a therapeutic relationship with a sense of curiosity about what specifically feels traumatic. Just because someone says they were upset by something they read or heard in a college class does not mean they have not been traumatized, though I would agree that the specific "trigger" may not be a trauma. However, triggers can feel traumatic as they can remind people of more severe and dangerous episodes in their lives. We should try to understand the meanings of people's concerns. In other words, I agree with the criticisms about the overuse of the word trauma and the way the word has lost some meaning in our lexicon. Yet, people do get triggered by material that reminds them of something terrible and frightening that happened to them. If we look at statistics, even just on how many people experience sexual assault, they are sobering. According to the Centers for Disease Control (Smith et al. 2018), more than one in three women and nearly one in four men have experienced sexual violence involving physical contact at some point in their lives.

Nearly 1 in 5 women and 1 in 38 men have experienced completed or attempted rape in their lifetimes. That's pretty striking. On the other hand, although 70% of the US population experiences at least one traumatic event in their lifetime, only approximately 6% develop PTSD (Breslau 2009; Pietrzak et al. 2011). This implies that we are incredibly resilient. Most of us do not develop PTSD from a single traumatic event. But traumatic events do have meanings that are woven into people's personalities. For example, I recall events in recent history in which public figures were accused of or actually admitted to sexual assault. Following those revelations I had many clients, some of whom I'd known for years tell me stories of similar things that had happened to them. They never considered themselves victims, they thought it was normal and that it happens to everyone, or they simply "forgot" about it. In fact, it's important to remember that many people who experience sexual assaults, abuse, and many other devastating traumatic events often don't advertise this. Shame quiets people.

As therapists, we should take an open and accepting stance about anything people want to describe, no matter how they label it. I also don't feel that we should define experiences for our clients. Although we may think of something as traumatic, we need to see if our clients feel that way. As I'll discuss in the chapter on dissociation, we have seen the damage done from therapists defining a client's experience before they are ready to fully understand their histories. Whenever we purport to know more than a client about their history, we engage in a kind of identity theft. A client's history is theirs to tell, understand, and think about, if they want to. Complex PTSD already robs people of their identities, and if we tell people who and what they are and how they came to be, it reenacts experiences of someone exploiting their power and control. Basing psychotherapy on a relational model allows therapists and client to discover together the meanings and nuances of different life events.

In writing this book and describing trauma, I am going to talk about people who have been repeatedly subject to traumatic and adverse experiences. As we'll see, childhood trauma predicts adult trauma because of a number of complex variables and mechanisms. I'll describe the plight of veterans who often have histories of childhood maltreatment or neglect and go on to multiple deployments based on extended wars and conflicts. I'll discuss the damaging nature of extended periods of neglect in childhood and how this can be a form of trauma in children who do not have the developmental capacity to handle demands associated with emotionally or physically caring for themselves. Likewise, physical and sexual assaults in both childhood and adulthood force people to confront terror, confusion, and helplessness. I'll describe the impact of traumas experienced by adults who work as first responders, police officers, and emergency workers after natural disasters or violent community events and by those in countries in which there is sectarian violence, as well as alienation and discrimination based on gender, sexual orientation, race, ethnicity, and religion.

In other words, I will discuss situations in which the aggregate of hurtful, frightening, and out of control experiences leaves people with a variety of emotional problems that meet criteria for PTSD and cPTSD. I am not advocating a position of people externalizing blame for their problems. Indeed, most people I see with backgrounds of trauma blame themselves. They feel responsible for the fact that they don't have better lives, that they have "let themselves" be victimized (which is not true, but a way to maintain a sense of agency and control). They feel confused about whether or not they are entitled to be treated well and they don't know if their thoughts and perceptions are realistic or not. I'm not too worried about clients overusing the term trauma largely because many people with complex trauma histories with PTSD want to avoid talking about what has happened to them. But when people do describe trauma, it's important to believe them, even though stories and feelings about trauma can shift over a lifetime and even over the course of treatment.

The remainder of this chapter will go on to distinguish differences between PTSD and cPTSD, and the rest of this book will describe the healing of wounds following multiple traumatic events.

Difficulties in the Study of Complex Trauma

Trauma survivors are an incredibly diverse group of people, and to use the language of researchers, heterogeneity is the enemy of clean research. Trauma experiences involve veterans in war scenarios, immigrants, and refugees who struggled to get to a safe country and spent time in camps, victims of childhood slavery and sex trafficking, and even those who, in some countries, experience violence related to being attacked for being part of some religious, racial, or sexual or gender minority groups. In addition, people who develop severe, life-threatening illnesses can experience PTSD symptoms, as well as people in traumatic accidents, victims of domestic violence, and people who were abused or neglected as children. This latter group may be the most complicated of all to treat and study for several reasons. First, people abused as children (and those with chronic traumatic experiences) are harder to treat with less successful outcomes. This makes sense, as childhood trauma can disrupt the ability to form a cohesive self that includes the ability to manage anxiety, stress, disappointment, and whatever adverse events that may be experienced throughout the lifespan. No matter what one's theoretical orientation, I think most of us agree that a safe and protected childhood, and one in which people feel loved, allows people to enter the world with a good ability to tolerate difficult emotions and the stress of life in general. I think of a secure childhood as creating a scenario for the development of a good relationship with one's mind and the presence of internal resources. Stress of any kind requires us to go inside of ourselves and to be able to know what we think and feel, as well as what we need. It also allows us to trust our feelings, an important skill especially in relationships, as it gives us confidence to be assertive and set limits. Trauma truncates our ability to think, but childhood trauma can create a paucity of internal resources and can limit the ability to recognize vital thoughts and feelings, and this creates a different starting place in psychotherapy. As I've argued (Greenberg 2016), we often expect that traumatized clients have access to basic thoughts and feelings. If they do not, it can make psychotherapy more challenging.

Data supports these observations. Karatzias et al. (2019) reviewed the efficacy of interventions for cPTSD and found that childhood abuse was found to impact outcomes across all types of PTSD treatments, suggesting that "those with a history of childhood trauma may experience less improvement, and that current treatments for this patient population can be improved" (p. 10). Research suggests that the effects of trauma are cumulative. For example, Breslau et al. (1999) found that the development of PTSD symptoms from exposure to any traumatic event increased the risk that future trauma would result in PTSD. This finding has been explained as the stress sensitization hypothesis and supports that the cumulative effects of multiple traumas increase the likelihood of a more extreme response to future traumatic events (McLaughlin et al. 2010).

I'll talk a lot more about the influence of childhood abuse throughout this book. For now, however, it's also important to emphasize the sheer complexity of human adaptation and resilience, as well as the ubiquitous nature of traumatic experiences. That said, clinical research suggests that there is a continuum of PTSD and cPTSD, as we humans rarely fall into neat categories of diagnostic criteria. However, it's important we discern the distinction of PTSD and cPTSD and the clinical implications.

PTSD vs. cPTSD: Important Distinctions

Although there is often overlap between PTSD and cPTSD diagnoses, the qualitative distinction between PTSD and CPTSD symptomatology has been supported in different groups (Brewin et al. 2017), including those experiencing interpersonal violence (Cloitre et al. 2013), rape, domestic violence, traumatic bereavement (Elklit et al. 2014), and refugees (Hyland et al. 2018). The distinction between PTSD and cPTSD has also been confirmed in samples of young adults (Perkonigg et al. 2016). The World Health Organization will likely include cPTSD as part of the 11th edition of the *International Statistical Classification of Diseases and Related Health Problems* (ICD-11). Based on the papers from the aforementioned authors, as well as Rosenfield et al. (2018), the general consensus is that cPTSD involves more severe symptoms; PTSD is often thought to involve "discrete traumatic events or set of traumatic events" (p. 364).

People who have experienced trauma exist on a continuum of "simple" PTSD to cPTSD, with the latter tending to reflect what we often consider as persons who not only have classic PTSD symptoms but with significant disorders of self-regulation, dissociation, depersonalization, suicidal behaviors, substance abuse, relational instability, and self-injurious behaviors. In terms of our diagnostic criteria, however, these lines are becoming blurry. Note that for the first time, the DSM-V included a category for people with PTSD who have dissociation (APA 2013). Given the complex nature of trauma, the ways people with trauma histories in childhood often go on to experience trauma as adults, as well as complex factors included in adult development, it can be difficult to tell the difference between PTSD and complex PTSD. However, complex PTSD does seem to affect attachment and relational development in a way that PTSD does not. To put a finer point on this, let's consider a case of PTSD in someone who does not have symptoms of cPTSD:

Ted, 26, was injured as a passenger in a ride-sharing service car. He was on his way to work on a dreary and foggy Tuesday morning in San Francisco and he was in a rush. The car he entered did not have a working seat belt. He mentioned this to the driver and the driver said there was nothing he could do. Ted had to make a quick decision. Should he risk the relatively low probability of getting into an accident or be late for work where he had an important meeting? He chose to stay in the car. While coasting through a green light, his driver's vehicle was hit by another car racing through the intersection. Ted was hit and sustained damage to his bladder, ribs, and right lung, but after a brief hospitalization was discharged. When I met Ted, he was in a great deal of pain, but had gone back to work. He had nightmares about the incident and reported that he kept seeing the face of the driver whenever he felt relaxed. He noted he had become "jumpy," and though he began walking to work so he could avoid taxis or ride-sharing services, he felt "afraid all of the time" that he would get hit by a car. He noted he had never felt this "helpless" before. Yet, Ted reflected that his husband had been "incredibly supportive" and his family who resided in another state offered to fly to California to help him if he needed it. Regarding his upbringing, Ted said that he felt very loved by his mother and father, one of whom was a college professor. Although coming out was difficult for him, he found his parents supportive, as one of them had a sibling who was gay. He had experienced some bullying in high school, which he said may have been linked with his sexual orientation. However, he found his parents as well as a school counselor to be supportive, and he utilized their support during this time. He was receptive to therapy and said he would do whatever he needed to get better. In our first couple of sessions, I noted how terrifying his experience was and just how hard it must be to have felt so out of control and at the mercy of a random event. These conversations helped after just a few sessions. He still continued to have intrusive thoughts and nightmares, however, and I discussed a referral to a trusted colleague who does EMDR for people with acute PTSD. I explained that EMDR was a kind of exposure therapy and that he would be pushed to think about some of difficult thoughts he was experiencing, but at a pace he could handle, all while the therapist kept note of his level of distress. We agreed to keep meeting during his EMDR treatments. Our meetings did not last long. He noted after two sessions of EMDR that he felt much better and "stronger." He met with me a couple more times and the EMDR therapist just three times more and left treatment with few residual symptoms.

As is clear from Ted's case, he had PTSD (not cPTSD) and was able to utilize the internal and external resources available to him to help him move on. Of course, exposure therapy can take shape in many forms, including what we may think of as traditional psychotherapy where someone talks about his or her experience of the trauma. But Ted was eager to get help quickly and "get back to normal." He seemed safe and secure in his life before this accident and felt genuinely happy. He found talking with me helpful, but EMDR seemed to be an appropriate referral, as he was ready to confront his intrusive ideations about the accident.

Ted is an excellent example of how certain people can utilize an array of short-term exposure-based treatments to deal with a relatively straightforward case of PTSD. He had an integrated sense of self, had navigated considerable obstacles before the car accident, had strong interpersonal relationships, and had a secure sense of himself intact. The trauma of his accident did not leave him with a sense of shame about his decision not to leave the car; rather, he was able to see his situation as the result of bad luck. Not only that, he had an appropriate, yet not outsized, feeling of anger toward the driver of his car. In other words, he experienced his PTSD symptoms as a problem that could be solved with the help of people he could trust.

In contrast, people with cPTSD may be less unquestioning of our help and may require considerable time to develop trust in the therapeutic relationship in order for us to begin to find a way to help. Although avoidance is a symptom of PTSD, in my experience, there is a certain variation of avoidance, which is seen most often among people who have cPTSD. This symptom is one that may be quite irritating to therapists as the kind of evasion I am describing is one that can manifest itself in anger toward the therapist or a kind of numbing, which makes us feel that anything we offer will not help. People with a lot of avoidance sometimes have defenses that allow them to seem as if they can tolerate therapy, but this idea should not be taken for granted. Sometimes, we assume we can proceed with therapy utilizing whatever approach we are most comfortable with, only to find that this does not work. Let's consider the beginning of Melanie's treatment:

As Melanie had come from an intensive outpatient program, she had a psychiatrist managing her medicines, a combination of an SSRI and a low dose of an antipsychotic medicine to take in the evening. Melanie reported that she felt her meds were helping, as she was not having panic attacks and she was able to get out of bed. But she was not looking for a job and she was doing little else. She was unable to tell me much about how she spent her days. As is the standard of practice, we discussed exercise, and I suggested the meditation app I recommend for people with cPTSD, one that uses guided meditation. In addition, I offered her the option to reinforce dialectical behavioral therapy DBT techniques she learned from her outpatient hospitalization program, which includes my preferred DBT workbook. Melanie accepted these suggestions without protest, but in subsequent sessions, said she found no use in these ideas. She was not angry with me, exactly, but she kept focusing on how it was not her fault that she lost her last job and how messed up the tech world was. While I was in agreement with Melanie about the difficulties for any young woman in the Bay Area technology industry, I was not convinced that all of her problems were solely external. Yet, we were in a bit of a quandary. In addition to not being thrilled with the techniques I had offered her, she made it clear to me that she was not interested in talking about her family, told me very little about current relationships, and seemed to have little access to an internal life that I could have access to. If we were not to engage in behavioral and cognitive behavioral therapies, what do we do to help stabilize her symptoms and make her feel safe?

As we will see for people such as Melanie, we need to figure out how to provide something for them in therapy when they literally see no use in cognitive behavioral techniques and are not interested in techniques such as mindfulness or other cognitive approaches to help them soothe themselves. At this point, it's ill-advised to use what many of us think of as classic psychodynamic techniques, as talking about early or family life is often off the table (and, in my opinion, contraindicated). Yet, they do want something from us. In my experience, many people who come to therapy are just not interested in *techniques*. Sometimes it is the case they have had therapies focused on techniques before and found these methods minimally helpful. Some clients rally against how simple certain tools seem. Others are less sure why they don't want specific tools, but I think that is because they are wanting something more meaningful and connected. They are looking for an attachment, warmth, and understanding. In terms of technique then, we need to talk with clients about whatever we can get them to talk with us about. In these times in the beginning of therapy, I often tell clients to tell me what interests them. If it's baseball or details of their work or their pets—especially in the beginning, when people feel more guarded and not sure how to use therapy, the actual content matters less than the action of relating. Focusing on the therapeutic relationship is what is most helpful and provides a needed foundation for everything else we do.

Therapeutic Efficacy and the Therapeutic Alliance

All bona fide treatments for trauma have roughly equal efficacy. We are left then to consider what ingredients are necessary for therapy success and in particular for those who have experienced trauma. This leads us to the decades of research on the therapeutic relationship. As all of us in clinical practice are aware, there just are certain clients we just feel more connected to. In my own experience, it's not just that people might have positive ideas of me in the beginning of treatment and vice versa; it's usually when I have empathy toward them, in which I may or may not be aware of the reasons. It may be that our mother's shared similar traits (a fact that I may find out a year after meeting someone) or that we both came from lower-class or working-class backgrounds. It could be any number of things. Sometimes I never really understand why, but for some people there is a sense that I more easily "get them" and can imagine their internal lives and situations. Also, I often find that clients feel more comfortable in the beginning of therapy when they tell me something that induces them shame with a worry that I will judge them, only to realize that I consider most "confessions" of this sort a clinical data point that we can be curious about and look at together. The fit between client and therapist is also largely about the environment we create in the therapeutic encounter.

Michael Lambert (quoted as a personal communication in Miller et al. 1997) stated: "When you watch good therapy being done, you know it and it has a lot of commonalities… Good cognitive therapists and good behavior therapists, psychodynamic therapists act an awful lot alike" (p. 23). Six decades of research supports that the therapy relationship is the most important factor in therapy outcome, more than the technique used (e.g., Henry 1998; Norcross and Wampold 2019a, b). These latter authors point out that the relationship is at the heart of healing trauma, yet they estimate that 90% of federal research grants for psychotherapy research, outcome studies, treatment guidelines, and continuing education on trauma therapy focuses on particular methods and not the relationship.

Those of us of a certain age, in the relatively early days of psychotherapy relationship research, learned that relationship factors constitute about 30% of psychotherapy outcomes, while techniques (the method of therapy conducted) account for 15% of outcomes. What the client expects from therapy was thought to be about 15%, and other factors were 40% of the estimated variance of how people were thought to get better (Miller et al. 1997).

The relationship between client and therapist is thought to contribute more to therapeutic change than the techniques we employ. This research has become more sophisticated in the last few decades. Recent data focuses more specifically on "alliance" factors, via one popularly used measure, the Working Alliance Inventory (Horvath and Greenberg 1989), and measures such aspects of therapy including agreement on goals and tasks of therapy and the bond between client and therapist. One study estimated that evidence-based relationship (EBR) variables account for up to 12% of the variance in treatment outcome (Laska et al. 2014). Norcross and Lambert (2019) have moved to describing aspects of the therapeutic relationship under the umbrella "common factors." They describe their understanding of the research this way as illustrated in Fig. 1.1.

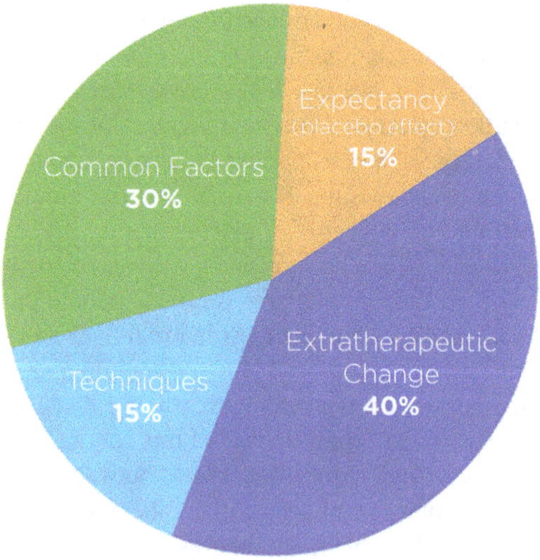

Fig. 1.1 Current explanation of therapy outcomes. (Adapted from Norcross and Lambert 2019)

> Common factors, variables found in most therapies regardless of theoretical orientation, probably account for another 30%. The therapy relationship represents the sine qua non of common factors, along with client and therapist factors. Technique factors, explaining approximately 15% of the variance, are those treatment methods fairly specific to prescribed therapy, such as biofeedback, transference interpretations, desensitization, systematic exposure, or two-chair work. Finally, playing an important role is expectancy—the placebo effect, the client's knowledge that he/she is being treated and his/her conviction in the treatment rationale and methods. These four broad factors account for the explained outcome variance. (pp. 11–12)

Relationship factors have been replaced with common factors as the authors stated above. Note that "extratherapeutic factors" in this model refer to self-change, spontaneous remission, the influence of social support, etc. In a second analysis of their research, the aforementioned authors include unexplained factors—accounting for the fact that, similar to medicine and medical research, we actually cannot account for all factors related to success or failure of our treatments. In the second model, unexplained variance accounts for 35%, patient contribution 30%, therapy relationship 15%, individual therapist contributions 7%, and other factors 3% of the outcome in therapy (Norcross and Lambert 2019). Treatment method accounted for only 10% of the variance of therapeutic outcome.

Some psychotherapists consistently have better outcomes with clients than other therapists (Baldwin and Imel 2013; Wampold and Imel 2015). Therapists account for around 5–10% of *unexplained* variance in patient outcomes, with 8–9% being most commonly reported (Saxon et al. 2017). Therapist effects are complicated and involve things such as empathy or number of sessions. Regarding empathy, Moyers et al. (2016) investigated therapist effects and therapist empathy in a randomized study of behavioral treatment during an alcohol reduction program. Results showed that 11% of outcome variance (i.e., alcoholic drinks per week) was associated with therapist behavior. Therapists rated as more empathic during sessions was associated with larger decreases in drinking. In a review of studies looking at therapist effects, some therapists were consistently more than twice as effective as other therapists (Johns et al. 2019). In this review there was also evidence that patients assessed as having more severe symptoms at intake experienced larger therapist effects.

It occurs to me that what may make therapists more effective goes beyond empathy. I know many therapists who are deeply sympathetic and empathetic, yet they do not necessarily have a good assessment of their clients, beyond DSM Axis I diagnoses. People's character, personality traits, and vulnerabilities matter in terms of thinking about how to relate to them. For example, if someone is suspicious, I'll tend to be especially transparent in my thinking with them. I make a concerted effort to say, "While you were talking, I was thinking…." If someone has issues related to grandiosity or narcissistic vulnerably, I more actively remind them of their strengths. If someone is avoidant or obsessional, I will be more measured and less directive. These interventions are based on character assessment. We can use the DSM as a guideline for thinking about personality traits, we can think about attachment styles and defenses related to certain cognitive processes, or we can use principles within psychodynamic therapy. It really does not matter how we think about character and personality, but it's important that we do. How we intervene is not just based on Axis I symptoms but on how someone's personality adapted to the world around them.

Although the alliance and therapeutic relationship are vital, it's also important to keep in mind client contribution to psychotherapy outcome is greater than that of either the particular treatment method or the therapy relationship (Lambert 2011, 2013; Wampold and Imel 2015). When it comes to trauma, there are questions regarding how well trauma survivors are able to attach to a therapist to get what they need. For example, Laska et al. (2014) suggested that a treatment alliance is more difficult to establish with trauma survivors than in a general treatment population.

It's not entirely clear that this is the case, though keep in mind published studies on therapeutic alliance do not report on the characteristics of people who drop out of studies. It could be they can't tolerate the intervention in the study; it could also mean these folks want a different kind of treatment and go on to find it. It could mean they seek no other treatment at all. Additionally, in therapy outcome studies, the measurement of alliance takes place in the third or fourth session (Wampold 2015). I was surprised to learn this, as three to four sessions may not be enough time for clients to develop a sense of trust in their therapist. Many people go to therapy because they think it's better than not being in therapy, but that does not necessarily mean that they have a full "buy-in" to the process. In considering people who have been hurt, which often occurs in the context of a relationship, I would expect that people would need a great deal longer than three to four sessions to develop a sense of safety or to even make a decision about their experience of the therapist and treatment.

To date, several studies have found that the therapeutic alliance is predictive of a reduction in symptoms among people who have traumatic backgrounds. In a review of 19 studies representing 1623 study participants, researchers found that in studies using a variety of techniques, including several cognitive behavioral therapies as well as interpersonal therapy (IPT), therapeutic alliance was associated with lower scores on depression measures, decreased trauma symptoms, and increased self-acceptance (Ellis et al. 2018). Their analysis also included four studies of prolonged exposure therapy, and though two of these studies had high dropout rates, of those participants who stayed in therapy, therapeutic alliance did predict increased likelihood of completing homework.

Treating people with trauma backgrounds and cPTSD symptoms involves therapists having to tolerate a great deal of uncertainty, including not knowing if we may be helpful or how long it will take to be. As we have seen in the discussion of the research on therapeutic alliance and therapeutic effects, our impact still involves relatively small effect sizes and percentages of the variance. There really is so much that we still do not know. Yet, the fact that some therapists consistently have better outcomes with clients can give us some reason for optimism. It may be this ambiguity that explains, in part, why many clinicians in our field focus on specific techniques and theories with the hope that one approach can be the one that helps some of the more challenging people we see. My own sense of this dilemma, however, is that we need as many tools in our tool box as possible to help people. As someone trained in several CBT approaches, as well as psychodynamic techniques, I have benefited from not feeling overly loyal to one theory. In fact, I've criticized some psychoanalytic colleagues for being too zealous in assuming that there is only one way to help people, particularly clients who are complicated and those with traumatic physical and psychological problems (e.g., Greenberg 2016). Given the overwhelming research that all genuine therapies have about equal efficacy, it's worth thinking about how we can tailor what we do. By this I mean switching approaches when needed, not assume a blind loyalty to one or two approaches and appreciating the rich and varied methods that are available to us.

Multiple Treatments, Equal Efficacy

Not only are there multiple ways to treat trauma, all of the common authentic therapies we are familiar with have about equal efficacy in treating people who have experienced trauma (Benish et al. 2008; Frost et al. 2014; Gerger et al. 2014a, b; Powers et al. 2010; Tran and Gregor 2016; Norcross and Wampold 2019a, b).

Yet, there is considerable disagreement among researchers and clinicians regarding which theories and techniques are best suited for the treatment of PTSD. There is less research on the treatment of complex trauma, but based on the overlap of PTSD and cPTSD, it makes sense to start with what we know about the recommendations for PTSD treatment. The recent American Psychological Association (APA) Guidelines to the Treatment of Trauma (2017) has faced considerable resistance among clinicians for its biomedical emphasis and neglect of the therapeutic relationship, which is the most robust indicator of therapeutic outcome (Norcross and Wampold 2019b). Courtois and Brown (2019) argue the same point and add that the APA guidelines fail to take into consideration cultural issues, developmental complications related to childhood trauma, as well as the neurobiology of trauma and how this may impact treatment choice. Further, critics have noted that randomized controlled trials (RCTs), on which APA exclusively relied on in the development of the guidelines, have limited utility in studying psychotherapy. This is particularly true for people with complicated psychological problems (Shedler 2017). Additionally, another major limitation in RCTs is that it measures patients in treatment for short periods of time. For many people who have PTSD and cPTSD, longer-term treatments are often the norm. Finally, dropout rates in CBT studies using exposure are extremely high.

With the above caveats in mind, the present APA guidelines strongly recommend cognitive behavioral therapy (CBT), cognitive processing therapy (CPT), cognitive therapy (CT), and prolonged exposure therapy (PE) and "conditionally" suggest the use of brief eclectic psychotherapy (BEP), eye movement desensitization and reprocessing (EMDR), and narrative exposure therapy (NET) in the treatment of PTSD. These recommendations are largely, but not entirely, consistent with those of various other organizations, with the exception of the recommendations by the International Society for Traumatic Stress Studies, which I will discuss below.

What follows is a brief review of the major treatments with evidence of their efficacy with traumatized populations. Not all are included in the APA guidelines. I will provide these treatments in alphabetical order, and I'll comment on their established efficacy in work with people with both PTSD and cPTSD symptoms (when possible). Keep in mind the limits to the research. First, people with PTSD are more likely to have other current or past psychiatric diagnoses with lifetime psychiatric comorbidity rates of around 80% (Fairbank et al. 2001). Further, cPTSD is associated with disruptions in work, social functioning, and physical health, adding to diagnostic complexity. The construct of cPTSD is still relatively new, not to mention more difficult to study because of the relational aspects of the cPTSD symptoms as well as the presence of disturbances of self-regulation. Many of the treatments I will describe and the research supporting them are based on models of short-term therapy and are based on randomized clinical trials. One reason the APA practice guidelines are controversial for some is that the research APA used for their recommendations does not include the thousands of other studies on therapy for people with histories of trauma (e.g., Norcross and Wampold 2019b). Finally, as clinicians we know that many clients go on to receive ongoing therapy after a completion of shorter-term, structured treatments.

Cognitive Behavioral Therapies (CBT)

CBT is often touted as the most effective treatment for PTSD (e.g., Bradley et al. 2005). CBT is fixed specifically on the relationship between thoughts, feelings, and behaviors. It focuses on specific symptoms and asks patients to record and keep track of various thoughts and related mood states. Given how wide and nuanced various CBT approaches have become, this approach used can vary, with some clinicians emphasizing cognitive versus behavioral aspects. The APA (2017) discusses certain underlying theories under the umbrella of CBT. For example, they highlight emotional processing theory (Rauch and Foa 2006), which focuses on changing associations to the traumatic event. Social cognitive theory (Benight and Bandura 2004) focuses on adjusting maladaptive beliefs that are associated with traumatic events. It should be noted that more recent publications blend even more techniques into the category of CBT. For example, prolonged exposure (PE) and cognitive processing therapy (CPT) with and without exposure, cognitive therapy, as well as eye movement desensitization and reprocessing (EMDR) have all been subsumed under the category of CBTs.

Prolonged exposure therapy (Foa et al. 2007) has a great deal of RCT evidence that supports its efficacy and is considered by some to be the gold standard for CBT treatment (Dorrepaal et al. 2014). Prolonged exposure therapy (PE) addresses the symptom of avoidance. Advocates of this approach believe that avoiding reminders of the trauma increases the traumatic event's strength for clients, because fear is reinforced. Exposures are initiated early in treatment with the idea that clients can learn that cues and thoughts related to the traumatic event are not inherently dangerous. A meta-analysis by Powers et al. (2010) of PE found this treatment to be very effective, both at posttreatment and at follow-up compared with control conditions (placebo or wait list). Treatments that were categorized as psychological placebo included supportive counseling, relaxation, present-centered therapy, time-limited psychodynamic therapy, and treatment as usual. Though the authors note that, "Consistent with previous meta-analyses, there was no significant difference between PE and other active treatments (CPT, EMDR, CT, and SIT)," where SIT refers to stress inoculation training, CT refers to cognitive therapy, EMDR is eye movement desensitization reprocessing, and CPT is cognitive processing therapy. Despite the idea that PE is the gold standard, this study supports that most of the commonly utilized CBT treatments are efficacious for those who participate in CBT studies.

Cognitive processing therapy, like prolonged exposure therapy, has a great deal of support through randomized controlled trials (Cukor et al. 2010). This therapy reduces the amount of exposure time clients need to endure while focusing on altering "unhelpful" beliefs related to the trauma.

Cognitive therapy is similar to CBT, though the focus is more on changing perceptions that are considered pessimistic and the aim is to alter ideas of the traumatic event. Cognitive therapy for PTSD was found to be better than emotionally focused supportive therapy (Ehlers et al. 2014) and is also strongly recommended by the APA 2017 guidelines.

Eye movement desensitization reprocessing is thought by some to be a kind of exposure therapy, and its efficacy has been found to be comparable to exposure treatments (Seidler and Wagner 2006). EMDR is said to work by enhancing the processing of the trauma because of new connections that are made when focusing on a vivid image while pairing this with eye movements, tones, tapping, or other kinds of tactile stimulation (e.g., Shapiro 2001).

A review of 51 randomized controlled trials on treatments for cPTSD found CBT, exposure therapy alone, and EMDR were effective when compared with various controls of usual care (Karatzias et al. 2019). These authors note however that few of the studies reported effectiveness on affect regulation, which is common in cPTSD.

Brief Eclectic Psychotherapy (BEP)

Like the name suggests, BEP is designed to be short-term and incorporates elements of CBT and psychodynamic methods. BEP for PTSD has been found to be as effective as other "trauma-focused treatments" (which frequently means CBT therapies) that are concentrated "on the expression of strong emotions like sorrow and anger which stem from the traumatic event and on learning the way in which the event has changed someone's life" (Gersons et al. 2015, p. 255).

Dialectical Behavior Therapy for PTSD (DBT-PTSD)

DBT was developed as a stand-alone treatment for people with borderline personality disorder (Linehan 1993) and has been particularly helpful for people who are suicidal or engaging in self-harm (DeCou et al. 2019). DBT has been described as a useful adjunct treatment for people with PTSD (Sears and Chard 2016). As people diagnosed with borderline personality disorder often have histories of complex trauma, there has been a movement to apply DBT techniques to those who have PTSD. This research is still in its infancy, but studies have found DBT-PTSD to be effective for client with histories of child sexual abuse who have both PTSD and difficulties regulating emotions (Steil et al. 2011, 2018; Bohus et al. 2013). DBT-PTSD focuses on distress tolerance, mindfulness, self-harm, and exposure.

Narrative Exposure Therapy (NET)

NET has been used most often with people with complex, multiple traumas and those who have escaped political turmoil, such as refugees. The idea is to create a cohesive narrative about the traumatic events and involves re-experiencing the emotions associated with traumatic experiences while being grounded in the present. For example, one study found that for refugees still living in unsafe conditions, people receiving NET had dramatically lower PTSD symptoms as compared with those who received psychoeducation or supportive counseling (Neuner et al. 2004).

Psychodynamic Therapy

There is some research that modern approaches to psychoanalysis are helpful for people with PTSD and cPTSD, though there is not the same level of evidence as the aforementioned approaches in terms of randomized controlled trials. This is perhaps, in part, due to the fact that psychodynamic therapies are often long term and the practice of this treatment may not fit the basic criteria for RCTs. That said, Russell Carr designed an effective approach for soldiers who did not benefit from CBT (Dingfelder 2012; Carr 2011). His method involved dealing with shame and isolation and sense of meaning among combat veterans. An interesting technique that Carr employed was being empathic toward the soldier's thoughts, even when these thoughts could cause some therapists to feel horror (e.g., aggressive thoughts toward others).

A randomized controlled trial (Brom et al. 1989) compared a short-term psychodynamic treatment to systematic desensitization and hypnotherapy. Brom et al. (1989) found that 60% of clients in each group (psychodynamic, systematic desensitization, and hypnotherapy) improved and found that psychodynamic psychotherapy resulted in greater reduction of avoidance symptoms.

Looking more broadly at the research, psychodynamic therapies are found to be as effective if not more effective for people with complex problems, including those with personality and relationship difficulties with significant symptom reduction for those with borderline personality disorder (Shedler 2010; Fonagy et al. 2005). In addition, the authors of these analyses found that people in psychodynamic treatments tend to have sustained gains in improvement.

Three-Stage Models

The International Society for Traumatic Stress Studies (ISTSS) (2012) recommends three phases of treatment for cPTSD. Although a three-stage model of treatment was initially suggested by Herman (1992), ISTSS describes that Phase 1 focuses on ensuring the individual's safety, reducing symptoms, and increasing emotional and social competencies. Phase 2 focuses on processing the unresolved aspects of the individual's memories of traumatic experiences so that these are integrated into a representation of self, relationships, and the world. This is achieved through using standard or adapted methods taken from conventional trauma-focused cognitive behavioral therapy. Phase 3 involves consolidation of treatment gains to facilitate the transition from treatment into a greater engagement with the outside world. Trauma expert Laura Brown (personal communication, 2019) describes creating safety using a three-stage model as decreasing biological activation (specifically HPA-axis functioning, which I will discuss in more detail in Chapter 2), creating boundaries with others and how to live in the presence of constant or frequent suicidality and shame reduction. There is evidence supporting the three-stage model. For example, Cloitre et al. (2010) compared a stage-based treatment (skills training followed by memory processing) as compared to an exposure-focused treatment and a skills-focused treatment. Results of this study indicated the superiority of the phase-based approach as compared to the exposure-focused condition.

Commonalities Among All Approaches

As we think about the many options we have for treating trauma, it's important to return to the discussion on therapeutic alliance. As we've seen, some of the aforementioned methods are more technically based, meaning the therapist overtly teaches certain skills or offers a preferred method. This is where the therapeutic relationship comes into play, as some clinicians may assume that they can jump into the techniques without adequately preparing the patient or, perhaps, even assessing the client's ability to tolerate certain techniques. In my experience, I have seen well-meaning colleagues assume their approach can work but may not have assessed the patient's readiness. This seems to be very true for exposure therapies, but I have seen psychodynamic clinicians do this as well. I do some exposure treatment for people with acute PTSD (not with cPTSD), and I refer to colleagues who are skilled at EMDR. But in both cases, I spend a considerable amount of time thinking with clients about what this will be like for them. I also describe the risks of exposure treatments and that it may increase their levels of distress (e.g., Morris 2015; Najavits 2015). Similarly, when I use a more psychodynamic approach, I prepare people for that as well. I suggest that it might be useful to talk about certain traumas but that we consider doing so if/when the client is ready and I also mention how destabilizing it can be to talk about trauma. Certainly for traumatized people with a lot of avoidance, they *already know* on some level how disorienting and frightening it is to discuss traumatic experiences. Yet, there is something soothing and stabilizing about saying this out loud. In addition, it places the control in the hands of the client and not the therapist. This is just one way we can strengthen the alliance in the therapeutic relationship, and I'll have a lot more to say about that throughout this book.

Another interesting similarity among all of the therapies described is that exposure is a common technique. Every theory discussed assumes that at some point, the client would benefit from talking about and thinking about the traumatic experience(s). I am not convinced that this is true for all people with complex PTSD, as the extent and numbers of traumatic events could be too overwhelming to discuss. Particularly when people are extremely dissociative, processing of memories may not be realistic. Indeed, this is why some clinicians have come up with thoughtful hybrid approaches to treatment that focus on creating stability and safety first and emphasize the therapeutic alliance (e.g., Courtois and Ford 2015; Herman 1992). Even these theories assume that discussing traumas at some point is needed for healing. This issue is complicated for people with cPTSD as there may be difficulties in the formation of memories when people are severely anxious or dissociated. We may need to temper our expectations. I'll talk in more detail about the risks and benefits of processing of memories in Chapter 3.

The Therapy Relationship and Clinical Hypothesis Testing

All bona fide therapies offer help for those with PTSD and cPTSD. We also know that the therapeutic relationship is important, vital even, for our clients to get better. Yet, this is complicated. How do we enhance the therapeutic relationship? It starts with having an authentic discussion with the client about what we are doing and why as well as genuinely setting shared treatment goals. I also think it's helpful to describe to clients how we think psychotherapy works, especially if they are curious about this. This is also necessary when people like Melanie seem unsure regarding the therapeutic process and may not even have a lot to talk with us about, at first. Before I get back to Melanie, there is the question of how we choose what approach is best. Let's say we live in a world where we do not have to pledge allegiance to any one theory and we can agree that certain techniques work for people at specific times. These times may involve discrete periods in treatment or even differences that occur in one therapeutic hour. How do we know what to do when? I wrestle with these questions every day as I am trying to help traumatized people. And while I don't know all of the answers, what has worked best for me is the teaching I got in graduate school about clinical hypothesis testing.

Clinical hypothesis testing is what was taught to me in graduate school about how to think as a psychotherapist. I assume the term was borrowed from the use of the scientific method and it goes roughly like this: When I am with a client, I say something or do something. Sometimes the thing I am doing is *not* doing something like creating space or allowing silence. I then watch to see how the person responds. If they do not respond in a way that seems to indicate that I'm being helpful, I change what I am doing. The idea is, "At this moment, the client needs X. That did not work, let me try Y." I'm certain that many therapists do this intuitively, but my suggestion is that we apply this more consciously. It involves trying a technique, method, and interpretation, noticing its effect, and then we either keep going or change course. The emphasis is to *shift away from interpretations when they do not work* and the idea that I am not the authority on the client's mind. Clinical hypothesis testing is a process that involves the client, where we work together to understand the nature of how their mind works. It's relational. Together we see what works and what doesn't. To be clear, I am not saying that we should never expect that clients experience anxiety. They may be, and sometimes it's, necessary when considering new thoughts and feelings. However, for people with cPTSD, I see it as our job to protect them from too much anxiety and overstimulation. For example, a client who sought me out specifically for psychodynamic therapy was recently talking to me about how something at work she was involved in required a great deal of competition. She came from a family in which there was only one person who could ever be seen as a winner. It was her mother. This client describes her mother as a "Queen Bee" who "ate her young whenever it suited her." As a smart young girl, my client could never feel important or special. In other words, she could never win. In the context of discussing this situation at work, which required a great deal of competition, she was very anxious in the session and clearly wanted me to help her find a way to feel less anxious. I tried to help her with her anxiety by connecting the fact that she came from a family that was akin to a Gladiator competition. There was no way to feel like competing did not lead to someone's demise. I saw my comment was not helpful in the moment. She began tapping her foot and looked at the floor. Though she could intellectually acknowledge this was true, it was too stimulating for her at that time. She appeared more anxious and disorganized. So I said, "Well, that may be true, I'm not sure, but let's pivot and think about who you feel specifically worried about at work right now and what you can do about it." We then went on to discuss the details of whom and what she was focused on at work. That proved to be more soothing as she clearly became calmer and could think with me about how to take care of herself. The issue of "kill or be killed" that was so prevalent in her family and in her mind did get eventually addressed, but we needed to do so when she was less intensely anxious and not as focused on an acute situation which she felt on some level was psychologically life-threatening to her. What I am describing is also akin to what advocates of mentalization suggest. Mentalization will be discussed in more detail in Chapter 3, but proponents of this way of working suggest it helps to build trust with people who have histories of trauma (Fonagy and Allison 2014).

The other key part of the approach of clinical hypothesis testing, as I have adapted it, is that I say to my clients what I am thinking about what they are saying, how I am viewing their situation, and what I think an overarching theme might be. For example, a woman was telling me about her considerable difficulty at work in setting limits with colleagues. She viewed herself as a "doormat" and felt considerable shame about this. As we were talking, I recalled (though it's often on my mind) that she had been involved in an accident as a teenager that involved the injury of a peer. She felt responsible for the teen's injury. She was clear that she did not want to talk about it. But in the context of discussing her considerable difficulty at work, I said, "I know you don't want to talk about this and that's fine, but I wanted to mention that I have an idea that some of your difficulties are related to the accident. It's not something we have to discuss, but it might be linked to the difficulty you are having with setting limits. It might help at some point if we could talk about this a little more." As someone who appeared to like me a lot and I think wanted to please me, she said, "We can talk about it!" though she appeared tense as she said this, and her gaze went out my window. I wondered if what I said felt like pressure to her and suggested we *think* about talking about it first. She relaxed her shoulders and said, "Let's think about it." I told her it was just a hypothesis (I often use that word) and it does not mean that I am right. The topic did not come up again for another year, but I held it in mind, knowing that I might have pushed her a bit too much, which of course is probably how she feels all the time at work. I present my hypotheses to people and am transparent with how I am thinking, as long as I don't feel I am being too overstimulating. Transparency is a key part of work with all people, but especially those who have experienced trauma, as is providing a sense of control over the process. It's important for people to feel involved in what we are doing and that they have a sense of agency in the process. Other clients may need a clearer sense that they are guiding the discussion.

Negotiating the Beginning of Therapy

Melanie was not interested in the techniques I had offered her in the beginning of therapy. I later learned that she ultimately found DBT to be a little pejorative, even though she did feel she had learned techniques that helped her manage her suicidal thoughts when she had this treatment in her outpatient program. However, she had been able to see me four times and had essentially not changed since our first meeting. Unlike many people who come from the relatively difficult (if not traumatizing) event of having been suicidal, she did not seem to have a sense of relief about being in therapy with me. I felt worried about this as this often seems to me to be a poor prognostic indicator of how the treatment will go. During the fourth session, I talked with Melanie about how hard it seemed for her to be in therapy. And I noted that maybe she felt a bit guarded. She agreed and said that she has actually always been a suspicious person. As she was from a nonwhite ethnic group, I asked her if she thought that maybe her wariness was partly cultural. She smiled slightly and said no, that others in her ethnic group would say she's "paranoid." I laughed. She seemed slightly more at ease. I told her that I thought then that therapy has to be hard, as we don't know each other and she really has no reason to trust me. Nor should she, until she has enough data to know that I am okay. I went on to say that we were in a bit of a bind, as therapy involves talking, especially in the setting of her not being interested in CBT approaches. I wondered if maybe she would be interested in us thinking about how she could go about finding a job, as she likely needed that security before she could do much else in therapy. She said she could get on board with that, and for the first couple of months of her therapy, we talked about looking for jobs and at one point, I even looked at her resume (she was not interested in a referral for a career counselor). Though it took a while for her to eventually get a job, the sheer concrete nature of the beginning of our work allowed her to begin to trust me. And it was a lot longer after that that I understood how she came to be so guarded.

The beginning of therapy is always a negotiation. I find that even if a client and I seemingly get along well in the beginning, for traumatized people, the world is never a safe place. The psychic ground is always shifting. As we'll see more throughout this book, we need to be flexible with our techniques and methods, and clinical hypothesis testing allows us an informal though valuable and organic way to assess our impact on clients.

Conclusion

I am convinced that we can offer more to people with cPTSD symptoms, but there are no concrete answers and no one technique that is a panacea for most people who have experienced multiple traumas. I think this ambiguity and uncertainty is important and should be embraced. It mirrors the reality of what our patients experience, and it reflects the helplessness many clinicians feel. Being a therapist is difficult, and the amount of pain and distress we have to bear trying to treat people can throw us into a number of vulnerabilities we may bring to our work, including our own histories of trauma. I imagine these difficulties, as well as the clinical uncertainties in our work, are what lead some clinicians to become "religious" about specific theories and methods. But no theory has it all. We have some help from what we know about the therapeutic alliance, but there is no easy answer. And though it may come down (somewhat) to the fit between client and therapist, I am going to do my best throughout this book to outline how to think about the work, with some ideas about what to do with the vexing clinical issues we face. Thinking, however, is key. It's what I was taught in grad school in the 1990s, even though I was trained at a

CBT therapist. Back then, there was not the same emphasis on technique. In fact, the foundation of clinical hypothesis testing was centered on learning how to think about clinical work, and not as reliant on specific techniques or what we do. It was about just sitting in a room with a client and connecting with them. Understanding someone is at the heart of what I learned psychotherapy is, and it's my hope that the rest of this book can bring some of those concepts back, as well as the need for all of us to feel like we have multiple ways to help complicated and traumatized people.

References

American Psychiatric Association. (2013). *Diagnostic and statistical manual of mental disorders* (5th ed.). Washington, DC: Author.

American Psychological Association. (2017). *Clinical practice guideline for the treatment of PTSD*. https://www.apa.org/ptsd-guideline/ptsd.pdf.

Baldwin, S. A., & Imel, Z. E. (2013). Therapist effects: Findings and methods. In M. J. Lamber (Ed.), *Bergin and Garfield's handbook of psychotherapy and behavior change* (6th ed., pp. 258–297). New York: Wiley.

Benight, C. C., & Bandura, A. (2004). Social cognitive theory of posttraumatic recovery: The role of perceived self-efficacy. *Behaviour Research and Therapy, 42*(10), 1129–1148.

Benish, S. G., Imel, Z. E., & Wampold, B. E. (2008). The relative efficacy of bona fide psychotherapies for treating post-traumatic stress disorder: A meta-analysis of direct comparisons. *Clinical Psychology Review, 28*(5), 746–758.

Bohus, M., Dyer, A. S., Priebe, K., Krüger, A., Kleindienst, N., Schmahl, C., et al. (2013). Dialectical behaviour therapy for post-traumatic stress disorder after childhood sexual abuse in patients with and without borderline personality disorder: A randomised controlled trial. *Psychotherapy and Psychosomatics, 82*(4), 221–233.

Boulanger, C. (2007). *Wounded by reality: Understanding and treating adult onset trauma*. Mahwah: The Analytic Press.

Bradley, R., Greene, J., Russ, E., Dutra, L., & Westen, D. (2005). A multidimensional meta-analysis of psychotherapy for PTSD. *The American Journal of Psychiatry, 162*(2), 214–227.

Breslau, N. (2009). The epidemiology of trauma, PTSD, and other post-trauma disorders. *Trauma, Violence, & Abuse, 10*, 198–210.

Breslau, N., Chilcoat, H. D., Kessler, R. C., & Davis, G. C. (1999). Previous exposure to trauma and PTSD effects of subsequent trauma: Results from the Detroit area survey of trauma. *American Journal of Psychiatry, 156*, 902–907.

Brewin, C. R. (2019). Complex post-traumatic stress disorder: A new diagnosis in ICD-11. *BJPsych Advances*. https://doi.org/10.1192/bja.2019.48. Published online by Cambridge University Press: 08 Aug 2019. Accessed on 16 Aug 2019.

Brewin, C. R., Cloitre, M., Hyland, P., Shelvin, M., Maercker, A., Bryant, R. A., et al. (2017). A review of current evidence regarding the ICD-11 proposals for diagnosing PTSD and complex PTSD. *Clinical Psychology Review, 58*, 1–15.

Brom, D., Kleber, R. J., & Defares, P. B. (1989). Brief psychotherapy for posttraumatic stress disorders. *Journal of Consulting and Clinical Psychology, 57*, 607–612.

Carr, R. B. (2011). Combat and human existence: Toward an intersubjective approach to combat-related PTSD. *Psychoanalytic Psychology, 28*(4), 471–496.

Cloitre, M., Stovall-McClough, K. C., Nooner, K., Zorbas, P., Cherry, S., Jackson, C. L., et al. (2010). Treatment for PTSD related to childhood abuse: A randomized controlled trial. *American Journal of Psychiatry, 167*, 915–924.

Cloitre, M., Garvert, D. W., Brewin, C. R., Bryant, R. A., & Maercker, A. (2013). Evidence for proposed ICD-11 PTSD and complex PTSD: A latent profile analysis. *European Journal of Psychotraumatology, 4*. https://doi.org/10.3402/ejpt.v4i0.20706.

Courtois, C., & Brown, L. S. (2019). Guideline orthodoxy and resulting limitations of the American Psychological Association's clinical practice guideline for the treatment of PTSD in adults. *Psychotherapy, 56*(3), 329–339.

Courtois, C., & Ford, J. (Eds.). (2009). *Treating complex traumatic stress disorders. An evidence-based guide*. New York: Guilford Press.

Courtois, C., & Ford, J. (2013). *Treating complex trauma: A sequenced relationship based approach*. New York: Guilford.

Courtois, C. A., & Ford, J. D. (2015). *Treatment of complex trauma: A sequenced, relationship-based approach* (Reprint edition). New York: The Guilford Press.

Cukor, J., Olden, M., Lee, F., & Difede, J. (2010). Evidence-based treatments for PTSD, new directions, and special challenges. *Annals of the New York Academy of Sciences, 1208*, 82–89.

DeCou, C. R., Comtois, K. A., & Landes, S. J. (2019). Dialectical behavior therapy is effective for the treatment of suicidal behavior: A meta-analysis. *Behavior Therapy, 50*(1), 60–72.

Dingfelder, S. (2012). A psychodynamic treatment for PTSD shows promise for soldiers. *APA Monitor, 43*(3), 11.

Dorrepaal, E., Thomaes, K., Hoogendoorn, A. W., Veltman, D. J., Draijer, N., & van Balkom, A. J. L. M. (2014). Evidence-based treatment for adult women with child abuse-related complex PTSD: A quantitative review. *European Journal of Psychotraumatology, 5*, 1–18.

Ehlers, A., Hackman, A., Grey, N., Wild, J., Liness, S., Albert, I., et al. (2014). A randomized controlled trial of 7-day intensive and standard weekly cognitive therapy for PTSD and emotion-focused supportive therapy. *The American Journal of Psychiatry*. Accessed on 7 July 2019 at https://doi.org/ajp.psychiatryonline.org, https://doi.org/10.1176/appi.ajp.2013.13040552.

Elklit, A., Hyland, P., & Shevlin, M. (2014). Evidence of symptom profiles consistent with post-traumatic stress disorder and complex posttraumatic stress disorder in different trauma samples. *European Journal of Psychotraumatology, 5*. https://doi.org/10.3402/ejpt.v5.24221.

Ellis, A. E., Simiola, V., Brown, L., Courtois, C., & Cook, J. M. (2018). The role of evidence-based therapy relationships on treatment outcome for adults with trauma: A systematic review. *Journal of Trauma & Dissociation, 19*(2), 185–213.

Fairbank, J. A., Ebert, L., & Caddell, J. M. (2001). Posttraumatic stress disorder. In P. B. Sutker & H. E. Adams (Eds.), *Comprehensive handbook of psychopathology* (pp. 183–209). New York: Kluwer Academic/Plenum Publishers.

Foa, E., Hembree, E., & Rothbaum, B. (2007). *Prolonged exposure therapy for PTSD: Emotional processing of traumatic experiences, therapist guide*. New York: Oxford University Press.

Fonagy, P., & Allison, E. (2014). The role of mentalizing and epistemic trust in the therapeutic relationship. *Psychotherapy, 51*(3), 372–380.

Fonagy, P., Roth, A., & Higgitt, A. (2005). The outcome of psychodynamic psychotherapy for psychological disorders. *Clinical Neuroscience Research, 4*, 367–377.

Ford, J. D., & Courtois, C. A. (2014). Complex PTSD, affect dysregulation, and borderline personality disorder. *Borderline Personality Disorder and Emotional Dysregulation, 1*, 9. https://doi.org/10.1186/2051-6673-1-9.

Frost, N. D., Laska, K. M., & Wampold, B. E. (2014). The evidence for present-centered therapy as a treatment for posttraumatic stress disorder. *Journal of Traumatic Stress, 27*, 1–8. https://doi.org/10.1002/jts.21881.

Gerger, H., Munder, T., & Barth, J. (2014a). Specific and nonspecific psychological interventions for PTSD symptoms: A meta-analysis with problem complexity as a moderator. *Journal of Clinical Psychology, 70*, 601–615.

Gerger, H., Munder, T., Gemperli, A., Nüesch, E., Trelle, S., Jüni, P., & Barth, J. (2014b). Integrating fragmented evidence by network meta- analysis: Relative effectiveness of psychological interventions for adults with post-traumatic stress disorder. *Psychological Medicine, 44*, 3151–3164. https://doi.org/10.1017/S0033291714000853.

Gersons, P. R. B., Meewisse, M., & Nijdam, M. J. (2015). Brief eclectic psychotherapy for PTSD. In U. Schnyder & M. Cloitre (Eds.), *Evidence-based treatments for trauma-related psychological disorders*. Cham: Springer.

Greenberg, T. M. (2016). *Psychodynamic perspectives on aging and illness* (2nd ed.). New York: Springer.

Haslam, N. (2016, August 15). The problem with describing every misfortune as 'trauma.' *Chicago Tribune*. Accessed online on 5th Jan 2020 at https://www.chicagotribune.com/opinion/ct-trauma-microaggressions-trigger-warnings-20160815-story.html.

Henry, W. P. (1998). Science, politics and the politics of science: The use and misuse of empirically validated treatment research. *Psychotherapy Research, 8*, 126–140.

Herman, J. (1992). Complex PTSD: A syndrome in survivors of prolonged and repeated trauma. *Journal of Traumatic Stress, 5*, 377–391.

Horvath, A. O., & Greenberg, L. S. (1989). Development and validation of the Working Alliance Inventory. *Journal of Counseling Psychology, 36*(2), 223–233. https://doi.org/10.1037/0022-0167.36.2.223.

Hyland, P., Ceannt, R., Daccache, F., Abou Daher, R., Sleiman, J., Gilmore, B., et al. (2018). Are Posttraumatic Stress Disorder (PTSD) and complex-PTSD distinguishable within a treatment-seeking sample of Syrian refugees living in Lebanon? *Global Mental Health (Cambridge, England), 5*, e14. https://doi.org/10.1017/gmh.2018.2.

International Society for Traumatic Stress Studies. (2012). *The ISTSS Expert consensus treatment guidelines for complex PTSD in adults*. Accessed on 17th Aug 2019. https://www.istss.org/ISTSS_Main/media/Documents/ISTSS-Expert-Concesnsus-Guidelines-for-Complex-PTSD-Updated-060315.pdf.

Johns, R. G., Barkham, M., Kellet, S., & Saxon, D. (2019). A systematic review of therapist effects: A critical narrative update and refinement to Baldwin and Imel's (2013) review. *Clinical Psychology Review, 67*, 78–93.

Karatzias, T., Murphy, P., Cloitre, M., Bisson, J., Roberts, N., Shevlin, M., et al. (2019). Psychological interventions for ICD-11 complex PTSD symptoms: Systematic review and meta-analysis. *Psychological Medicine, 49*, 1–15. Accessed 1 July 2019. https://doi.org/10.1017/S0033291719000436.

Lambert, M. J. (2011). Psychotherapy research and its achievements. In J. C. Norcross, G. R. VandenBos, & D. K. Freedheim (Eds.), *History of psychotherapy* (2nd ed.). Washington, DC: American Psychological Association.

Lambert, M. J. (2013). The efficacy and effectiveness of psychotherapy. In M. J. Lambert (Ed.), *Bergin & Garfield's handbook of psychotherapy and behavior change* (6th ed., pp. 169–218). New York: Wiley.

Laska, K. M., Gurman, A. S., & Wampold, B. E. (2014). Expanding the lens of evidence-based practice in psychotherapy: A common factors perspective. *Psychotherapy, 51*, 467–481.

Linehan, M. (1993). *Cognitive-behavioral treatment of borderline personality disorder*. New York: Guilford Press.

McLaughlin, K. A., Conron, K. J., Koenen, K. C., & Gilman, S. E. (2010). Childhood adversity, adult stressful life events, and risk of past-year psychiatric disorder: A test of the stress sensitization hypothesis in a population-based sample of adults. *Psychological Medicine, 40*, 1647–1658.

Miller, S. D., Duncan, B. L., & Hubble, M. A. (1997). *Escape from Babel: Toward a unifying language for psychotherapy practice*. New York: Norton.

Morris, D. J. (2015, July 21). Trauma post trauma. Slate. Accessed online 13th July 2019, at https://slate.com/technology/2015/07/prolonged-exposure-therapy-for-ptsd-the-vas-treatment-has-dangerous-side-effects.html.

Moyers, T. B., Houck, J., Rice, S. L., Longabaugh, R., & Miller, W. R. (2016). Therapist empathy, combined behavioural intervention, and alcohol outcomes in the COMBINE research project. *Journal of Consulting and Clinical Psychology, 84*, 221–229.

Najavits, L. M. (2015). The problem of dropout from "gold standard" PTSD therapies. *F1000Prime Reports, 7*, 43. https://doi.org/10.12703/P7-43.

Neuner, F., Schauer, M., Klaschik, C., Karunakara, U., & Elbert, T. (2004). A comparison of narrative exposure therapy, supportive counseling, and psychoeducation for treating posttraumatic stress disorder in an African refugee settlement. *Journal of Consulting and Clinical Psychology, 72*(4), 579–587. http://dx.doi.org.ucsf.idm.oclc.org/10.1037/0022-006X.72.4.579.

Norcross, J. C., & Lambert, M. J. (Eds.). (2019). *Psychotherapy relationships that work. Volume 1: Evidence-based therapist contributions* (3rd ed.). New York: Oxford University Press.

Norcross, J. C., & Wampold, B. E. (2019a). *Psychotherapy relationships that work. Volume 2: Evidence-based responsiveness* (3rd ed.). New York: Oxford University Press.

Norcross, J. C., & Wampold, B. E. (2019b). Relationships and responsiveness in the psychological treatment of trauma: The tragedy of the APA clinical practice guideline. *Psychotherapy, 56*, 391. Advance online publication, Accessed 29 June 2019. https://doi.org/10.1037/pst0000228.

Perkonigg, A., Höfler, M., Cloitre, M., et al. (2016). *European Archives of Psychiatry and Clinical Neuroscience, 266*(4), 317–328.

Pietrzak, R. H., Goldstein, R. B., Southwick, S. M., & Grant, B. F. (2011). Prevalence and Axis I comorbidity of full and partial posttraumatic stress disorder in the United States: Results from Wave 2 of the National Epidemiologic Survey on alcohol and related conditions. *Journal of Anxiety Disorders, 25*, 456–465.

Powers, M. B., Halpern, J. M., Ferenschak, M. P., Gillihan, S. J., & Foa, E. B. (2010). A meta-analytic review of prolonged exposure for post- traumatic stress disorder. *Clinical Psychology Review, 30*, 635–641. https://doi.org/10.1016/j.cpr.2010.04.007.

Rauch, S., & Foa, E. (2006). Emotional Processing Theory (EPT) and exposure therapy for PTSD. *Journal of Contemporary Psychotherapy, 36*(2), 61–65.

Saxon, D., Firth, N., & Barkham, M. (2017). The relationship between therapist effects and therapy delivery factors: Therapy modality, dosage, and non-completion. *Administration and Policy in Mental Health and Mental Health Services Research, 44*(5), 705–715.

Sears, R. W., & Chard, K. M. (2016). *Mindfulness-based cognitive therapy for posttraumatic stress disorder*. West Sussex: Wiley.

Seidler, G., & Wagner, F. (2006). Comparing the efficacy of EMDR and trauma-focused cognitive-behavioral therapy in the treatment of PTSD: A meta-analytic study. *Psychological Medicine, 36*(11), 1515–1522.

Shapiro, F. (2001). *EMDR: Eye Movement Desensitization of Reprocessing: Basic principles, protocols and procedures* (2nd ed.). New York: Guilford Press.

Shedler, J. (2010, February–March). The efficacy of psychodynamic therapy. *American Psychologist, 65*(2), 98–109.

Shedler, J. (2017, November 19). Selling bad therapy to trauma victims. *Psychology Today Online*.

Smith, S. G., Zhang, X., Basile, K. C., Merrick, M. T., Wang, J., Kresnow, M., & Chen, J. (2018). *The National Intimate Partner and Sexual Violence Survey (NISVS): 2015 data brief – Updated release*. Atlanta: National Center for Injury Prevention and Control, Centers for Disease Control and Prevention.

Steil, R., Dyer, A., Priebe, K., Kleindienst, N., & Bohus, M. (2011). Dialectical behavior therapy for posttraumatic stress disorder related to childhood sexual abuse: A pilot study of an intensive residential treatment program. *Journal of Traumatic Stress, 24*, 102–106.

Steil, R., Dittmann, C., Müller-Engelmann, M., Dyer, A., Maasch, A. M., & Priebe, K. (2018). Dialectical behaviour therapy for posttraumatic stress disorder related to childhood sexual abuse: A pilot study in an outpatient treatment setting. *European Journal of Psychotraumatology, 9*(1), 1423832. https://doi.org/10.1080/20008198.2018.1423832.

Tran, U. S., & Gregor, B. (2016). The relative efficacy of bona fide psychotherapies for post-traumatic stress disorder: A meta-analytical evaluation of randomized controlled trials. *BMC Psychiatry, 16*, 266. https://doi.org/10.1186/s12888-016-0979-2.

Van der Kolk, B. A. (1994). The body keeps score: Memory and the evolving psychobiology of posttraumatic stress. *Harvard Review of Psychiatry, 1*(5), 253–265.

Van der Kolk, B. A. (1996). *The complexity of adaptation to trauma: Self-regulation, stimulus discrimination, and characterological development*. New York: Guilford Press.

Van der Kolk, B. A., McFarlane, A. C., & Weisæth, L. (2012). *Traumatic stress: The effects of overwhelming experience on mind, body and society*. New York: Guilford Press.

Wampold, B. E. (2015). How important are the common factors in psychotherapy? An update. *World Psychiatry, 14*, 270–277.

Wampold, B. E., & Imel, Z. (2015). *The great psychotherapy debate* (2nd ed.). Mahwah: Lawrence Erlbaum.

Chapter 2
How Trauma Stokes Fear: Clinical and Neurobiological Considerations in Beginning of Therapy

The Neurobiology of Trauma

The bodies and brains of people who have experienced repetitive trauma are different than those who have not. I'll review some of the major findings and how to think about frightened people who seek our help. Considering our traumatized clients through the lens of what happens in the body and brain is important, as clients who appear difficult to help are often repeating patterns that are quite literally neurological patterns. My hope is that by focusing on the neurobiology of trauma, we can get an appreciation for how it's imperative to create a sense of safety, promote healthier defenses, and increase social support before delving into memories of traumatic experiences or what some people vaguely refer to as "trauma work." Everything we do is trauma work, whether or not we are talking about memories in detail. I'll argue we may need to temper expectations regarding the latter. Complex PTSD is different than PTSD in terms of the ability to deal with the recollection of traumatic events while still maintaining a sense of safety and integrity regarding psychological functioning. Additionally, since the past always informs the present, we can deal with vexing clinical issues, particularly when they involve relationships, in the here and now. Emotions, especially when they live in the body, are dynamic and active constructs that have no idea of what is past, present, or future.

As we all know from experience, stress is both physical and emotional. Stress triggers the body's fight/flight response by activating the sympathetic branches of the autonomic nervous system. The activation of this response had evolutionary value; it allowed us to be able to respond aggressively or to leave situations when we were in danger (e.g., being attacked by a predator). When our senses indicate risk, a signal is sent to the amygdala, which is specialized for threat detection (Whalen et al. 2001). This activation may be more so when threat detection is automatic, like we see in people with PTSD or cPTSD. Involuntary threat attention tends to activate the amygdala, while voluntary attention tends to activate the superior temporal and anterior cingulate cortex (Vuilleumier 2002). This suggests that we

T. M. Greenberg, *Treating Complex Trauma*,
https://doi.org/10.1007/978-3-030-45285-8_2

can be activated and not even be consciously aware of it. It occurs to me that one example of this are people who have an exaggerated startle response but are literally not aware of it. I have known colleagues and clients who experience this. Something unexpected happens and they physically jump. Their body registers fear, but they cannot voice this.

Activation of the amygdala triggers outputs to many other areas, including the hypothalamus which controls the autonomic nervous system and physical functions such as breathing, blood pressure, blood flow, etc. The hypothalamus is a very basic part of our brain and is linked to survival. The hypothalamic–pituitary–adrenal (HPA) axis is a hormonal response system in which cortisol levels are impacted via neurological responses to stress. Hypothalamic activation of the HPA-axis is modulated by a variety of brain signaling systems, particularly neurotransmitters. The actions of this system are normally tightly regulated to ensure that the body can respond quickly to stressful events and return to a normal state just as rapidly. The main determinants of HPA-axis activity are genetic background, early-life environment, and current life stress (Stephens and Wand 2012). The hypothalamus sends a signal to the adrenal glands which release stress hormones (such as epinephrine, norepinephrine, and cortisol). This creates a feedback loop within the hypothalamic–pituitary–adrenal axis (HPA-axis) which has further consequences on mood and physical functioning (National Institutes of Health 2002). While the release of these stress hormones is helpful to manage stressful situations in the short term, living in a state of chronic stress weakens the body. At the very least, prolonged activation increases inflammation, which is implicated in both physical and psychological illnesses. As I'll discuss in Chapter 7, the HPA-axis response is one hypothesis for understanding the increases in medical illnesses among people who have experienced child abuse and/or chronic stress and chaos in early life (Fig. 2.1).

Neurological changes in response to trauma involve far more than the amygdala and hypothalamus. Many parts of the brain are implicated, and it's important to keep in mind that the brain is designed so that different parts communicate with each other. For example, flashbacks activate the limbic brain, indicating their intensely emotional nature, and the visual cortex, indicating the visual aspect of the flashback experience, while the brain's area for speech production (Broca's area) shows decreased activation (Rauch et al. 1996). This shutting down of the areas of the brain responsible for speech might explain why words are so elusive for traumatized people. As the main technique in traditional therapy is talking, this might be why body-oriented and somatic therapies are emphasized by some in working with cPTSD clients, but as I'll discuss, there are limitations to these approaches for people with histories of complex trauma.

Others have hypothesized that PTSD can affect the hippocampus which is partly responsible for memory. Reduced hippocampal volume is seen in many neurologic and psychiatric disorders, including PTSD (O'Doherty et al. 2015). Several studies have found that people with depression have lower hippocampal volume (Sheline 2011) and may impact people with cPTSD who experience chronic or recurrent depression. The physiological experience of being in traumatic situations affects how and if memories of the event are formed. The secretion of glucocorticoids (via

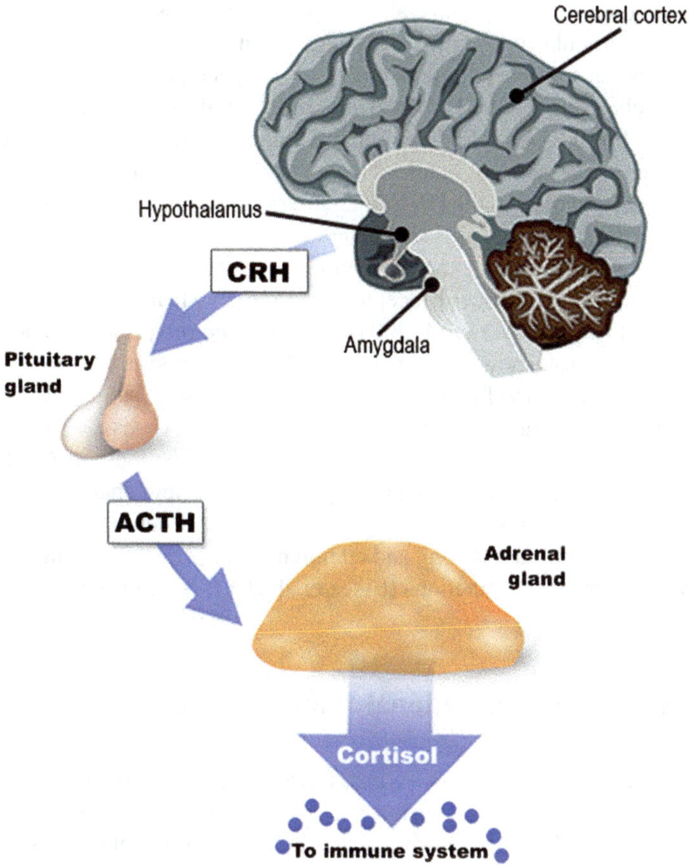

Fig. 2.1 Relationship between the amygdala, hypothalamus, and the HPA-axis. Cortisol levels are affected, which is thought to be related to increases in inflammation and possibly alterations in immune functioning

ACTH) and norepinephrine disrupts episodic and explicit memory (e.g., LeDoux 1996; Solms and Turnbull 2002), often making it difficult for people to have access to many details of traumatic events, particularly when they are chronic. This finding reinforces the idea that details of some memories, particularly in childhood, may not be able to be fully recalled and discussed in psychotherapy.

Several authors have described that the neurological effects of trauma are what makes it difficult for some traumatized people to have a cohesive narrative of not only their traumatic experiences but of their lives (e.g., Siegel 2003; Schore 2003; Van der Kolk 2014). For example, van der Kolk (2014) presented functional magnetic resonance imaging (fMRI) of a woman who was in a severe car accident, in which she was trapped. The woman he was describing, Ute, experienced severe dissociation as one component of her PTSD. Her fMRI showed decreased activation in almost all areas of her brain while in a dissociated state, suggesting how trauma can limit the ability to think, in a very basic sense.

Our genes themselves cannot be altered, but their expression is influenced by our environment, particularly when we are young. Chemical tags on the DNA sequence tell the cells when and where to make more of one gene product and less of others, often utterly changing the final result. There is data in the epigenetics literature that both maternal behavior and childhood maltreatment impact HPA-axis responses via changes in the expression of genes as measured through gene expression that are produced by methylation of the DNA. Increases in DNA methylation is an indicator of increased HPA-axis responses, meaning the organism is more stressed and activated. For example, rats that experience more soothing behaviors from their mothers express more glucocorticoid receptors and are less fearful than rats raised by indifferent mothers (Weaver et al. 2004). Also in rats, offspring that have experienced early life stress show an increased HPA-axis response to stress (Liu et al. 1997). In people, childhood maltreatment is associated with increased DNA methylation of the glucocorticoid receptor gene, increased HPA-axis activation, and the presence of symptoms of borderline personality disorder symptoms (Radtke et al. 2015). Children exposed to stress in early childhood show changes in the DNA methylation of many genes, including some related to neuronal patterning and development, neuronal functioning and communication, stress hormone production, and many other important functions (Essex et al. 2011; Naumova et al. 2011).

Evidence for Intergenerational Trauma Effects

Maternal responses to trauma involve unresolved states of loss or abuse experienced by parents and how these states can have second-generation effects on their children (Hesse et al. 2003). The mechanism is thought to be via fear and role inversion in cases of traumatized parents who were not overtly maltreating their children but did have symptoms of a disorganized attachment style because of their own loss/abuse. Disorganized attachment is a now-common term used to describe the effects of fear states and fearful interactions between parents and children. Young children with disorganized attachment styles exhibited a "collapse of attentional and behavioral strategies" when reunited with their mothers after separation (Main and Hesse 1992). In young children, Ainsworth's "strange situation" saw children who exhibited behavioral disorganization or disorientation in the form of wandering, confused expressions, freezing, undirected movements, or contradictory and unorganized patterns of interaction with a caregiver (Ainsworth and Bell 1970). Disorganized attachment is not just a clinically interesting phenomenon relating to the ability to feel safe in the presence of others. Disorganized attachment predicts suicide attempts, as will be discussed in Chapter 4, as well as dissociation, which will be discussed in Chapter 5. Hesse et al. (2003) note the simple presence of a loss in mothers did not predict the development of a disorganized attachment among their infants. However, mothers who had a loss that remained unresolved and disorganized did have infants who exhibited disorganized attachment styles. In their research, Hesse and his colleagues relied on slippages in speech that indicated mothers who were disorganized/

dissociative themselves. In such cases, their children were more frightened. In addition, the children of these mothers, again, who had experienced no known maltreatment, were found to have recurring catastrophic thoughts, more controlling behaviors, and "cognitive confusion or blank spells" (Hesse et al. 2003; Liotti 1993), suggesting the powerful effects that fear in a parent can have on their children.

In another study, maternal PTSD predicted child PTSD, and emotional abuse predicted higher levels of cortisol among children of Holocaust survivors (Yehuda et al. 2001). Maternal PTSD can increase the risk for emotional reactivity and difficulty with emotional regulation in children as early as infancy (Bosquet Enlow et al. 2011). In a study of low-income African American women with high incidents of trauma, emotional dysregulation among mothers was significantly associated with greater PTSD symptoms in the child independent of the child's own trauma exposure or emotion regulation difficulties as well as independent of the mother's trauma history and psychiatric symptoms (Powers et al. 2020).

Although many of us can imagine PTSD to be passed down to offspring as intellectually true among some of the second- and even third-generation trauma survivors, it can be hard to put into focus how something like this can manifest. I'll describe one case in which this scenario seemed probable:

Janice was raised by two parents who had escaped violent political traumas and genocide in their country of origin. She was vaguely aware that one of her parents endured situations in which she was hungry and had to "beg" for food from neighbors. She was proud of her heritage, could still speak the language her parents spoke, and named her child with an ethnic sounding name, even though her parents never talked about where they came from. She felt strongly she had not been abused as a child. In fact, she felt that her mother, especially, went to great lengths to give her a good life in America. This latter fact did result in Janice being left with multiple and different caregivers for prolonged periods as a child as her parents had to work multiple jobs to support her. Yet, Janice insisted she had been well cared for. For example, her parents only left her with people they knew well, and there was no overt evidence of abuse or neglect.

One day during a stressful event in her life involving problems with her partner of over two decades, Janice was at the mall looking for clothes. She wandered into a cosmetics store and very uncharacteristically for her, she thought about shoplifting. She reported later that she was not sure why she thought about this; she had never done anything like this before. While she eyed some skin care products, she thought seriously about putting an expensive moisturizer into her bag. She thought she could do it without anyone noticing. She decided against it but noticed that a man had started following her around the store. On one level, Janice knew rationally that she had not done anything wrong; she thought about stealing, but she did not. Yet, this man who turned out to be a loss prevention employee followed her; she became more and more anxious and she ran out of the store. A security guard followed her and she ran through the mall to the parking garage. She said she felt panicked, as if her life were in jeopardy, though on one level, she knew this made no sense. She stopped a passing car and told the driver she was being attacked (Janice realized this was a lie and not based on the reality of her circumstance), and the woman in the car, assuming that she was being harassed, or worse, allowed her into the car. The thoughtful and unassuming woman in the rescue car waited with Janice for 15 minutes until Janice thought it safe to go back to her car. The woman took Janice to her car, but the security guard was waiting nearby with a police officer and stopped her and brought her back to the detention office in the mall. Janice was accused of shoplifting. After a search, Janice was released as she had no unpaid merchandise in her possession.

Janice had little insight as to what had happened to her or why. She knew she ran from the security guard, and it felt as if she was "running for her life." But her reaction was deemed quite outsized by both of us at that time. I'd been seeing Janice for several years at this point, and though it was clear that disorganized attachment and dissociation were part of her clinical picture, this event was striking and alarming to both of us. As Janice had no real narrative of the history of her parents, except she did know her father did have to steal in order to keep himself alive, we wondered about an intergenerational legacy as part of the story of what happened.

As we can see, trauma creates fear, but of the primal kind. To be clear, it was never obvious what happened to Janice as she fled treatment shortly after this event. I don't know if this was because of the separation of her primary relationship and there were very real financial limitations she was deemed to endure. However, something about her behavior was alarming to her, and I have wondered if this was the real reason she left. At the time of this event, she had gotten closer to thinking about her parents and what they might have had to do to endure and survive their trauma histories. Perhaps there was more to Janice's experience as well. It was not clear she was ready to think about these things even though she brought it up and a part of her wanted to talk about it.

Under stressful situations, our bodies and minds may relive our own traumas and possibly those of our caretakers, though it seems more research is needed to understand the links from our actual pasts to those of our parents. Whether it's actually genetically epigenetic or metaphorically so, we do live the lives of our caretakers to some extent. If our parents are traumatized, we will attach deeply to this, whether we want to or not.

Fear: Known, Unknown, and Acted Out

Fear as a result of trauma is not often the kind of fright where someone can come to therapy and say, "I realize I am afraid of everything." Some people with acute or simple PTSD can do this if they had good enough and safe enough backgrounds, and their minds work in such a way that they can generally distinguish what is safe from what is not. Complex PTSD not only challenges several aspects of neurological functioning, the repetitive nature of trauma serves to remind the mind and the body that it can never be safe. This may be true because the world is dangerous, and some people who have been traumatized are more likely to be victimized again. It can also be true if we are primed to consider that threats exist everywhere we go.

This is something many people are not even aware of until they are in therapy and can think about this in the presence of another person in which such ideas can really be known. Let's return to Melanie, whom I described in Chapter 1:

As Melanie settled into therapy, she got a new job. It was not as prestigious as her previous positions but seemed like a good fit. She had a manager who really saw the extent of her abilities, which had always seemed to me to be quite impressive for a young woman of her age. Her manager worked quickly to give Melanie more responsibility and this was when the problems started. Melanie became so anxious that she started to work from home, even though this was frowned upon by her employer. I felt alarmed, as this was obviously a red flag, but could not get a sense of what was troubling to her. I wondered if maybe being taken seriously made her anxious, as she was used to a world in which people diminished her potential. I considered if she worried this was too good to be true. These observations offered no traction in the treatment and her mood worsened, and she became very angry at her place of employment, though I could not discern why. Eventually, she told me that one of her colleagues was very upset about her role. Melanie imagined that he perceived her as "too young." This colleague was a man and one she had relatively little contact with. Yet she worried all of the time about his impressions of her. She thought this guy had the power to take away her position, though there was no rational reason for her thinking this. She considered whether or not she should be moved to a different team, so she could avoid contact with him altogether. I felt even more concerned upon hearing this, as she had lost previous jobs because of impulsive decisions and angry outbursts related to people she did not like. Yet, I felt I had no real say, as I did not know the details except that she seemed scared and agitated. In addition, I felt worried about her becoming aware of the extent of my concern, as it was unclear to me that our relationship could tolerate this kind of overt or subtle discloser. I did not want to be experienced by her the way she felt her "panicked" parents seemed. Once I could organize these thoughts in my mind, I realized that it was pointless to try to get a logical explanation about what was happening at work. Finally, I said to her, "I can't quite get a sense of what is going on here, but it's clear you are scared. Of what, I am not sure. Can you wait a bit before transferring teams so we can see if we can figure out what is driving your fear? I'm sure this guy is challenging, but maybe we can try to think about what is best for you." In addition, she allowed me to help her concretely in terms of the tone of her emails to members of her team, which had been already escalating and exposing her state of burgeoning anger.

Since I had mentioned a few times early in the therapy (even when we were concretely thinking about looking for jobs) that fear must have some place in her previous problems at work, she agreed to wait before being transferred. I suggested if she could try to tell me more about this man at work. He was older, of a similar ethnic background as she and her family. She had not mentioned this before, and I remarked that being around someone who may have better understanding of her cultural background did not seem soothing. This appeared to wake her up, almost as if she had been jarred awake from a deep sleep. She said, "No! Oh, God, no!" I let her know that I thought maybe I was starting to get it. She was unable to say more dur-

ing that session. The next week she said, "He's like someone I knew growing up. My parents used to have him watch me. Bad things happened." I did not ask for detail. I said, "There were bad things and you weren't safe." She looked down and nodded slowly. I mentioned that it may be hard sometimes to know if she can trust her perceptions about things and so her anxiety was a marker that something did not feel right. She took this in a very concrete way and said, "So you think I should transfer teams?"

As a result of trauma and the incredible ways some people adapt and are resilient, many people I meet in therapy have little to no conscious recognition of fear. This is in large part due to the fact that they simply are not in their bodies or aware of a lot of content in their minds. Intense anxiety just brings a lot of noise and not really access to thoughts or feelings. Although many people who have been traumatized are anxious and have excessive anxious rumination, this is not the kind of access to one's mind I am referring to. I remember suggesting to another young woman with extreme anxiety that she may not always know what is on her mind, and she shot back with, "Of course I do!" And she listed all of her worries that had little to do with own her mind, but her worries about what was on other's minds, including how others viewed her. Trauma causes people to be outside of their own minds. Hypervigilance requires that people pay attention to what is going on outside (not inside), and survivors of trauma harness their hyperawareness to try to read the thoughts and motives of others.

Clinical Hypothesis Testing and Thinking About Fear with Our Clients

Many people who have had repetitive experiences of trauma are disembodied or dissociated from many physical and psychological states. Melanie had been seeing me for over 6 months when we had the conversation about her co-worker, and it was the dawn of her realizing that her hatred of this man was a manifestation of a kind of abject fear. I often consider a goal of therapy with people who have experienced complex trauma to bring their sense of fear into their awareness. We have to be careful with this, as anger or being numb often feels safer than fear. To return to the idea of clinical hypothesis testing, I may develop an idea that someone is fearful and not just angry. Whether or not I say something about this has to do with how they are seeming to me in the moment. For example, a woman with a sexual trauma history was telling me about how her boyfriend was playfully trying to get her to lie down on their bed. She had a panic attack, which led to rage at her boyfriend. She told him he was trying to "assault" her. Her boyfriend was confused, as their sex life had involved far more explicit activities related to submission than him trying to get her into bed. After I let her finish her fairly long diatribe about her boyfriend, I mentioned that maybe she felt scared. She bristled at this and said, "This might apply to other people, but not me. I am not scared." She seemed angry at me and was likely disappointed that I missed her emotions at that moment. I immediately backed off.

Although the evidence seemed pretty strong to me that she was frightened, she was not ready to see it. I focused then on what she felt in terms of her anger and I wondered with her about why she did not seem to feel she could set boundaries. It was after 20 minutes of discussing this that she calmed down and seemed less angry in general. It was important that I let go of my idea of fear and meet her where she was consciously at. She then said, "I suppose I could have felt fear. Is that what you think?" I told her that I had an idea about it but that I may have been wrong. She paused, "I'm not sure." I said, "What's in your mind is more important. You don't have to take care of me by agreeing."

It's important to pivot if we have a thought that does not fit. In this instance, the client's state of mind could not have allowed her to feel fear. I jumped in too soon with my hypothesis. And while this woman did eventually realize how fearful she was during sex with her boyfriend (as well as during many other interactions with him), she did not feel safe enough to acknowledge her fear and I needed to respect that.

Despite extreme disembodiment, in my experience, people with cPTSD don't often do well with bodily focused therapies as this can feel like a forced entry into their physical selves and they feel out of control. As one client put it to me, "I was told to breathe into my body and I was like, 'Are you fucking kidding?!'" Another woman said something similar when she recounted an experience with a somatic therapist, though with more expletives. Neither of these women were conscious of feeling afraid; they remarked that they felt "frozen" or "dead." They were so terrified, they dissociated when being told to pay attention to their bodies. Even less dissociated individuals with cPTSD experience paradoxical anxiety when people try to relax, meditate, or even become aware of their bodies. For many of these clients, lessening arousal not only strips them of the benefits they feel they get from hypervigilance, it makes them more anxious. Behaviorally, this reinforces that they should not try to relax at all because relaxation leads to panic.

As I've suggested, anger is the counterpart to fear. If the choice is fight or flight, "fight" can feel safer. Sometimes in the beginning of therapy, often later when someone feels secure, clients like Melanie tell me they have gotten feedback that they have "anger issues." These problems with anger are often complicated. It's true that some people, including Melanie, seem angry, but anger is often the go-to emotion for people who have little access to their minds. Anger is organizing; it allows us to delineate good people vs. bad people, and it allows us to know where we stand. We can feel clear if we feel that someone else is being "bad"; it resolves confusion. Yet, the expression of anger often carries a high price. So much so that an entire chapter of this book is devoted to anger and aggression. Even in people who insist they are comfortable with their expressions of anger (and this is more socially acceptable for men), there is usually some kind of discomfort if someone feels that they overreacted or were too harsh. They may not have the words to say it, but they tend to not sleep well at night, or they have physical concerns not rooted in objective medical findings. One man I am thinking of with these issues would spend literally hours trying to convince me he had the right to act as angry as he did. Yet, if he was really okay with his aggression, why did I need convincing? I'm pretty sure it was not me he was trying to convince, but himself.

It's these kinds of anger responses and the subsequent difficulties in relationships that often lead us to assume that people such as Melanie have a personality disorder. I'm not so sure this is true. I think, as therapists, we have difficulty sorting out how to deal with anger. We often have an immediate aversion to it, and I think this causes us to have missed opportunities for people who can benefit from understanding the complex relationship between anger and fear and just how literally amped up their bodies are. I'll say more later in this chapter about dealing with angry people, especially in the beginning of therapy, and all of Chapter 8 is devoted to discussing anger. First, I will describe the strains caused by the way many of us have learned to consider cPTSD as a euphemism for personality disorders.

The Unhelpful Link Between cPTSD and Personality Disorders

Most clinicians are aware that there is considerable overlap between the myriad of symptoms in people with cPTSD and personality disorders. For example, researchers have noted overlap between cPTSD and borderline personality disorder (Ford and Courtois 2014), as well as the link between personality disorders and attachment disturbances in the context of early trauma (Mills 2005).

However, personality disorders are notoriously difficult to diagnose, because of considerable overlap of symptoms used to identify these disorders. This is an issue that has plagued the last several editions of the DSM (e.g., Pfohl et al. 1986; Oldham et al. 1992; Widiger and Trull 1998; Grant et al. 2005). This has led to researchers suggesting that the DSM simply does not represent so-called categorical phenomena (Haslam et al. 2012).

There is a deep divide between how clinicians and researchers diagnose and understand personality functioning (Westen 1997; Thylstrup et al. 2016). The debate around personality disorder criteria commonality is explained by some researchers as categorical versus dimensional classifications. Proponents of a dimensional classification of personality disorders argue that the symptoms of personality disorders exist on a spectrum of *normal to abnormal* as opposed to the presence or absence of specific symptoms (Gøtzsche-Astrup and Moskowitz 2016).

Additionally, many of us have been taught that the hallmark of someone with a personality disorder is that their symptoms are *ego-syntonic*. The classic way of describing this is that the symptoms of someone with a personality disorder (which aren't really symptoms at all; "symptoms" is a term used to describe our subjective experience of suffering) don't bother the patient, but they bother everyone else around them. I think it's more complicated than this. Of course, it's true that people who have challenges to their character and have interpersonal problems are difficult for the people around them. But it's simply not true that people with these diagnoses are immune to a sense of suffering. This has been observed most often in people who are thought to have borderline personality disorder (e.g., Mulder 2009). I have seen many people who could meet criteria for several different personality disorders in my work, and I am struck by the amount of suffering people endure. This includes people who are extremely paranoid and people who can be considered histrionic and even some people with narcissistic traits. The old teaching was if someone with a personality disorder comes to therapy, it's usually because someone else wants them to, and once they can appease the people who urged them to therapy, they quit. This does sometimes happen, but not always or even frequently in my work. As I have gotten older, I've found that if I can point out that certain personality traits actually do cause internal misery (not to mention external interpersonal problems), there can be a way to get a buy-in for them to engage in therapy. However, this is not true for people who are extremely antisocial or sociopathic, as these individuals never get therapy, usually unless it's mandated by law enforcement. That said, there is clinical data that some people with personality disorders are not simply clueless as to their suffering and even their impact on others.

Personality functioning and the impact of trauma on identity are often at the heart of what we treat when we try to help people with cPTSD. Certainly, dimensional categories of personality disorders also fit right in with a trauma approach to care. In such an approach, we tend to evaluate clients while thinking about development; for example, why do people develop the coping strategies they have? We assume, based on the reality of traumatic environments, that these strategies once worked well. For example, consider the plight of a 9-year-old girl who is being molested by her father. Her mother is aware of this abuse however vaguely, but she certainly notices that her husband (the father of the abused girl) gives the child more attention than the mother thinks is warranted. Some mothers in this situation hate their daughters and imagine that their daughters are seductive and a threat, as opposed to being able to see the situation for what it is, that a child is being exploited and abused. As this (abused) girl grows up, she might find that the only way to feel safe and not hated is by gaining the attention of men. As one woman who grew up in this exact situation told me, "I learned that women were jealous, and I could only find attention from men. If I don't have that, I am starving emotionally." As an adult, she had been diagnosed with borderline personality disorder. She was fired by every female boss she had but was able to work with men, but this sometimes required her to act "flirty" (her word) in ways that felt all too familiar. She hated herself for acting this way, but felt she knew of no other way of responding. She figured out the only way she could to keep herself from terrifying isolation and continued to use this way of coping. When we think about this situation through this lens (albeit focusing on just one symptom), it's not clear that a personality disorder diagnosis fits. Though her behavior was not helpful for her as an adult, as a child, it made sense, because she had to get love and attention, somehow.

How Trauma Can Lead to Incorrect Diagnoses

When the term complex trauma is thought of as a euphemism for personality disorders, this creates a kind of bias. We are all entitled to have preferences about with whom we work, and I am not suggesting that any of us take on clients we don't feel we can help. But I have wondered if sometimes clients are not given adequate chances to connect. What may look like intractable pathology or someone who will be unable to form an attachment with us may be a mask for an extremely traumatized state.

Consider the case of Thomas:

Thomas is a 76-year-old retired policeman who had a successful career and had never received therapy or had mental health problems before, though one of his children mentioned that he was a "big drinker." He was referred for therapy at the urging of his son following the sudden death of his wife in a car accident in which he had been driving. Thomas had a number of medical problems, which were exacerbated following his wife's death. He initially saw a psychoanalyst for psychotherapy. They met three times, but the analyst concluded that he was "unsuitable" for therapy as reported to me by his children. I met with Thomas shortly thereafter, as his son felt strongly that his father needed "someone to talk to." Thomas was pleasant enough and initially in our first session denied both psychological symptoms and the need for therapy. In fact, he simply stared at me. I felt awkward and found myself adjusting my body position in my chair. I realized that part of my discomfort was that I could get no read on Thomas's affect. His face just seemed frozen and he had a blank stare.

I then asked him where he was from. He answered my question but was more curious to know the same about me, and I replied that I came from the same region. I then asked about his hobbies, and he told me of an active life involving a certain sport. Since I was especially familiar with the sport, I talked with him about my own experience and briefly discussed how my father had pursued similar sports-related interests. We talked for nearly 30 minutes about these topics when he spontaneously became tearful and talked all about his wife. He described his disabling despair and told me he had been considering suicide and that he had a plan involving firearms in his home for carrying this out.

Thomas was in a traumatized state when I met him, and like many people in this situation, he was blank, dissociated, and disembodied. I had no initial inkling that he was planning suicide. But I knew he had lost his partner of 50 years and I guessed he felt responsible. Additionally, I was familiar with the high rates of vicarious trauma and PTSD among police officers (e.g., Hartley et al. 2013). It seemed imperative to try to reach him.

Because Thomas was used to being "in charge" of many different situations, it seemed crucial in that first session that I could provide an environment that allowed him to maintain control. At the same time, it was also vital that I convey a sense of confidence and authority that would match his sense of control in order for him to feel safe and assured of my ability to be of help to him. I needed to offer an environment where I could be flexible with my use of self-disclosure and could talk about seemingly unrelated or concrete (nonemotional) topics. Although I felt hesitant in discussing aspects of my personal experience, especially my father, it became clear that this disclosure was essential to his feeling comfortable with me. Though to some extent I feel that I took a risk (as is always the case with self-disclosure), I could tell by Thomas's reluctance to talk with me that if I did not participate in a concrete conversation, and one that acknowledged some shared interest, I would have not seen him a second time. Could this be evidence of some narcissistic trait? Absolutely. I imagine some colleagues might suggest that I colluded with his narcissism by emphasizing a similarity. But it worked and we never once talked about my life again, except when we wanted to know where I went on vacation.

Thomas continued therapy weekly for 2 years. He seemed very suited for treatment. As I came to know Thomas and his perception of why his first experience in therapy did not work, it seemed as if his previous therapist wanted Thomas to address narcissistic aspects of his illnesses and possibly expected that Thomas talk openly and right away about the death of his wife. Thomas explained that his therapist had made interpretations about his anger and his feelings of unfairness about being "left" by his wife, as well as having to endure his medical problems and limitations. This sounded to me like pretty standard interpretations one might make to someone who is perceived as narcissistic. I don't know how narcissistic Thomas was, versus what could be considered understandable defenses or even just shock and horror. In this case it really did not matter. Thomas had experienced a horrible trauma and loss and I was able to help him with that. He did not need to take control of the ending of his life. He felt like he could go on with life, as shocked and bewildered as he was in the depths of traumatic grief. An additional factor in that first session was not what we talked about but rather the fact that I was willing to discuss something other than the obvious topics, his grief, his sense of responsibly for the accident, and his worsening medical problems. I respected his need for avoidance.

When we meet people who seem like they have a personality disorder, we are quick to assume they can't benefit from therapy. Certainly with Thomas, his traumatic state made it seem like he was not accessible. This was not the case. He just needed a flexible therapeutic approach to get help.

People who experience severe traumas and have cPTSD live in a world they know none of us get. This is a unique hallmark of trauma, the realization that no one else can really live inside of you and know how horrible something is. Pain and suffering are unique to all of us. Additionally the random nature of trauma exacerbates the experience of shock and isolation. David Morris in his 2016 book, *The Evil Hours: A Biography of Post-Traumatic Stress Disorder*, describes his war trauma this way:

> The lesson taught by the war was clear: to be human is to be small, powerless, and subject to the forces of randomness. (p. 5)

This description fits the experience of many trauma survivors and serves as a reminder of just how much care we need to employ in our work with traumatized clients. We can never truly know the extent of another's suffering, but we can try. I think the therapeutic action, what makes people get better, is in the trying. The less we pathologize people, the easier this is.

Assessing Character Style

Although I have advocated that we think about trauma reactions first and foremost in our work with clients, it's important that we think about the effect of trauma on character development in the case of childhood trauma and the impact on identity in the case of adult trauma. No matter which technique we choose to employ in psychotherapy, knowing someone's character style can guide us in choosing our interventions. By character style I am referring to a wide range of internal and external characteristics, such as coping behaviors, affect regulation, the ability to connect and get help from others, comfort with depending on others, general defenses, the tendency to internalize or externalize, attachment patterns, learning style, how they soothe themselves when anxious, the nature of cognitions and beliefs, etc.

There are many ways to assess someone's character. Obviously, the DSM gives us some guidelines for thinking about styles that when operating excessively can lead to the construct of a personality disorder or personality disorder traits. As I've stated, I think there are limitations to this approach, especially if we assume that if someone meets criteria for an Axis II diagnosis, we can't help them. Another avenue of understanding personality style is formal training in assessment. I realize that a small percentage of us actually perform formal personality testing, but this training is vital to understanding character and personality functioning. Years ago, when I used to teach graduate students in personality and intellectual assessment, I could always count on a few students who grumbled at learning about assessment. They wanted to be therapists and therefore saw no benefit in learning testing. I was taught that training in assessment is less about learning to test people but more about learning how to think about different facets of human functioning. It's a valuable foundation, and I learned a lot about how to think about many facets of personality and symptoms, even in my program which emphasized cognitive behavioral therapy.

A good assessment of character style allows us to choose interventions and more importantly can inform how we connect with our clients. As we've seen, how we relate to clients and our relationship with them is a powerful predictor of therapeutic outcome. Therefore, if someone I am seeing is more dramatic, I match this and will tend to use more hyperbolic speech. If someone is more obsessional, I will be more measured and cautious regarding how I speak. If someone is suspicious, I actively explain what I am thinking about what they are saying. A lot of us do this intuitively, but it involves matching, to some extent, the language and emotional styles of our clients.

Regarding techniques, a combined approach to treating trauma means that we tailor our interventions to their character style. For example, if someone comes with specific complaints about anxiety and wants immediate relief, I suggest some CBT approaches as a concrete option to reduce symptoms. I then wait to see how these ideas land. Sometimes people readily endorse the idea of CBT and are eager to do homework. More often, however, people come back saying they put off doing recommended CBT approaches. Instead of interpreting resistance, I wait instead to see if there is something else on their mind they want to talk about. In a recent example of this, a man came back offering reasons why he did not exercise and attempt the guided meditation we had discussed. It was clear he needed to tell me about his mother and how hostile she was and how he felt that his main problem was not anxiety at all, but his anger. This led us in a different direction. His anxiety was an issue but was often a sign that he was feeling angry. Further, I also guessed based on his comments that a more directive treatment might not be suited for him, given his communication about his anger at his mother, and I was another woman in a position of authority.

If someone seems suspicious, I think with them about ways for them to feel safe with me in therapy and let them know it can take a long time to get to know me. If someone presents with problems with emotional regulation, I imagine that their trauma history has led to an intense sense of fear, and I focus issues on present relationships (which are often something myself and my client can understand quickly) and work toward containment. If someone is more obsessional, I'm likely to start with behavioral approaches as they can provide a quick and practical way to control symptoms and can also be organizing. Sometimes people who are more obsessional enjoy homework or assignments, and I am happy to provide that.

In terms of formal learning about character assessment, I have found psychoanalytic ideas regarding personality helpful. Specifically I have appreciated the first and second editions of *Psychoanalytic Diagnosis* (McWilliams 2011). This text offers an in-depth look at psychoanalytic diagnosis but is extremely practical and is a great introduction to understanding character, even if psychodynamic therapy is not the treatment of choice. In addition to reviewing major defenses, McWilliams also describes different character styles, including paranoid, depressive, manic, dissociative obsessional, and histrionic styles. David Shapiro's books, *Psychotherapy of Neurotic Character* (Shapiro 1999) and *Neurotic Styles* (Shapiro 1973), are classic texts addressing ideas of character functioning, though the latter may feel a bit dated for a modern audience, as there are descriptions of gender stereotypes that I have found a bit hard to digest when I have gone back to this book. That said, *Neurotic Styles* provides some key concepts related to different character traits.

The other helpful idea from psychodynamic therapy that I find useful is the idea of anxiety. Literally thousands of pages in psychoanalytic literature on anxiety have been published, but put simply, we can better access what a client's conflicts are if we understand what makes them anxious, particularly in relationships. In Freud's (1926) theory, anxiety is regarded as a compromise between a threatening impulse and what we do to ward off feelings or thoughts we don't want to have (defenses). In this way, anxiety is a distraction but also signals the danger of unwanted thoughts or feelings. Again, I am simplifying over a century of analytic ideas on anxiety, but for clients who are slow to engage in therapy or who may be guarded, I use this idea and weave it into informal CBT techniques. For example, with Melanie, she said she simply felt bad. Although she was anxious and having panic attacks, these were not connected in her mind with anyone or anything. She just thought something was wrong with her. As she started to have more problems at work, I asked her to keep track of who or what at work caused her the most anxiety. It was then I found out about the man who reminded her of the caretaker who had abused her.

People familiar with psychoanalytic theory likely realize that these aforementioned references and ideas are geared toward people with what is referred to as *neurotic* functioning. In older psychoanalytic ideas, neurotic functioning was thought not to encompass people with complex trauma histories or people who could be deemed challenging in terms of personality structure. For many of our complex PTSD clients, it is not always the case that we can address anxiety in the ways I have described above. This is often an evolution in therapy when people feel safe. With Melanie, I learned she had been diagnosed as having depression with every therapist before myself. When her therapy really started to gain traction, she realized the extent of her anxiety. She said, "I have spent my whole life thinking about my depression. It was not until now that I understand how anxious I feel around other people." Anxiety, when we can see how it is connected with relationships, is a needed part of therapy for most people, particularly people who have experienced trauma. It can take a while for these kinds of conversations to develop as people with cPTSD are often hesitant to think in this way in the beginning of therapy.

Managing Fear in the Beginning of Therapy

As I have suggested so far in these first two chapters, I think we need to be flexible with technique and avail ourselves what the client needs. This takes place in the context of a good assessment, though I often conduct these assessments informally. In fact, I have found that most of what I learned about diagnostic interviewing really did me little good when seeing therapy clients for the first few sessions because of the tendency for them to be overwhelmed by questions, particularly surrounding abuse and trauma. Therefore, it's imperative that initial meetings are not intrusive. I am aware that in many clinic settings, especially ones that involve training, there is an emphasis on screening for appropriate matches with clinicians. I respect the need for this, but in situations in which there has been aggressive screening, it's important for the therapist to ask the client how they felt about the intake process. Some people with trauma histories are sensitive to these kinds of intrusions, though I imagine many people are. There are limitations to tests and screening methods; at the very least, they don't capture nuances of people's experience.

Even if I suspect someone has been traumatized, I begin all therapies with the idea that we will work in the here and now. The reasons for this include the following:

1. Most of the time clients come to therapy with concerns about the present.
2. When cPTSD is a likely diagnosis, they may not even be thinking about traumatic events, and if they are, they may not see how these events have any link to the present.
3. When clients are aware of trauma, they may simply not want to talk about it in detail.

4. Since trauma impacts relationships, as well as the common tendency to find people in life who may represent features of those who have caused harm, discussing relationships in the present is a way to get at relational and attachment traumas but without being overstimulating.

Therefore, the beginning of therapy is about developing a good therapeutic relationship. Proponents of three-stage models (Herman 1992; Courtois and Ford 2013) emphasize safety as well, but I think, in comparison, I find myself less directive about labeling trauma in the beginning of therapy. Many traumatized people are resilient because they have not thought about traumas. As I'm getting to know someone, I might notice a pattern that looks like cPTSD, but I will say something after several sessions of observing their patterns and behaviors, especially with others. When I do talk about it, I talk about it through the lens of symptoms and behaviors. For example, I might say, "I notice you are super concerned about what others think, so much so that it's really hard to know what is in your mind. It's a little like hypervigilance, like we see sometimes in people with PTSD. I don't know if that's exactly what you have, but there is this way you can't ever relax and it seems important." I rarely overtly link current situations to traumas people have told me about.

In the beginning of therapy, clients sometimes want to tell me their traumas, but not in a way that we have been able to really digest. For example, one client who clearly met criteria for cPTSD (e.g., she was currently cutting herself when anxious, had an eating disorder, and was significantly dissociative) told me in the beginning of therapy, "I just want you to know, and I don't want to talk about it, that I was raped in college and someone tried to abduct me when I was a teenager; also my sister died." Given the current chaos in her life, we spent a lot of time talking about current relationships, which proved fruitful as she was reenacting some of the chaos of her past in the present and I could help her think about these current emotions. I did offer her DBT, as that could have been helpful with her self-harm, but she was not interested. Talking about her current relationships and dealing with a problematic boyfriend proved to reduce her need to hurt herself. She also got better control over her eating disorder.

I am not convinced that people with cPTSD need to go back and "process" all past traumas, certainly not in the beginning of therapy where safety is the primary goal. I'll discuss this in more detail in the next chapter. Pragmatically speaking, for people with cPTSD, there simply may be too many traumas. Additionally, as I have discussed in this chapter and will discuss in the chapter on dissociation, thinking about past traumas may be impossible because extreme anxiety and dissociation can interfere with the development of memories and thus render this goal impossible. I think the ultimate aspects of therapeutic action lie in our ability to hold and contain the emotions of others and with the ability to imagine or get "inside of" the emotions of clients, particularly fear (e.g., Slade 2014). In the next chapter, I operationalize these ideas more in talking about mentalization as another probable indicator of therapeutic success.

Many people with cPTSD think there is something wrong with them: they don't think the thing wrong is what has been done to them. Additionally, I am always careful to not take up one side of the traumatized person's ambivalence. What I mean by this is that I think an approach that solely emphasizes what has been done to someone can take away their personal agency for the ways they do have control over their lives. This is especially true in persons who do act in ways that are alienating toward others. Further, an idea of being more powerful than we are is a crucial defense among people who have been traumatized. Feeling responsible for trauma has a high cost, but it diminishes a sense of helplessness. Although it is a fact that trauma causes a sense of helplessness, it's important that clients become aware of this when they have enough external supports and internal resources to deal with this kind of terrifying emotion. In my thinking with clients, I am always walking a careful balance between doer and done to (Benjamin 2004[1]). A client taking up a position of feeling victimized too soon can lead to them feeling helpless. Hypervigilance is a defense that offers a sense of control in the minds of clients. I want to help them find other ways to feel in control before thinking too much about the ways in which they have been hurt or exploited, in the present or the past.

Because traumatized patients have been so controlled, I work especially hard to give them control over what we talk about. This is particularly true if someone mentions that they have been abused. I always start with the suggestion that trauma may or may not be something they wish to discuss. I respect avoidance and appreciate that this has kept them from becoming overwhelmed, or worse.

Conclusion

The bodies and minds of people who have experienced trauma are primed to feel fear and experience constant physical and psychological activation. People who have experienced multiple traumas, especially those that start in childhood, have developed ways of coping that made sense while they were being victimized. It behooves us to remember that patterns that may be viewed as maladaptive worked at one point. In addition, the powerful neurobiology at play requires us to help people feel safe and to learn they are not in danger now. Thinking about people with difficulties in relationships or excessive fear or anger as personality disordered does not match with current thinking about dimensional categorizations of character and personality functioning, which is that most behaviors exist on a continuum of normal to excessive. We have cheated ourselves and some of our clients out of getting needed help by emphasizing pathology and not trauma. That said, considering

[1] Benjamin does an admirable job of describing the ways that not thinking about our participation in some of our difficulties can lead to a sense of helplessness. However, this model is somewhat at odds with a trauma model that focuses on the reality of childhood and some adult situations of victimization. In my opinion, some psychoanalytic clinicians have not focused enough on the realities of victimization because of an attempt to encourage patients to see their involvement in current difficulties.

character structure and functioning is also important and can help us tailor our style of relating and interventions to what our clients need and may be more likely to respond to.

Initial Goals in the Beginning of Therapy for People with cPTSD

- Establish a good relationship. Determine what the client needs to feel safe and grounded in the present.
- The relationship we have with clients is dependent on them having a mind that understands them. A vital approach to both creating safety and increasing emotional confidence is to develop a series of hypotheses of overarching themes about what troubles them. This involves identifying triggers but really is more about establishing the sense that the therapeutic dyad is all about understanding how the client's mind works.
- Match some aspects of a client's personality style; temper language and speaking pace that fits theirs.
- If someone seems especially angry, acknowledge that while they certainly have the right to feel angry, it may also be that their anger is the flip side of the fight/flight response. They may feel fear at times. Ask them to try to notice this outside of therapy.
- Wonder if there are sensations they can notice before they get angry. Certain clients can be urged to try to notice if they feel anything physically, like a nervousness in the stomach, or feeling hot, or feeling shaky, etc.
- Avoid intense inquiry about trauma history in the beginning unless a client expects otherwise.
- If a client does want to discuss trauma, monitor emotions and affect regulation. Particularly when people are dissociative, they can seem fine when discussing traumas but may become overwhelmed later.
- When asking questions about trauma, allow the client to feel in control. I frequently will say something like, "If you feel comfortable, it might be helpful to discuss when you were raped on college. We don't have to, but when you are ready, it might be helpful."
- Sometimes clients need to tell us about trauma, but then don't want to talk more about it. We can hold onto their experience until they are ready to discuss further.
- Unless someone is really keen on "getting into their bodies," avoid somatic therapies or therapies that force people to relax. I find it's better to leave this as something optional. I suggest noticing body sensations as a cue that might signal other emotions. If someone is not interested in this, I don't press it.
- Embrace humility. Even if we are experts, we don't know someone's unique story until they tell us.
- Remember that brittle defenses and clients who seem difficult are using what has worked with them in the past.

- If recommending meditation, suggest guided approaches, but consider paradoxical anxiety which occurs in people who are very hypervigilant. Some people I see find even guided meditation to be too anxiety provoking. Unguided meditation leaves clients too alone with their minds, and this can risk overstimulation or an increase in intrusive thoughts and flashbacks.
- Allow content in the sessions to be related to the here and now. How are they functioning? How suicidal are they? What are they doing for enjoyment? What are the benefits of current relationships?
- Make sure clients have an idea of how you see them and make sure this is reflected in the goals the two of you set out to treat. For example, with Melanie I said, "I think part of the issue is you get stressed and overwhelmed, but since it's hard to know what's on your mind, you can get confused about what is happening. The first step might be trying to figure out what some of your thoughts and even feelings are."
- Be transparent in your thoughts. People with cPTSD have no real reason to trust anyone, especially us. So it's important to say things like, "While you were talking, I was thinking about your suicide attempt and how that happened. It was like a dream that you can't quite remember. Maybe that is important, that you get overwhelmed and can't quite keep track of yourself."
- Make a "new friend" in the first few sessions, with the caveat that it's extremely important not to be overly familiar with clients, as that rings false or can lead to a worry about boundaries being maintained. But be yourself. Don't be overcontrolled. Remember that people who have survived trauma are experts in sensing interactions that are inauthentic. Use humor if that is natural and not alienating to clients, and ask questions about their current lives, with genuine curiosity.
- Work toward understanding the presence of anxiety in relationships, which is often present when there are things the client does not want to see or think about.

References

Ainsworth, M. D., & Bell, S. M. (1970). Attachment, exploration and separation: Illustrated by the behavior of one-year-olds in a strange situation. *Child Development, 41*, 49–67.

Benjamin, J. (2004). Beyond doer and done to: An intersubjective view of thirdness. *Psychoanaltic Quarterly, 73*(1), 5–46.

Bosquet Enlow, M., Kitts, R. L., Blood, E., Bizarro, A., Hofmeister, M., & Wright, R. J. (2011). Maternal posttraumatic stress symptoms and infant emotional reactivity and emotion regulation. *Infant Behavior & Development, 34*, 487–503.

Courtois, C. A., & Ford, J. D. (2013). *Treatment of complex trauma: A sequenced, relationship-based approach*. New York: The Guilford Press.

Dohrenwend, B. P., Yage, T. J., Wall, M. M., & Adams, B. G. (2013). The roles of combat exposure, personal vulnerability, and involvement in harm to civilians or prisoners in Vietnam war-related posttraumatic stress disorder. *Clinical Psychological Science, 1*(3), 223–238.

Essex, M. J., Thomas Boyce, W., Hertzman, C., Lam, L. L., Armstrong, J. M., Neumann, S., et al. (2011). Epigenetic vestiges of early developmental adversity: Childhood stress exposure and DNA methylation in adolescence. *Child Development, 84*(1), 58–75.

Ford, J. D., & Courtois, C. A. (2014). Complex PTSD, affect dysregulation, and borderline personality disorder. *Borderline Personality Disorder and Emotional Dysregulation, 1*, 9. https://doi.org/10.1186/2051-6673-1-9.

Freud, S. (1926). Inhibitions, symptoms and anxiety. In J. Strachey (Ed.), *The standard ed. of the complete psychological works of Sigmund Freud* (Vol. 20, pp. 12–66). London: Hogarth Press.

Gøtzsche-Astrup, O., & Moskowitz, A. (2016). Personality disorders and the DSM-5: Scientific and extra-scientific factors in the maintenance of the status quo. *Australian and New Zealand Journal of Psychiatry, 50*(2), 119.

Grant, B. F., Stinson, S. F., Dawson, D. A., Chou, P., & Ruan, J. (2005). Co-occurrence of *DSM-IV* personality disorders in the United States: Results from the National Epidemiologic Survey on alcohol and related conditions. *Comprehensive Psychiatry, 46*(1), 1.

Hartley, T. A., Violanti, J. M., Sarkisian, K., Andrew, M. E., & Burchfiel, C. M. (2013). PTSD symptoms among police officers: Associations with frequency, recency, and types of traumatic events. *International Journal of Emergency Mental Health, 15*(4), 241–253.

Harvard Health Publishing. (2019). Understanding the stress response. Accessed online at https://www.health.harvard.edu/staying-healthy/understanding-the-stress-response.

Haslam, N., Holland, E., & Kuppens, P. (2012). Categories versus dimensions in personality and psychopathology: A quantitative review of taxometric research. *Psychological Medicine, 42*, 903–920.

Herman, J. (1992). Complex PTSD: A syndrome in survivors of prolonged and repeated trauma. *Journal of Traumatic Stress, 5*, 377–391.

Hesse, E., Main, M., Yost Abrahms, K., & Rifkin, A. (2003). Unresolved states regarding loss or abuse can have "second generation" effects: Disorganization, role inversion, and frightening ideation in the offspring of traumatized non-maltreating patients. In M. F. Solomon & D. J. Siegel (Eds.), *Healing trauma: Attachment, mind, body and brain*. New York: W.W. Norton & Company.

LeDoux, J. (1996). *The emotional brain: The mysterious underpinnings of emotional life*. New York: Touchstone.

Liotti, G. (1993). Disorganized/dissociative attachment and dissociative experiences. An illustration of the developmental-ethological approach to cognitive therapy. In H. Rosen & K. T. Kuehlwein (Eds.), *Cognitive therapy in action*. San Francisco: Jossey-Bass.

Liu, D., Diorio, J., Tannenbaum, B., Caldji, C., Francis, D., Freedman, A., et al. (1997). Maternal care, hippocampal glucocorticoid receptors, and hypothalamic-pituitary-adrenal responses to stress. *Science, 277*, 1659–1662.

Main, M., & Hesse, E. (1992). Disorganized/disoriented infant behavior in the strange situation, lapses in the monitoring of reasoning and discourse during the parent's adult attachment interview, and dissociative states. In M. Ammaniti & D. Stern (Eds.), *Attachment and psychoanalysis*. Rome: Guis, Lateza & Figili.

McWilliams, N. (2011). *Psychoanalytic diagnosis: Understanding personality structure in the clinical process* (2nd ed.). New York: The Guilford Press.

Mills, J. (2005). *Treating attachment pathology*. Oxford: Roman & Littlefield Publishers.

Morris, D. J. (2016). *The evil hours: A biography of post traumatic stress disorder*. Boston: First Mariner Books.

Mulder, R. (2009). Is borderline personality disorder really a personality disorder? *Personality and Mental Health, 3*, 85. Accessed online on 2nd Aug 2019 at https://onlinelibrary.wiley.com/doi/pdf/10.1002/pmh.80.

National Institutes of Health. (2002). *Stress system malfunction could lead to serious, life-threatening disease*. Accessed on 25th July 2019 at https://www.nichd.nih.gov/newsroom/releases/stress.

Naumova, O. Y., Lee, M., Koposov, R., Szyf, M., Dozier, M., & Grigorenko, E. L. (2011). Differential patterns of whole-genome DNA methylation in institutionalized children and children raised by their biological parents. *Development and Psychopathology, 24*(1), 143.

O'Doherty, D. C., Chitty, K. M., Saddiqui, S., Bennett, M. R., & Lagopoulos, J. (2015). A systematic review and meta-analysis of magnetic resonance imaging measurement of structural volumes in posttraumatic stress disorder. *Psychiatry Research, 232*, 1–33.

Oldham, J. M., Skodol, A. E., Kellman, H. D., Hyler, S. E., Rosnick, L., & Davies, M. (1992). Diagnosis of DSM-III-R personality disorders by two structured interviews: Patterns of comorbidity. *American Journal of Psychiatry, 149*, 213–220.

Pfohl, B., Coryell, W., Zimmerman, M., & Stangl, D. A. (1986). DSM-III personality disorders: Diagnostic overlap and internal consistency of individual DSM-III criteria. *Comprehensive Psychiatry, 27*, 21–34.

Powers, A., Stevens, J. S., O'Banion, D., Stenson, A. F., Kaslow, N., Jovanovic, T., & Bradley, B. (2020). Intergenerational transmission of risk for PTSD symptoms in African American children: The roles of maternal and child emotion dysregulation. *Psychological Trauma: Theory, Research, Practice, and Policy*. Advance online publication. Accessed online on 22nd Jan 2020 at https://doi.org/10.1037/tra0000543.

Radtke, K. M., Schauer, M., Gunter, H. M., Ruf-Leuschner, M., Sill, J., Meyer, A., & Elbert, T. (2015). Epigenetic modifications of the glucocorticoid receptor gene are associated with the vulnerability to psychopathology in childhood maltreatment. *Translational Psychiatry, 5*(5), e571.

Rauch, S. L., van der Kolk, B. A., Fisler, R. E., et al. (1996). A symptom provocation study of posttraumatic stress disorder using positron emission tomography and script-driven imagery. *Archives of General Psychiatry, 53*(5), 380–387.

Schore, A. (2003). *Affect regulation and the repair of the self*. New York: W.W. Norton & Company.

Shapiro, D. (1973). *Neurotic styles*. New York: Basic Books.

Shapiro, D. (1999). *Psychotherapy of neurotic character*. New York: Basic Books.

Sheline, Y. I. (2011). Depression and the hippocampus: Cause or effect? *Biological Psychiatry, 70*(4), 308–309.

Siegel, D. J. (2003). An interpersonal neurobiology of psychotherapy: The developing mind and the resolution of trauma. In M. F. Solomon & D. J. Siegel (Eds.), *Healing trauma: Attachment, mind, body and brain*. New York: W.W Norton & Company.

Slade, A. (2014). Imagining fear: Attachment, fear and psychic threat. *Psychoanalytic Dialogues, 24*(3), 253–266.

Solms, M., & Turnbull, O. (2002). *The brain and the inner world: An introduction to the neuroscience of subjective experience*. New York: Other Press.

Stephens, M. A., & Wand, G. (2012). Stress and the HPA axis: Role of glucocorticoids in alcohol dependence. *Alcohol Research: Current Reviews, 34*(4), 468–483.

Thylstrup, B., Simonsen, S., Nemery, C., Simonsen, E., Noll, J. F., Myatt, M. W., & Hesse, M. (2016). Assessment of personality-related levels of functioning: A pilot study of clinical assessment of the DSM-5 level of personality functioning based on a semi-structured interview. *BMC Psychiatry, BMC Series, 16*, 298.

Van der Kolk, B. A. (2014). *The body keeps score: Brain, mind, and body in the healing of trauma*. New York: Penguin.

Vuilleumier, P. (2002). Facial expression and selective attention. *Current Opinion in Psychiatry, 15*, 291–300.

Weaver, I. C., Cervoni, N., Champagne, F. A., D'Alessio, A. C., Sharma, S., Seckl, J. R., et al. (2004). Epigenetic programming by maternal behavior. *Nature Neuroscience, 7*(8), 847–854.

Westen, D. (1997). Divergences between clinical and research methods for assessing personality disorders: Implications for research and the evolution of axis II. *American Journal of Psychiatry, 154*(7), 895–903.

Whalen, P. J., Shin, L. M., McInerney, S. C., Fischer, H., Wright, C. I., & Rauch, S. L. (2001). A functional MRI study of human amygdala responses to facial expressions of fear versus anger. *Emotion, 1*(1), 70–83.

Widiger, T. A., & Trull, T. J. (1998). Performance characteristics of the DSM-III-R personality disorder criteria sets. In T. A. Widiger, A. J. Frances, A. Pincus, R. Ross, M. B. First, W. Davis, et al. (Eds.), *DSM-IV sourcebook, 4* (pp. 357–373). Washington, DC: American Psychiatric Association.

Yehuda, R., Halligan, S. L., & Grossman, R. (2001). Childhood trauma and risk for PTSD: Relationship to intergenerational effects of trauma, parental PTSD, and cortisol excretion. *Development and Psychopathology, 13*, 733–753.

Chapter 3
Nurturing the Therapeutic Alliance: Mentalizing and Maintaining Emotional Safety

Characteristics of Therapists Who Have Good Outcomes

We've seen so far that the therapeutic relationship is the primary factor in therapeutic outcome, and all therapies have roughly the same effect in the treatment of trauma, no matter what technique is used. In addition, we've seen that the neurobiology of trauma creates states of fear and heightened emotional states that require a lot of attention to help people feel safe. Heightened physiological states may also explain patterns and behaviors that may make some people with cPTSD more difficult to reach. The reality is that for many of our clients with cPTSD, therapy takes a long time and that we need to embrace a flexible use of combined approaches. In this chapter I will describe more about the common factors associated with good therapeutic outcomes as this lies at the heart of how we help create emotional safety. Mentalization captures one facet of how successful therapists act and think as well as a probable explanation of therapeutic action, or what makes clients better.

Before I describe mentalization in detail and how we can use this approach to help, I want to review the main qualities that make us good at our job. There are certain traits and honing of skills that we possess or can learn in order to create a sense of safety and security for the people seeking our help. As our individual selves are the main device in the treatment of our clients, it's worth thinking more about what skills are associated with better clinical outcomes. Wampold (2020) described 14 qualities of successful therapists. Below, I'll summarize some of his ideas and add my thoughts and emphases, some of which were described in Chapter 1. I urge the reader to see Wampold's many publications in this area of research for an in-depth reading. Below is a summary of therapist skills that appear to be associated with better outcomes.

T. M. Greenberg, *Treating Complex Trauma*,
https://doi.org/10.1007/978-3-030-45285-8_3

The Effective Therapist Has Sophisticated Interpersonal Skills

Wampold emphasizes that the effective therapist is kind, perceptive, trusting and open, and accepting and empathic. They tend to be warm, with good verbal skills, and can create a trusting environment with a wide range of clients. Therapists think of their clients as complicated individuals from diverse social and contextual backgrounds. They work collaboratively with clients and involve them in thinking about treatment goals. Initial trust should be built upon and I add to this that trust should not be taken for granted. Particularly with people who have histories of complex trauma, the ground can shift in terms of feelings of security within moments.

The Effective Therapist Has an Ability to Explain a Client's Distress and Takes the Client's Unique Experience into Account

One way I think of this quality involves a focus on being transparent with clients about the thinking in the therapist. Wampold emphasizes that clients need to know why they are suffering and such explanations must be acceptable and accepted by the client. Treatments are adapted for clients and require flexibility in changing treatment course when current methods are not helpful. Wampold also notes the importance of explaining how clients can get better. The explanation provides a means by which the client can overcome difficulties while being mindful of race, ethnicity, socioeconomic status, and other client issues. My added emphasis to these ideas is that we not keep our clients in the dark about what kinds of techniques and methods we think might be useful, including the importance of the therapeutic alliance. In other words, it's not uncommon in my practice that I explain how and why the relationship with myself and my client matters. I explain how it's a source of healing and repair.

The Effective Therapist Is Persuasive About Treatment Ideas and Monitors Progress in an Authentic Way

Wampold states that it's important that the therapist provide a sense of hopefulness to clients through being influential about methods agreed upon. However, he notes that progress must be continually monitored and that the therapist can be flexible when needed to switch approaches that do not seem helpful. Most importantly, he emphasizes that effective therapists are particularly attentive to evidence that their clients are deteriorating.

The Effective Therapist Can Deal with Difficult Material While Communicating Hope and Optimism

In my mind, these qualities involve a kind of heartiness in a therapist who can handle strong emotions—the hearing of painful traumatic events—and who limits defensive overintellectualizing to move away from emotions. Wampold states that when the difficult material involves the relationship between the therapist and the client, the therapist emphasizes the interpersonal process and deals with difficult material in a therapeutic way. I think of communicating hope and optimism as vital when times are tough. For example, when a client is thinking about aspects of their lives or personality that seem unflattering, I remind them of their progress and point out we all have limitations. It's important to emphasize that we all are fallible and need to work on ourselves.

The Effective Therapist Is Keenly Aware of Their Own Psychology

Wampold describes this quality as a therapist who does not infuse his or her own material into the therapy process unless such actions are deliberate and therapeutic. The effective therapist is reflective and tries to understand strong emotions elicited by clients and their meaning of what may be related to the client versus therapist issues.

The Effective Therapist Stays Aware of Relevant Research and Strives to Continually Improve

My ideas on these qualities are that we need to be aware of the limits of our abilities and competencies. Good therapists are cognizant of their limitations and get consultation and training before taking on clients they are not experienced with. Wampold notes that understanding the biological, social, and psychological bases of the disorder or problem experienced by the client is crucial to providing good care.

As we can see from the above qualities, any qualified therapist using any reliable empirically validated technique or techniques can be helpful to clients. Through this lens good therapies look roughly the same. Consider the following comment:

> [Work] with traumatized and suicidal patients should always emphasize the therapeutic relationship and can take years. Healing takes place in the context of the therapeutic relationship—our job as therapists is to have a different kind of relationship with clients because so many relationships before us have hurt them. And a key part of helping patients is the regulation of our own affect. (David Rudd, personal communication, September 2019)

At first glance you might have assumed that the author of this quote is a psychodynamic clinician. In fact, Rudd is a CBT therapist and quite a notable one, affiliated with the Department of Veterans Affairs. In this time of tribalism and therapy wars, it's vital to remember that good therapists have more similarities than differences.

Rudd's words about the need for us to regulate our own affect fit neatly in this chapter on maintaining emotional safety. Next, I'll highlight the approach and philosophy of mentalization to treatment as this way of working was designed with cPTSD clients in mind and optimizes the ways we can be connected to people who are suffering. In many ways, I have already described aspects of mentalization; it's something a lot of clinicians do naturally.

Trust and the Mentalizing Therapist

The ability of the therapeutic relationship to create safety and a secure attachment is a part of what makes healing possible. Mentalization, or the ability to understand what may be going on in the mind of another, has become a widely used way to describe important elements of therapeutic action. Mentalizing is a form of imaginative mental activity that allows us to perceive and interpret mental states, including needs, desires, feelings, and beliefs (Fonagy and Allison 2011). It must be imaginative because we have to conjure up what is going on in the mind of the other person. Allen et al. (2008) describe how they apply aspects of secure attachment (as described by Main and Goldwyn 1984) to their approach to mentalizing. Features of secure attachment and what we should strive for in our relationships with clients involve the following (adapted from Allen et al. 2008):

- Reflectiveness
- Lively consciousness
- Freshness of dialogue
- Little self-deception
- Ability to alter one's views
- Compassion
- Comfort with imperfection

Although our clients may not come to us with all of these qualities, as clinicians we can model them in terms of how we conduct ourselves, with the ultimate goal of helping clients develop their own mentalizing capacities. Trying to picture what is going on inside the mind and the body provides a crucial sense of stability and safety and helps to develop trust at the beginning of therapy (Fonagy and Allison 2014). The goal is for the client to feel that we are attuned to them. At the heart of this way of being with clients is our ability to imagine or "get inside" of what they are experiencing. Especially with people who have complicated relationship histories, they may have ideas or experiences that I find I need to try extra hard to imagine. The following difficult and extreme example suggests how this might work.

Someone I will call Susan who had been seeing me for just over a year following a hospitalization for suicidality told me about the brutal way she imagined killing herself. She'd researched it and could name celebrities who had done something similar. It was at a time when she felt acutely suicidal and we developed a crisis plan (which will be described in Chapter 4). However, she did not need hospitalization, I think in part, because I could not only tolerate what she said, I was able to imagine her ideas about suicide. I asked questions about the method. Why that method of suicide and not something else? I even tried to imagine how it would be if I was thinking of ending my life in the same way. This was difficult because I have never seriously considered suicide, especially with the method she discussed. I finally concluded that her way of thinking about the end of her life was meant to express just how helpless, afraid, enraged, frustrated, and disorganized she felt about people who had disappointed her in the past and present. There are not things I discussed with her all at once; at the time the majority of the work was what I was doing in my mind. She later told me that no one else had seemed to "get it," though she had not ever told anyone the details about how she thought she deserved to have her life end.

Susan likely could tell me about her ideas because a foundation was created for her to sense that I would try as hard as I could to understand the nuances of what she was feeling and thinking, especially since she had an awareness that there were aspects of her mind that seemed unusual and out of control to her. Mentalizing is not just sympathy or empathy, though it involves aspects of both. Much of Susan's therapy did involve many different CBT and mindfulness techniques for stabilization. She also sometimes brought up issues regarding her family and one particularly disorganized and sadistic caretaker, but this was mostly for background information she thought I needed and I think initially because she thought she should be talking about her family. But what I really wanted to know, especially in that first year, was how her mind worked.

Bateman and Fonagy (2010) describe elements of the mentalizing stance and how we should conduct ourselves as therapists: "The therapist's mentalizing therapeutic stance should include: a) humility deriving from a sense of 'not-knowing'; b) patience in taking time to identify differences in perspectives; c) legitimizing and accepting different perspectives; d) actively questioning the patient about his/her experience—asking for detailed descriptions of experience ('what questions') rather than explanations ('why questions'); e) careful eschewing of the need to understand what makes no sense (i.e., saying explicitly that something is unclear)" (p. 13).

Mentalizing is about the relationship and developing a place where people can feel like thinking about what is on their minds is manageable in a very basic sense. I find the emphasis on "what questions" very valuable. As opposed to "why questions" which promote intellectualization and imply that we expect clients to have rational reasons for their ideas and beliefs, what questions imply curiosity and neutrality. The disorganizing nature of trauma and its aftermath is anything but rational. Clients who try to be over-rational may be dissociated with their emotions. So much so that it is hard to know what is really bothering them.

Stephanie had been in therapy with me for over a year, and yet I felt I knew little about her. She came to therapy at the urging of her physician, who thought that therapy could help with her management of an autoimmune disease. Yet, her medical treatment seemed to be under control, and she kept coming to therapy with complaints about her work environment as well as problems with her partner of 15 years. However, even though these common complaints often can develop a sense of traction in therapy, with Stephanie, I was often left confused. I literally could not understand the nature of her distress, despite endless explanations of people she said she was upset with. I assume this was partly so because she literally never stopped smiling when she was complaining. My comments about the disconnection between her affect and words were met with an acknowledgment; she'd heard this before. After discussing this extensively (and probably because I was asking "why" there was a disconnect between her words and facial expressions), there was still no change in her smiling while offering at best vague descriptions about people who she was supposedly angry or disappointed with. At the end of an exhausting session (for me) when she was quasi-complaining about something at work, I said, "I try so hard to imagine what work must be like for you and I often think to myself, what is it that I am not getting?" Stephanie showed a slight smile and not of the kind she often uses to hide her true emotions. I went on, "I have a sense of the culture of start-ups and how it can seem like people are not really paying attention to what others need and I imagine that this could really be difficult. Because you feel then that you have to take care of everyone around you, which you've been doing your whole life. Am I beginning to understand what is going on?" It was at that point that she could tell me in detail about many experiences of her work environment that felt toxic to her, with specific examples of how she felt mistreated and ignored. In fact, although she had talked about one man in her workplace several times before, I was not aware that he had been engaging in all kinds of subtle but inappropriate behavior. Suddenly her descriptions felt alive to me, and I could get a much better sense of her understandable frustrations and fear with an appreciation of how her history could leave her vulnerable and unable to take care of herself.

Stephanie illustrates a key way that mentalizing works in therapeutic practice. She was someone who had spent years with different therapists, with little benefit, as she smiled her way through her complaints and likely made it difficult for even skilled clinicians to have access to her. I, too, thought that I would be one of the therapists who had failed to help her, but it was in the moment described above that seemed to change things in her therapy: *"I try so hard to imagine what work must be like for you and I often think to myself, what is it that I am not getting?"* This was actually a last-ditch effort on my part (not to be confused with therapeutic skill, per se!), as I felt Stephanie slipping away, with a hopeless sense that no one could ever get her. It was the end of a long day, she was my last client, and I was desperately trying to find a way to make our connection seem more alive. But after this comment, she suddenly became more real in the sessions. Nothing changed in terms of me knowing aspects of her early history, which seemed extremely neglectful and possibly abusive, at least to some of her siblings in what seemed to be an incredibly chaotic environment. Indeed, I had tried in vain to make comments about her past and how this linked to her present state of not feeling cared for. When I made these interpretations, I was met with her ever-present smile and change of subject. Yet, when I could say out loud just how hard I was struggling to know her, she relaxed and felt safer. Then, we could at least deal with emotions, including fear, that were available to her in the present.

Another model of this imagining is clearly described by Slade (2014) where she applies attachment theory to concepts of imagining the fear our clients have felt when in states of fearful arousal when they were children. Slade notes the clinical utility of this as such:

> This attunement begins, on our part, with the attempt to imagine our patients' experiences of fearful arousal in the past and attend to their dynamic efforts to regulate fear and threat in the present. For example, when I imagine an adult patient's past, I try to imagine early threats to her safety. What happened when she was fearfully aroused, threatened, or needy? What did she find in the eyes and minds of those she most relied upon? Did she have to adapt the expression of her needs in a way that minimized the threat of losing the protection of even the most limited or barren intimacy? How did she do this? What do I imagine were the outcomes of early efforts to maintain proximity when threatened, either by external dangers or the parent's unavailability? And how are these reflected in the present? (p. 259)

A large part of mentalizing is what we do with our minds while we are with clients. I find with some clients with cPTSD that it can take a great deal of time to accurately imagine how things work in their minds and what it may have been really like during their difficult or traumatic experiences. Yet, the process of trying to think about them in a nuanced way is healing. For people who had abusive or neglectful early experiences, therapy may be the first time someone actually spends time trying to understand their thoughts, motives, behaviors, and feelings.

To this end, I also use clinical hypothesis testing and make my thinking fairly transparent in order to try to create a relationship with clients that involves shared goals. I think it's easy for us to forget just how terrified and (rightly) suspicious our clients are. Trust takes a very long time, even in situations in which therapist and client seem to genuinely like one another. By being transparent and stating ideas as hypotheses, I let clients know I am thinking about them in a complex way and that I am not harboring thoughts about them that could be construed or felt to be dangerous. Especially for people whom I might imagine to be suspicious, I frequently say something like, "While you were talking, I was thinking about…" People with cPTSD are sensitive to the thoughts others have about them, and I think can determine within a very short period of time if someone does not like them, can't empathize, finds them annoying, etc.

In addition, I tend to emphasize whatever strengths the client has. For example, with clients such as Susan, Stephanie, and Melanie (whom I'll discuss below), even though I may not know a ton of details about their childhood, I often imagine what it must have been like to be a kid in a family where they realized early on that their parents lacked some capacity for basic caregiving. This may be because their mother is depressed, in an unhappy relationship, or resents being a mother, and so on. Kids that are particularly attuned to their parent's emotional life may realize (though often out of conscious awareness) that a parent is not happy enough of the time in their caregiving role. Their adaptation takes into account the need to numb themselves from what does not seem right in their household, as well as experiences of blatant abuse (e.g., Miller 1997). The reality of their traumatic past lives on in less conscious ways. As clinicians, we are faced with a kind of "split screen" scenario. On one level, we are having a rational conversation with someone who is seeking our help, on the other, they are terrified and we need to provide a constant sense of security and reminders that they are not in danger.

Normalizing and Managing Shame

Another way I attempt to maintain safety is to normalize behaviors and thoughts that clients often feel ashamed about. Rarely do they admit shame, but certain clients have very clear ideas about what is wrong with them and often assume we will agree. Let's return to Melanie's treatment (whom I described in the previous two chapters) to illustrate the aforementioned ideas.

Although Melanie asked me if she should transfer teams, I was able to get her to hold off on this so we could understand more about what was frightening. After the disclosure that a man on her team reminded her of a man who had been violent with her in the past, she found herself being more aggressive with members of her team, and this led to a reprimand from her supervisor. I continued to imagine that as a smart kid in a home with two very unhappy parents, who by then I had learned had very difficult immigration experiences in the countries of their births, she felt angry and scared a lot. As we were discussing these issues, she mentioned that she was a controlling person. She said, "I am just a control freak. I need to control things and that is why I get so angry." I tried to convey a facial expression that expressed my surprise, sympathy, and confusion. And then I offered a different hypothesis. I said, "I don't experience you as controlling. You may be and perhaps I have not seen that side of you yet. But overall, control is a good thing. Who does not want to be in control?! The trick for all of us is just to know how to cope when we don't have control. Especially since you get so scared at work, and in other parts of your life, it makes sense you need to figure out the ways you can manage your environment. But that does not mean that something is wrong with you. It makes you just like the rest of us." She appeared stunned and changed the subject to what was happening with her boyfriend, as they had argued over the weekend, I think in part to provide more evidence of her controlling nature. She was worried that she had acted too aggressively, as she had yelled at him in a restaurant. We pivoted to her telling me what was happening with her boyfriend and my giving her some practical ways she could express herself to her boyfriend, without making her feel like she was being too aggressive. At the end of the session, I said, "Look, I think with these things at work and with your boyfriend, you have a thought or feeling that makes you really scared and then it's hard to think. I know we have not talked about your family much or what happened to you when you were younger, but I do wonder if there is a way you kind of know something's not right. You are very smart and I can imagine that when you were quite young you knew things were not right at home. And now, I think that can be true too. There is a sense that something does not feel right, but you're genuinely not sure if that is true or even how to organize your thoughts about this in a way that can be helpful for knowing what to do next."

This is a fairly typical representation in terms of how I work—weaving in and out of the past and the present and not getting too caught up (when I can) in worry about external behaviors (regulating my own affect) and finding a balance between normalizing and still considering the distress some behaviors cause the client. This latter point is important, because change seems more likely when clients view certain behaviors as problematic. I was well aware that Melanie's aggression had gotten her in trouble many times, but I was trying to decrease her shame about her difficulties modulating her affect. If we join in with what they think (critical self-appraisals) about their behaviors, this creates too much shame, which makes it impossible for clients to consider what they might do differently. More important, difficulty regulating emotions gets in the way of people being able to think about what is bothering them. When people become too aggressive, they then look like the "bad guy." The thing that they are upset about gets lost and often clients focus on how messed up they are, how extreme their reaction was, what others think of them, etc. These feelings of shame do little to change aggressive behaviors. Shame causes confusion and more difficulties with affect containment because they can't realistically think about what caused them to feel upset in the first place. Normalizing is one way I have found to soften shame so we can think together about different scenarios. With Melanie, I eventually learned that her boyfriend at dinner made an offensive comment to the waiter, repeatedly cut Melanie off when she was trying to talk, and made a derogatory comment about Melanie's appearance. Yet, she did not tell me any of this right away, she talked all about how aggressive she was. Once her shame was under better control, she was able to consider that while her aggression could be too much, often, she focused on her being a "control freak" as opposed to how others (e.g., her boyfriend) were at times not treating her well.

Further, it's important to add that we live in an increasingly aggressive culture; mixed messages regarding aggression abound. Role models of all stripes, especially on social media, express aggressive and even violence with wild abandon. I am mindful that this leaves people confused, especially if they struggle with aggressive feelings and thoughts. Never has normalizing anger been more realistic and aptly connected to the external world! I bring this up because it's an additional avenue that we can use to point out how aggression has become normalized (as troubling as that is). More so, normalizing things that many people assume, though popular psychology (or perhaps things that have been pathologized or critiqued by other therapists), allows clients to know they are not alone. The larger point, however, is that approaching our work with clients should indicate that we are also humans, with an implication that we too have struggled. That said, I rarely, if ever, talk openly with clients about my personal struggles. I find that I can speak to universal issues and provide an environment of understanding without taking the risk of being overstimulating (or worse, asking to be taken care of) to a client with self-disclosure. For example, I'll frequently say to women who are struggling with being assertive, "It's important for all of us that we figure out how to navigate our feelings of aggression. We live in a society that if we seem angry, it is assumed that we are crazy, so we have to become comfortable with our anger so we can assert ourselves and be confident in that." This is a tack I take at some point with most women I treat.

There is a caveat about normalizing, however. A young woman I will refer to as Becky, who was on disability and had several stays in psychiatric inpatient facilities for both suicidal ideation and psychotic thinking, had a history of trauma that involved a lot of sadism from multiple caretakers. She had also been a victim of a number of assaults as an adult. She was deeply worried about her own aggressive ideas, even though she never acted on them. Making her feelings about her aggression worse, though, was that she believed she had special powers involving the ability to read and control other people's minds. This level of omnipotence was neatly compartmentalized into a fantasy life that proved to be quite soothing and important to her. At the same time, she had internalized an idea of herself as a "psych patient" and saw herself as especially damaged. So when I commented at times that some of her struggles were normal, human issues that we all deal with, she overtly got angry with me. She told me I was wrong, not hearing what she said, and that I must not be listening to her at all. At times, she implied that I may have been poorly trained as a therapist. After a few times of this happening, I said to her, "I notice when I try to normalize your situation that it is not helpful." She initially seemed worried about this, and I think worried I would fire her as a client. I then told her I can find another way to be helpful, but I was just curious about what she thought about my clearly unhelpful attempts at normalizing her situation. It was then Becky went into more detail about her special powers and abilities and it occurred to me that she felt extremely positive about herself (her powers) and extremely negative (her sense of herself as uniquely damaged). She did not feel like the rest of us. I realized that she felt both subhuman and superhuman. Therefore the normal rules of humanity did not apply to her. For a while, we had to focus on the uniqueness of her situation. As that happened, she allowed me to have more contact with her in terms of understanding her mind, including what seemed to be a fairly active psychotic process that always operated alongside the more rational aspects of her psychology. Additionally, I eventually realized that my normalizing probably felt like I was trying too hard to have emotional contact with her, something that she likely experienced as terrifying given her history of being sadistically exploited. In this situation, I said to her directly that maybe my attempts to connect to her might be too aggressive. Interestingly, she noted that I seemed "masculine" at times. I took this to mean that I might be at least in the ballpark in terms of understanding her better and that my assertiveness (through normalizing) in the therapeutic situation could feel dangerous. I offered to literally talk less if that seemed helpful, but that we should also make sure she did not feel too alone if I remained quiet.

Creating Safety Though Respecting Avoidance

As I've described, every treatment, especially with those who have cPTSD, involves negotiation, which sets up the crucial structure of allowing the client to have a sense of control and agency. Herman (1992) described traumatic events as those that "overwhelm the ordinary systems of care that give people a sense of control, connection and meaning" (p. 33). Allowing clients to have control is vital to the setup of the therapeutic situation. If we think back to the discussion that some therapists consistently have better outcomes than others, it's likely the case that therapists that have more success are those who are good at mentalizing, with an ability to know what clients need in certain moments including when to let them take the lead. Successful therapists also have a capability to more successfully imagine what is going on in the mind of clients. Fonagy and Allison (2014) speculate that the "mentalizing therapist" is a universal constituent of effective psychotherapeutic interventions. Perhaps as key, though, is to repair ruptures when they happen and to pivot approaches when needed. It seemed to be the case that my thinking about how to work with Becky out loud with her was the thing that allowed her to stay in therapy, probably because I could admit that I had been unhelpful and that I wanted to learn how to connect with her in a way and at a pace that she could tolerate.

Talking specifically about trauma requires us to negotiate even further. Whenever I make a comment about past traumas, no matter how obliquely, I pay close attention to eye contact, facial expressions, and bodily movements and whether or not the client seems to become detached or dissociative. I rarely argue my point or observations with clients; this sets up a power struggle against the forces in the client to not see things they are not ready to see. Equally as important, I try to avoid a position in which I communicate that I am the authority of what is on the mind of the client, consciously or unconsciously. This is why clinical hypothesis testing is useful, because it presents ideas that can be thought about, challenged, or ignored.

Many clinicians feel that talking about traumatic events is what leads to eventual symptom reduction. This is clearly the case for clinicians who use exposure treatments. Psychodynamic or psychoanalytic approaches historically have not focused on behavioral symptom improvements in a formal way, but many psychoanalytic clinicians address trauma, along with unconscious material that is related with the hope that this will lead to healing. Trauma therapists, using a three-stage model, focus on treating emotional, somatic, attention, and behavioral dysregulation, and once dysregulation is under better control, they, too, have an expectation that they can process traumatic events (Courtois and Ford 2015).

No matter the theory, I'd argue that any time we speak with clients about trauma, we are doing a kind of exposure treatment. Different clinicians use exposure in different ways, but it's something all therapies have in common, the idea that talking about trauma is key to healing. Exposure may be woven into thoughtful treatments. It goes without saying that we need buy-in from our clients in order to achieve these goals, however. In addition, inherent in three-stage models, CBT models, as well as psychodynamic treatments, is that there is usually an overt verbal acknowledgment (usually later in psychodynamic therapies) that the client has been traumatized. Trauma therapists provide a psychoeducational approach to this by validating the reality of the traumas. This is important when clients are able to talk about traumatic experiences and believe that they have been victimized. Many people with cPTSD have difficulty with both of these, however. For example, I interviewed a number of clinicians at Veterans Affairs Medical Centers to ask about the issue of avoidance among vets who are often urged to receive exposure treatments. Some noted how humiliating it was for patients who could not tolerate exposure treatment and a feeling that they (the clients) had "failed." Our clients desperately want to get better, but if we therapists overtly state through our methods, or even just hold in mind that the path to getting better is talking about traumas, that might be setting them up for failure. In fact, many people I see with both adult and childhood traumas are not even sure their traumas are responsible for their current situation. Denial not only explains this phenomenon, dissociation (which will be described in detail in Chapter 5), associated memory problems, the need to feel responsible for being hurt, etc. leave some clients unsure of the extent to which they have been victimized. In Chapter 5, I'll describe a case in vivid detail in which this latter point is apparent.

Many of us have had the experience of linking a traumatic event to something in the present and have found this not helpful. Sometimes these interpretations (psychodynamic clinicians refer to them as genetic interpretations) offer intellectual understanding, but given that the experience of emotions for people with cPTSD can be so overwhelming and frightening, we need more than intellectual understanding. When someone is in crisis about a boss, a boyfriend, or even a basic feeling of whether or not it makes sense to continue to try and live when the world seems so fraught with disappointment, relating traumas to present intense emotions often carries little traction. In fact, it may even imply we want to get them away from their feelings. Dealing with affect is thought to contribute to therapeutic change (e.g., Spezzano 1993; Bateman and Fonagy 2010). Yet, talking about trauma does help some people for a variety of reasons. This raises the question of how much should we encourage the processing of memories and when.

How Much Should We Encourage the Processing of Memories?

As clients experience safety in therapy, most clinicians assume that the next part of therapy will involve some aspects of thinking about traumatic events. Although this can be helpful, I'm not sure it always is. For people with cPTSD, they have had repeated multiple traumas and/or neglect, often starting in early childhood. From a practical standpoint, there may simply be too many traumas to resolve, and given the prevalence of severe anxiety and dissociation in some, it may not even be possible to reconstruct many elements of the past. This is in contrast to what has historically been the ideal goal of trauma survivors, to come up with a coherent narrative.

Yet, stories are an interictal part of human existence. One of the major deprivations that occurs with repeated trauma is that it takes away our ability to have a tale to tell. Therapy can and should help clients develop this, but it's more realistic that part of the narrative involves a loss of coherence, the loss of a story. I think of the large numbers of clients I have met who tell me they don't remember much before high school or even college. It's not clear that these memories can come back. Memory for many who have cPTSD has jagged edges and missing pieces. This might be a big part of the chronicle for some.

As therapists, in almost any modality, we have learned to link the past with the present. Dynamic and trauma therapists may do this more directly, but CBT clinicians operate on the pretense that past experiences (e.g., the target of exposure therapies) impact the present. And though I agree intellectually with this, it's not always clear that this is what is connected to majority of therapeutic action—what really helps to make people better. Again, based on the data of therapeutic outcome discussed in Chapter 1, we are not really sure how people get better, except that a good empathic relationship offers much of what we can explain, and even that is not a high percentage of the variance. I am suggesting that we pause certain ideas that have come to define the way we work so we can not only rethink what is helpful but that our clients can let us know if and when they are ready to talk about trauma. I communicate to clients that I am very open to hearing about trauma, but that it is better when it comes up naturally and when the client has a secure foundation before doing so. This means social support, a good handle on emotional modulation, no or very limited suicidal thoughts, behaviors for self-care and self-regulation, and a real sense of physical safety. If someone does begin talking about trauma and begins to feel overwhelmed, especially with a return of nightmares, intense anxiety, hypervigilance, and/or dissociation, it's important that we don't power through with our will and agenda in terms of talking about trauma. For example, a client who had been the victim of attempted murder would begin talking about things related to the attack but would become extremely dissociated, which we could describe as "losing himself." When this happened, we returned to the techniques that worked for him to get these symptoms under control—grounding techniques, creating positive triggers and mindfulness, and asking his wife to help him—until he felt safe again and when he wanted to discuss some aspect of what he'd experienced in terms of his trauma background. This fits with a trauma model of care for people with PTSD. According to one expert, "Even when you've started with a lot of stabilization work people will dysregulate, either into hyper or hypo arousal, when they start going into dealing directly with the trauma. The foundation of providing stabilizing though, provides something the therapist and client can go back to when needed" (Laura Brown, personal communication, 2020).

Avoidance is a key feature of cPTSD and I think it's important to create space for clients to be in control of any discussions about trauma. It may be the first time they have felt as if they can have control. Many clients are terrified of becoming overstimulated by thinking about terrifying events or even becoming more aware of their thoughts. Dealing with memories can be more our goal than that of our clients. It seems to me that some of how we have been thinking about processing trauma may be incomplete, if not incorrect. For some people with cPTSD, it is often not possible to develop a coherent narrative, as the old teaching suggests. Trauma, disorganization, and not really being able to put it all together *is the story*, and I think we can still help people to live gratifying lives without having to relive many traumatic experiences. There are many risks involved when clients remember and relive traumatic events. Sometimes people can get so overwhelmed that the idea of continuing to live can seem unbearable. Dealing with suicidality will be the subject of the next chapter.

Conclusion

Providing safety for our clients with cPTSD involves a number of skills. Mentalization explains what may well be the mechanism of action in terms of how psychotherapy works. Creating safety involves authentically relating to clients, close monitoring of affect, speech and body language, and flexibility to shift our approaches whenever needed. We need to regulate our own affect and be ready for whatever difficult material we may hear. At the same time, it's vital that we respect avoidance. Clients should be entrusted to know when they can think about traumatic events. For people with cPTSD traditional ideas of processing of memories may not be realistic, but we can still help provide healing by piecing together aspects of a client's story and a full engagement and commitment to understanding how someone's mind works.

Interventions for Mentalizing and Maintaining Emotional Safety

- Balance authority with humility. Clients need us to be strong, but this means being able to take in negative feedback and shift our approach as needed.
- Be transparent and use clinical hypothesis testing. Let a client know what you are thinking. State interpretations as ideas that may or may not be true.
- We are always doing trauma work. Don't worry if a client can't talk directly about traumas. They may eventually or never. Be open to stories that are fragmented and lack an ideal coherent narrative.
- Provide an environment of curiosity about how our client's minds work, even when doing structured CBT approaches. Ask questions to clarify and be curious about the nature of complex feelings and motives.
- If you and a client have the shared goal of discussing trauma, make sure there are a number of techniques in place for stability first.
- If discussing trauma is too destabilizing, go back to techniques that allow the client to feel safe and enhance cognitive and emotional stability and regulation.

- Normalize (most of the time). Unless someone can't tolerate it, remind clients that so many of their struggles are issues we all face, without self-disclosing in a way that could be construed as asking for help or risking TMI (too much information).
- Repair rupture and missteps. Pivot approaches to something that works better if what we're doing does not work. Try to embrace feedback and complaints and be transparent about therapist motives when acknowledging something was not helpful.
- Imagine, imagine, imagine. Try to think about what it is like to be the person sitting across from you. Imagine fear until the two of you can think about it together.

References

Allen, J., Fonagy, P., & Bateman, A. (2008). *Mentalizing in clinical practice*. Washington, DC: American Psychiatric Press.

Bateman, A., & Fonagy, P. (2010). Mentalization based treatment for borderline personality disorder. *World Psychiatry, 9*, 11–15.

Courtois, C. A., & Ford, J. D. (2015, September 15). *Treatment of complex trauma: A sequenced, relationship-based approach* (Reprint edition). New York: The Guilford Press.

Fonagy, P., & Allison, E. (2011). *What is mentalization? The concept and its foundations in developmental research and social-cognitive neuroscience*. Accessed online on 9th Feb 2019 at https://pdfs.semanticscholar.org/995b/4ea80865b6bc4cbe89cf266d7c5a4299425e.pdf.

Fonagy, P., & Allison, E. (2014). The role of mentalizing and epistemic trust in the therapeutic relationship. *Psychotherapy, 51*(3), 372–380.

Herman, J. L. (1992). *Trauma and recovery*. New York: Basic Books.

Main, M., & Goldwyn, R. (1984). Predicting rejection of her infant from mother's representation of her own experience: Implications for the abused-abusing intergenerational cycle. *Child Abuse & Neglect, 8*(2), 203–217.

Miller, A. (1997). *The drama of the gifted child: The search for the true self.* New York: Basic Books.

Slade, A. (2014). Imaging fear: Attachment, threat, and psychic experience. *Psychoanalytic Dialogues, 16*(3), 253–266.

Spezzano, C. (1993). *Affects in psychoanalysis: A clinical synthesis*. New York: Routledge.

Wampold, B. (2020). *American Psychological Association Education Directorate. Qualities and actions of effective therapists*. Accessed online on 27th Feb 2020 at https://www.apa.org/education/ce/effective-therapists.pdf.

Chapter 4
The Therapeutic Alliance and Maintaining Physical Safety

Trauma, Suicidal Ideation, and Deaths of Despair

For people with trauma histories, thoughts of death can be an ever-present part of life. Suicidal ideation can also occur when people in therapy are discussing aspects of abuse or trauma. As therapists we need to keep a watchful eye on the impact of our discussions of trauma-related material, including knowing when to shift approaches if clients become overwhelmed. When trauma discussions are too much, we need to pivot to soothing and grounding techniques that hopefully have already been established in the treatment. This is why proponents of the trauma model of treatment start with stabilizing techniques, though, of course, many clinicians using a variety of different approaches create a sense of safety before discussing trauma in detail.

As I discussed in Chapter 3, I think everything we do as therapists with traumatized clients is trauma work, and although it can be helpful for some clients to talk about what has happened to them in detail, not all clients benefit from this. That said, people who have experienced trauma, especially when it is cumulative, blame themselves for their troubles. Thinking about trauma can decrease some of those beliefs and the shame associated with them. But we can acknowledge someone has had extreme difficulties while still working in the present. Healing can take place in the here and now and based on experiences in current relationships.

Risks of suicide go well beyond facets of psychotherapy, however. Suicide rates are increasing among many groups in general, including those previously not considered to be high risk. This complicated phenomenon behooves us to think about suicide as a cultural tragedy and one that we need to be prepared for in our work. Suicidal thoughts are a very common part of existence for many people and may come up for a variety of reasons.

T. M. Greenberg, *Treating Complex Trauma*,
https://doi.org/10.1007/978-3-030-45285-8_4

The Alarming Epidemic of Suicide

Suicidal thoughts are very common. An estimated 8.3 million adults in the United States or 3.7% of the adult US population reported having had suicidal thoughts in the past year during 2008–2009. Adults aged 18–29 years were more likely than their older counterparts to have had suicidal thoughts, made any suicide plans, and attempted suicide in a large sample studied (Crosby et al. 2011). About 1.4 million adults make a nonfatal suicide attempt each year in the United States (Piscopo et al. 2016).

Deaths by suicide have been increasing and are at epidemic levels. A suicide occurs in the United States roughly once every 12 minutes. After decades of decline, the rate of self-inflicted deaths per 100,000 people annually has been increasing sharply since the late 1990s (Menon 2019). Suicide is the tenth leading cause of death in the United States. The World Health Organization (2019) notes that globally, every 40 seconds someone dies of suicide. More people die worldwide from suicides than from homicides and wars combined.

Deaths of despair are also linked with substance abuse which has increased dramatically in the United States. I'll describe the high rates of substance abuse in Chapter 6, but it's important to state a few facts here as suicide and substance abuse share common characteristics, including a relationship with PTSD and cPTSD. Woolf and Schoomaker (2019) analyzed life expectancy data collected by the Centers for Disease Control and Prevention and all-cause mortality rates listed in the US Mortality Database from 1959 to 2017. These authors note that although life expectancy had been steadily rising, it decreased after 2014 related to an increase in mortality from specific causes (drug overdoses, suicides, organ system diseases) among young and middle-aged adults of all racial groups, with an onset as early as the 1990s and with the largest relative increases occurring in the Ohio Valley and New England. In many places in the United States, midlife mortality increased, caused by drug overdoses, alcohol abuse, suicides, and a diverse list of organ system diseases, related to substance use. Of course, it makes sense to partially blame the opioid epidemic, which has been plaguing the United States and Canada for a number of years. However, substance use overall has increased and combined with intentional suicides paints a dire picture of people engaging in several types of self-harm.

It's unusual that we are seeing increases in suicides in groups not known to be at high risk. Many of us learned, for example, that older white men had the highest risk for death by suicide. Although this group is still at high risk, there is an alarming rise in youth suicides, particularly among African Americans. In young people aged 10–19 years, suicide is the second leading cause of death with over 3000 youth who died by suicide. Increases in the suicide death rate of African American youth have seen a dramatic rise with young people under 13 years twice as likely to die by suicide compared with previous rates. African American males, 5–11 years, are more likely to die by suicide compared to their white peers (Watson Coleman 2020). This data challenges previously held notions; there were fewer deaths in young people and among African Americans until recently. It's unclear why this is so, though authors of the above report from the Congressional Black Caucus note that African American youth who are depressed receive less mental health care than their white counterparts.

I'll expand on the large number of risk factors for suicide below, but to state this now, PTSD is a risk factor for suicide attempt in those who have recurrent major depression, and people with cPTSD symptoms have a higher risk for attempted suicide (Stevens et al. 2013; Pinheiro et al. 2016). Hyperarousal symptoms are thought to be especially predictive of suicide (Panagioti et al. 2017). Symptoms of hyperarousal include difficulty sleeping and concentrating, being easily startled, irritability, anger, angry outbursts, agitation, panic, anxiety, and hypervigilance. Veterans have a 21% higher suicide rate than age-matched and sex-matched civilian cohorts (Editorial, *The Lancet* 2019).

However, the increased agitation that we think of with some people who have PTSD is not the only presentation I have seen in suicidal clients. Let's return to Thomas who I discussed in Chapter 2.

Thomas was a police officer who had been rejected for treatment by another clinician because he seemed too closed off for the other clinician to connect with. When I met him he did not do what we expect clients to do; he did not want to talk about himself. Yet, he had a clear suicidal plan. He was not agitated; he was quite clear and calm regarding his intentions. He had firearms in his home, which made his risk even higher. During our first meeting, I got him to agree to postpone his suicide attempt so that we could work together to see what may happen. After that, I had permission to talk with his children and his primary care doctor. I asked that all firearms were moved to a locked safe. An additional step was taken to lock up hard liquor, as Thomas was a heavy drinker. Thomas hated these interventions, especially the latter one, but he and his adult children worked out a system in which we could have a couple of small hard alcohol drinks each evening and a glass of wine with dinner. An important part of the initial therapy was to allow Thomas to discuss how infantilized he felt about these interventions by recognizing the reality of his complaint while also helping him to recognize that the motive for these interventions was to keep him alive, because people loved him. Thomas never quite got over the wish that he would die, which is common among many suicidal people, but he realized that he could wait to die and try to derive whatever pleasure he could in the meantime.

I'll say more about clinical management of a suicidal crisis, but one thing that has worked for me with some suicidal people is just to practically state how though it is true that suicide provides people with control over how they will die and may end current suffering, it is actually a very lonely and violent way to go. There has been something useful about just naming the reality that we all have to die; but doing so through suicide is often experienced as a negative way to end our time in this life. Data from survivors of suicide attempts report that as soon as they have completed the action intended to end life, they immediately regret it. For example, according to Firestone (2019), all 29 people who survived a suicide attempt by jumping off of San Francisco's Golden Gate Bridge said they regretted it as soon as they jumped.

Being empathic with a client's wish to die has been described as an important intervention with people considering suicide (Orbach 2001; Berglund et al. 2016). When I am having a discussion about the limitations of suicide, I am also communicating I can understand why a client might want to end their life. I have found these kinds of discussions about suicide helpful with clients who are used to having a great deal of control in their lives and/or when I imagine (though not expressly interpreted) part of suicidality is related to intense feelings of helplessness and anger. In my experience this is the case for older adults with chronic illnesses or people who genuinely never imagined aging and related limitations as part of their trajectory. It's as if people like Thomas are justifiably mad that the last chapter of life can be so hard. Note that I am describing situations when someone is suicidal, expresses some uncertainty, and there is space for me to think with them about their reasons for wanting to die. This technique is not helpful when someone is in a suicidal trance or suicidal mode, when there is very little ambivalence. In such a state of mind, people see suicide as the only way to end suffering. In these cases, securing safety is often only possible through hospitalization. That said, with Thomas's permission, I still worked with his family to provide him with a safe environment and limit his access to means.

Statistics regarding the number of clinicians who have had a client end their life through suicide are unclear. Indeed, given the scope of the problem, there is relatively little research on how many of us are impacted by these tragedies. For therapists who have had a client die by suicide, there can be a great deal of shame and embarrassment which may limit their willingness to talk about it. An article in *The Atlantic* by Sulome Anderson (2015) reported very different statistics about how often this impacts therapists. For example, one person Anderson interviewed suggested that 51% of psychiatrists lost a client to suicide, and another said it's as high as 80% of all people who work in the mental health field. I have heard from authorities that anywhere 5–25% of nonphysician therapists have a client die by suicide, which is a very large range. Two older survey-based studies with psychologists found that 22% and 28.8% indicated that they had experienced at least one client suicide (Chemtob et al. 1988; Pope and Tabachnick 1993). Other data suggests that almost half of the individuals who complete suicide in the United States are under treatment by a mental health professional (Goldsmith et al. 2002).

Avoidance and Therapist Feelings About Suicidal Clients

The strain regarding and fear of working with suicidal clients is often on the minds of mental health professionals. For example, a number of therapists simply state they do not want to work with suicidal people. It's not as if we can control this completely. Clients may not express suicidal thoughts until well into the therapy. They may become aware of suicidal ideas as life circumstances change. Whatever the reason, we can't always know if someone will become suicidal. Further, it's important to note that therapists consistently underestimate how suicidal clients are (Leenaars 1994).

Suicidal thoughts may be a part of what some clients with cPTSD think about every day. We often don't ask about these thoughts. In some cases, we may unconsciously communicate that we don't really want to know about them. This is not helpful, but understandable; most of us go into the field because we want to help people get better. Some clinicians worry if they bring up suicide that it might cause a client to consider suicide. This is not how it works—we therapists don't have that much power—but fear of discussing suicide is common, usually when we are younger in our careers. Additionally, it's also probable that some of us as therapists have been suicidal ourselves. For example, one study with psychologists found that 60% acknowledged being significantly depressed at some time during their careers, 29% reported having felt suicidal, and nearly 4% had attempted suicide (Pope and Tabachnick 1994). This issue could hit very close to home for many in our field.

Suicidal thoughts are not only frightening and hard to deal with, they also risk injuring the normal self-esteem-related identities we as clinicians hold dear. I suppose this could depend somewhat on our backgrounds. For example, if a clinician had a suicidal mother or has been seriously suicidal herself/himself, then this issue is likely much more vexing. For all of us, though, our self-worth as therapists involves a view of us being life-affirming, meaning that we can provide hope to our clients. One study found that 97% of psychologists worried that a client would die by suicide (Pope and Tabachnick 1993). When suicidal thoughts are present this can make us feel hopeless and that we have little to offer. Obviously, it can be terrifying to think that someone in our care could die by suicide. However, it's important that we remember our limits when dealing with clients who are suicidal. Kernberg et al. (1989) suggest that we remember that we may fail in our attempts to prevent suicide. This is not only true, it's valuable advice because it helps keep our own grandiosity in check, something that can be triggered by clients in these dire and distressing situations. It can also help increase our ability to feel empathy; if we get too caught up in our own perceptions of our control (or lack thereof), we can check out and leave suicidal people feeling too alone. It's about finding balance and realistic ways we can help while remembering our own limits.

For those of us in the helping professions, the effect of suicide has been described as "the ultimate narcissistic injury" (Gabbard 2003, p. 253). Tillman (2006) interviewed a number of therapists who had lost clients to suicide and noted themes of traumatic loss, difficulties in interpersonal relationships, as well as concerns about professional identity. One clinician reported that her loss irreparably changed her: "I think I have lost something as a clinician, the empathy. I can empathize with people to a point, but I quickly hospitalize people if I'm anxious. I think my patients are being cheated out of my being able to plumb the depths of their illness" (p. 171). The impact of client suicide is often traumatic for therapists which can lead to burnout and other problems that may interfere with our work and will be described in more detail in Chapter 10.

Dealing with facets of suicidality is a reality in our line of work and we need to manage our fears about the possibility of this tragedy. It's important that we do not take suicidal thoughts personally when they occur in the people we see and that we work as hard as we can to get inside of the minds of suicidal clients so we can appreciate and empathize with their suffering. Consider my struggles in doing so in the case of Rachel.

Rachel was in her fifties when her partner of 15 years left her for another younger woman at her workplace. Rachel was devastated and became increasingly suicidal. By the time she took an overdose of pills, she felt taken over by what is often described as a suicidal trance or suicidal mode. For weeks, suicide was the only thing on her mind. She imagined taking her own life continually and rehearsed the scene over and over. Additionally, she also heard voices telling her that she was worthless and should die, which led to a probable diagnosis of depression with psychotic features. I saw her for several years after her hospitalization and during various mood shifts, she never had psychotic symptoms again. Her dark mood persisted during much of the therapy, though we had a good relationship which we both experienced as warm and caring. One winter, when it was particularly dark and rainy, we recognized that my seeing her twice a week, even with her psychiatrist's support might not be enough to keep her from becoming seriously suicidal. We decided that she would attend an intensive outpatient program. I felt a sting of shame about this development. I initially worried that I was not doing enough for Rachael. Quickly though, I realized I had to get these feelings in check (and I did talk about them in consultation with a trusted colleague), because it would have been problematic if Rachel picked up on these feelings given her history with narcissistic and exploitive parents who never put Rachel's needs above their own. Rachel completed the intensive program for 3 weeks, and interestingly, despite her previous comfort with some of the techniques used in the program (Acceptance and Commitment Therapy and Dialectical Behavioral Therapy), she felt that she already knew much of this material and found these aspects of the program less helpful. Instead, she realized what she was longing for was more contact with people who had experienced severe depression. This led to a depression group referral, which was short term but offered the buffer she needed to get through this crisis.

Perhaps because Rachel and I had such a long relationship and a strong therapeutic connection, I was initially narcissistically wounded by her worsening mood and increase in suicidal thoughts. In other words, I made her symptoms about me. Fortunately, I was able to deal with the emotions I was having while also trying to think about what was working and what may need to be improved in her therapy. We were not discussing trauma-related material, as Rachel made it clear these topics were off the table, at least at that time. Yet I did consider if there were things I had not done that could have been more supportive to her and protective during times of increased suicidality. Rachel was already very familiar with a number of stabilizing techniques, but I had mentioned many times that I wondered if it might be good to have Rachel's partner (who had only been with her for 2 years at that point) come in for a session to discuss the impact and treatment of Rachel's depression and cPTSD. Rachel had never been open to this. I decided to push this issue, albeit gently, a bit more. Eventually, her partner came in and we talked about ways she could help Rachel when she was depressed. It proved to be very useful; Rachel's partner thought she was being helpful by giving Rachel "space" when she was isolating herself and the three of us talked about how alone that made Rachel feel, which of course, worsened her feelings of despair. Additionally, I realized I had fallen off a bit in terms of talking with Rachel about her meditation practice, which was very important to her but that she had also neglected, and it was clear that I had to be more assertive in terms of bringing that up in Rachel's therapy.

To be clear, people with histories of complex trauma and severe depression can become suicidal for any number of reasons which may or may not be related to the treatment we provide. As I said, clients who are suicidal can test our own feelings of self-responsibility. I don't know if the treatment with Rachel was lacking, but it seemed important to think about how I could be more helpful. People with cPTSD who are suicidal require our own intense work, introspect, and self-compassion. I did not beat myself up for being initially narcissistically involved—decent therapists, like good parents, should worry about how they are taking care of someone. But it's crucial that we shield our clients as much as possible from our issues in order to avoid them feeling that we need to be cared for.

The Trauma of a Suicidal Crisis

As seasoned clinicians know, a suicide attempt is itself a traumatic event for clients. People I have seen who have been so close to ending their lives experience terror that they could feel that way again. I think of suicide attempts as a form of trauma that becomes layered among previous traumas. Trauma results in confusion about our power. Both childhood and some adult traumas result in people feeling more powerful than they actually are. They believe that they are responsible for being injured, that something they have done or did not do is related to their victimization. When someone is seriously considering suicide or has made a suicide attempt, ideas of their own power and control become terrifyingly real.

For people with histories of multiple and chronic traumas, they likely felt that their lives were endangered at some point, either through the reality of a situation involving violence or the intensity of emotions which can feel so strong as to overwhelm and overtake their lives. And then to have this sense of danger felt internally—that they could put their own lives in jeopardy—is another cruel and terrifying facet of life and the aftermath of trauma. One client talked with me about this and expressed it very plainly. He said, "I don't want to kill myself now. But it's weird, you know? I could. I could simply choose to die at any time." This is a reality that most people try to distance themselves from, but it is true. It seems that once someone has come close to suicide, it changes them. It makes the idea of death seem ever-present and ever-possible. This becomes a part of the trauma story, spoken or unspoken.

It's important that we can name the traumatic nature of a suicidal crisis and express compassion for those in this situation. I think at times there is a way that we may want to move past suicidality and get on to the focus of living, but thinking about the meaning of suicidal thoughts, actions, and their consequences can be very helpful to some people, usually a while after having been acutely suicidal. It's part of dealing with the trauma of this terrifying event. Of course, it's also helpful to note for clients that although perhaps a part of them may have always wanted to die, a bigger part of them does want to live and we can hold both realities at once.

Risk Factors for Suicide

Turecki (2014) suggests an epigenetic theory about the risk of suicide (Fig. 4.1).

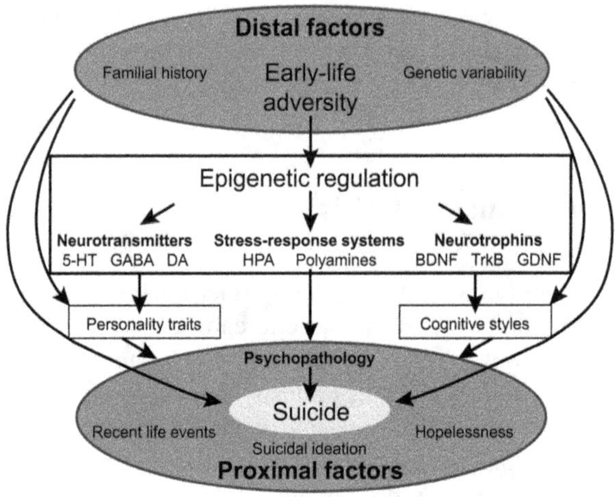

Fig. 4.1 Epigenetic theory of suicide risk factors. (Turecki 2014)

Early life adversity, family history of suicide, genetic vulnerability, as well as recent life events and the presence of mental illness in the last 6 months are risk factors for attempted suicide. Turecki notes the epigenetic data I discussed in Chapter 2, how early life trauma can regulate the response to stress. People who are prone to suicidality have heightened HPA-axis responses—meaning that the early environment, if it involves excessive fear, can make people more sensitive and reactive to stressful events. Additionally, people with reduced serotonin levels are found to have increased sensitivity to interpersonal relationships, increased distress, and potential suicidal thinking when there are problems in relationships (Mann 2013; Turecki 2014). In addition to low serotonin levels, alcohol use disorder constitutes an additional risk factor (Underwood et al. 2018).

Robust data on suicidality and childhood maltreatment comes from research from studies of over 17,000 patients at Kaiser Medical Centers in Southern California on Adverse Childhood Events, or ACEs. Dube et al. (2001) looked at adverse childhood experiences (childhood abuse [emotional, physical, and sexual], witnessing domestic violence, parental separation or divorce, and living with substance-abusing, mentally ill, or criminal household members) to the lifetime risk of suicide attempts. Adverse childhood experiences in any category increased the risk of attempted suicide twofold to fivefold. The more ACEs people experienced, the more likely they were to attempt suicide, and this was mediated by alcoholism, drug use, and depression.

People with anxious-ambivalent and insecure attachment styles are more likely to have suicidal ideation and attempts (Violato and Arato 2004; Wright et al. 2005). These attachment styles are punctuated by a desire to be around people, but difficulty obtaining comfort when others are present. A study by Stepp et al. (2008) found anxious attachment styles predicted interpersonal sensitivity, interpersonal aggression, and lack of sociability, which in turn were associated with suicide-related behavior.

As I've previously stated, PTSD and cPTSD are risk factors for suicide attempt. Simon (2006) lists additional primary risk factors for suicide:

- Depression
- Anxiety
- Panic attacks
- Psychosis
- Sleep disturbance
- Substance abuse
- Impulsivity
- Agitation
- Physical illness
- Work, family relationship stress
- Lethal means

McCall (2015) states that additional factors for risk of suicide are advancing age, male sex, and being white. He also emphasizes that insomnia has been associated with suicide for at least 25 years and adds specifically that nightmares and hypersomnia are risk factors that we often are unaware of. Self-harm, defined as a preoccupation with deliberately hurting oneself without conscious suicidal intent, is predictive of suicide attempts in adolescents, undergraduate students, and adults (Muehlenkamp 2005; Klonsky et al. 2013). Access to a firearm, particularly during stressful events, has been identified as a key factor increasing one's risk for completing suicide. States with higher rates of gun ownership have higher suicide rates than states with low gun ownership (American Public Health Association 2018).

Additionally, previous suicide attempt is a risk factor for suicide (Bridge et al. 2006), as well as contagion effects that occur in local communities, especially in schools in the aftermath of a death by suicide (Gould et al. 2003). Further lesbian, gay, and bisexual youth are at increased risk for suicide attempt (Rimes et al. 2019) as are transgender persons (Wolford-Clevenger et al. 2018).

Despite this dizzying list of factors associated with suicide, many of the cases of suicide I have heard of came as a shock to people who knew the victim. There is so much that we don't really know about what goes on in the minds of people who take their own lives. That said, there is a lot we can do to help our clients who feel suicidal.

Interventions for Suicidality

The high number of risk factors for suicide reminds us of the importance of making discussions of suicidal thoughts a normal part of therapy. Survivors of suicide attempts and others at high suicide risk appear to be more likely to drop out of mental health treatment than those not at elevated risk (Hom and Joiner 2017). Many of our clients are often as hesitant as we are to discuss suicidal thoughts, but clinical experience has taught me that it's very soothing for clients if ideas of suicide can be brought out into the open, even among people whom we may see as being at relatively low risk. For example, one client I worked with for two decades had stashed a number of lethal drugs in a drawer in the event she decided to try to end her life. I literally worked with her for 15 years before she eventually threw away her stash, her escape route from this life, but we discussed it routinely. I tried to convey genuine curiosity and respect for the fact that she needed the idea of self-inflicted death as a kind of solace when life seemed hard.

A recent study with 329 people who had survived a suicide attempt were asked what they thought could improve outcomes for people in their situation. Data analyses provided areas in which mental health treatment experiences might be improved for survivors of suicide attempts. These factors included clinicians who reduce the stigma of suicidality, express empathy, listen actively, and provide a range of treatment options, including those that don't involve medication, addressing root problems while also utilizing active coping strategies, and improving access to continuity of care (Hom et al. 2020). Again, any therapist using any modality can provide these factors, but it requires us to manage our fear in situations of clients who feel suicidal.

However, being open to discussing suicide is just a start when people in our care are seriously suicidal. I'm referring to clients who are deemed to be at risk but do not meet criteria for hospitalization; their suicidality is not imminent, yet. Many of us who are older learned that we should provide our clients with a "no harm" or "no suicide" contract in which we had clients contact us before they attempted to hurt themselves. These contracts are no longer the standard of care. Instead, they have been replaced by crisis response plans or safety plans. The idea of a crisis response plan is to collaboratively create a plan that a client can carry with them so that they know what to do if they get into a suicidal crisis. Craig J. Bryan, Executive Director, National Center for Veterans Studies, is credited with the following guidelines regarding suicide crisis planning or crisis response planning (CRP) (2019):

Crisis Response Plan

1. Explain rationale for CRP
2. Provide card to record CRP
3. Identify personal warning signs
4. Identify self-management strategies

5. Identify reasons for living
6. Identify social supports
7. Provide crisis/emergency steps
8. Verbally review and rate likelihood of use

Bryan's recommendation is that we provide clients with an index card in which we record the aforementioned information together in a session. I should add that for people who are accustomed to their smartphones, there are apps that can serve the same purpose. That said (and this could be my age-related bias talking), for many people there is something soothing about an index card that can be carried with them. It is a concrete reminder of something the therapist and client developed together and a kind of transitional object connecting the therapist and client, to use the language of Winnicott (1953). It also seems important to note that from a simple behavioral conditioning perspective, smartphones are associated with anxiety—social media alerts, email alerts, and texts—all things that could cause stress in a crisis situation that a simple index card may not. That said, clients should be able to tell us what will work best for them.

The CRP starts with explaining to clients that once they become suicidal, it can be hard to remember or access coping resources. Once a client is in a suicidal trance, they are often unable to remember why they want to live, what coping resources they can access, as well as whom they might contact to help. Therefore, I complete safety plans with clients before a suicidal crisis if there is a history of suicidality. I was recently with one client who tends to find the winter months unbearable and we were heading in to the colder and darker months. I suggested we do a safety plan, even though she was not currently suicidal. She remarked while we were doing it that it was soothing to think about this aspect of herself while in a non-suicidal state. Additionally, although I had known this woman for a long time, the crisis planning gave me much more details about whom she really thought were social supports and I learned more about her relationships.

Having access to a plan that clients carry with them can help them navigate a crisis and, equally as important, access the part of them that does want to live. Once the client agrees, the first task is having a client identify what their warning signs are. What are personalized warning signs that they might become suicidal? Having them write these down while we are with them is an important part of the intervention; the therapist and client do this together. Following that, what helps them manage suicidal thoughts? The idea is to remind clients what works for them when they are suicidal to get them out of that state of mind. I should add that I have found it incredibly valuable to label the suicidal trance or mode out loud with them because it's often confusing for clients when they are not suicidal to understand how they could have been so willing to end their own lives. Included in the CRP are reminders of reasons for living as well as people who can be a support. People who become suicidal can easily forget that there are reasons for living and that there are people who love them. Having such concrete reminders is crucial because in a suicidal mode, people genuinely believe that they are alone. Finally, putting in writing what emergency steps can be taken in the event of serious intent can help clients remember how to take care of themselves.

The Veterans Affairs Medical Center has recently updated their guidelines for the management of suicidality, available at https://www.healthquality.va.gov/guidelines/MH/srb/. A recent review of treatments for the prevention and management of suicide suggests that CBT and DBT (dialectical behavioral therapy) showed modest benefits in reducing suicidal ideation compared with treatment as usual or waitlist controls (D'Anci et al. 2019). Additionally, another novel intervention that has been associated with decreased incidence of suicide is sending postcards to people who have previously attempted suicides (Carter et al. 2013; NIH 2017). The postcards are emailed to people after emergency room visits for suicide attempts and are essentially a check-in and reminder that staff are thinking about them and hope they are doing okay.

Conclusion

There is so much we still don't understand about the phenomena of suicide. This should not encourage us to sit back and not actively help our clients. But remembering the limits of our control with suicidal clients has been helpful when I work with suicidal people. It allows me to access empathy and an ability to think. If we feel overly responsible and panicked with suicidal clients, we cannot be as present with them. People who want to die need us to hear what is on their minds about their thoughts of ending of own lives. I've noticed a lot of the writing and trainings on suicide sometimes emphasize risk management aspects of caring for people who want to end their lives. Of course, risk management is important, and we all need to follow legal guidelines regarding care as well as legally required documentation. However, I have sometimes worried that risk management approaches leave something out about the importance of relating in a compassionate way to people who are suicidal. Like we say to our clients, it's always helpful to remember the limits of our control. This has helped me when clients talk about the specific ways they want to die. I can slow the conversation down and just listen and find empathy. When people I see are suicidal, I find it terrifying and painful to sit in my office while having a seemingly reasonable conversation about how someone wants to die, but it is important that I do not recoil or suggest that a client is damaged because he/she has those thoughts. People who feel seriously suicidal have a great deal of shame that they are too much or, as one person put it, "too grotesque and hideous to be seen." We need to see them and presume that by viewing, holding, and containing these ideas, we communicate that they deserve to live.

Providing safety for our clients with cPTSD involves a number of skills. We need to regulate our own affect and be ready for whatever difficult material we may hear. Suicidal thoughts and actions are terrifying to us and our clients. We should strive not to take suicidality personally, but at the same time be ready to shift approaches if a client becomes suicidal. These approaches involve crisis plans but also techniques that reinforce coping defenses.

Interventions for Maintaining Physical Safety

- Ask every client about suicidal thoughts. Bringing it up won't give a client ideas about suicide unless it has already been on their minds.
- Engage in discussions about suicide in an active way.
- Try to provide empathy for the suicidal wish.
- Decrease stigma about feeling suicidal.
- Try not to make suicidality about you as the therapist. Our clients become suicidal for many reasons.
- If someone is suicidal after making sure the client is safe, consider what is working and what is not in treatment.
- If talking about traumas or other techniques have been too overstimulating, shift gears to interventions that reinforce healthy defenses and coping skills, as well as increasing social support.
- Manage expectations in terms of talking about past traumas. Respect avoidance. If someone can't talk about trauma, it does not mean therapy can't be helpful.
- Crisis plans or safety plans are the current standard of care. Give clients the tools they need to help themselves when suicidal.
- A suicidal crisis becomes woven into the trauma narrative, no matter how disjointed that narrative is. It's often helpful to discuss the terror and confusion associated with a suicidal crisis.
- If you have suicidal clients, get regular consultation with a trusted colleague.

References

American Public Health Association. (2018). *Reducing suicides by firearms. Policy Number: 20184*. Accessed online on 12th Oct 2019 at https://www.apha.org/policies-and-advocacy/public-health-policy-statements/policy-database/2019/01/28/reducing-suicides-by-firearms.

Anderson, S. (2015, January 20). How patient suicide affects psychiatrists. *The Atlantic*. Accessed online at https://www.theatlantic.com/health/archive/2015/01/how-patient-suicide-affects-psychiatrists/384563/.

Berglund, S., Åström, S., & Lindgren, B. M. (2016). Patients' experiences after attempted suicide: A literature review. *Issues in Mental Health Nursing, 37*, 715–726.

Bridge, J. A., Goldstein, T. R., & Brent, D. A. (2006). Adolescent suicide and suicidal behavior. *The Journal of Child Psychology and Psychiatry, 47*, 372–394.

Bryan, C. J. (2019). *Crisis response planning for suicide prevention*. Accessed online on 13th Oct at https://avapl.org/conference/pubs/2018%20Conference%20Presentations/Craig%20Bryan%20VA%20Leadership%20CRP.pdf.

Carter, G. L., Clover, K., Whyte, I. M., Dawson, A. H., & D'Este, C. (2013). Postcards from the EDge: 5-year outcomes of a randomized controlled trial for hospital-treated self-poisoning. *British Journal of Psychiatry, 202*(5), 372–380.

Chemtob, C. M., Hamada, R. S., Bauer, G., Torigoe, R. Y., & Kinney, B. (1988). Patient suicide: Frequency and impact on psychologists. *Professional Psychology: Research and Practice, 19*(4), 416–420.

Crosby, A. E., Han, B., Ortega, L. A. G., Parks, S. E., & Gfroerer, J. (2011). Suicidal thoughts and behaviors among adults aged ≥18 years—United States, 2008-2009. *Centers for Disease Control and Prevention, Surveillance Summaries, 60*(SS13), 1–22.

D'Anci, K. E., Uhl, S., Giradi, G., & Martin, C. (2019). Treatments for the prevention and management of suicide: A systematic review. *Annals of Internal Medicine, 171*, 334–342.

Dube, S. R., Anda, R. F., Felitti, V. J., Chapman, D. P., Williamson, D. F., & Giles, W. H. (2001). Childhood abuse, household dysfunction, and the risk of attempted suicide throughout the life span: Findings from the adverse childhood experiences study. *Journal of the American Medical Association, 286*(24), 3089–3096.

Editorial. (2019). Suicide risk in U.S. veterans. *The Lancet, 394*(10201), 805–894.

Firestone, L. (2019). Busting the myths about suicide. *PsychAlive*. Accessed online on 9th June 2019 at https://www.psychalive.org/busting-the-myths-about-suicide/.

Gabbard, G. O. (2003). Miscarriages of psychoanalytic treatment with suicidal patients. *International Journal of Psychoanalysis, 84*, 249–261.

Goldsmith, S. K., Pellmar, T. C., Kleinman, A. M., & Bunney, W. E. (Eds.). (2002). *Institute of Medicine (US) committee on pathophysiology and prevention of adolescent and adult suicide*. Washington, DC: National Academies Press.

Gould, M., Jamieson, P., & Romer, D. (2003). Media contagion and suicide among the young. *American Behavioral Scientist, 46*(9), 1269–1284.

Hom, M. A., & Joiner, T. E. (2017). Predictors of treatment attrition among adult outpatients with clinically significant suicidal ideation. *Journal of Clinical Psychology, 73*, 88–98.

Hom, M. A., Bauer, B. W., Stanley, I. H., Boffa, J. W., Stage, D. L., Capron, D. W., et al. (2020). Suicide attempt survivors' recommendations for improving mental health treatment for attempt survivors. *Psychological Services*. Advance online publication. https://doi.org/10.1037/ser0000415. Accessed online on 24 Feb 2020.

Kernberg, O. F., Selzer, M. A., Koenigsberg, H. W., Carr, A. C., & Appelbaum, A. H. (1989). *Psychodynamic psychotherapy of borderline patients*. New York: Basic Books.

Klonsky, E. D., May, A. M., & Glenn, C. R. (2013). The relationship between nonsuicidal self-injury and attempted suicide: Converging evidence from four samples. *Journal of Abnormal Psychology, 122*(1), 231–237.

Leenaars, A. A. (1994). Crisis intervention with highly lethal suicidal people. *Death Studies, 18*(4), 341–360.

Mann, J. J. (2013). The serotonergic system in mood disorders and suicidal behaviour. *Philosophical Transactions of the Royal Society of London. Series B, Biological Sciences, 368*(1615), 20120537. https://doi.org/10.1098/rstb.2012.0537.

McCall, W. V. (2015). The correlation between sleep disturbance and suicide. *Psychiatric Times, 32*, 9. Accessed online on 12th Oct 2019 at https://www.psychiatrictimes.com/special-reports/correlation-between-sleep-disturbance-and-suicide.

Menon, R. (2019). Suicide is becoming America's latest epidemic. *The Nation*. Published on 18th June. Accessed online on 17th Aug 2019 at https://www.thenation.com/article/suicide-rate-americas-latest-epidemic/.

Muehlenkamp, J. (2005). Self-injurious behavior as a separate clinical syndrome. *American Journal of Orthopsychiatry, 75*(2), 324–333.

National Institute of Health. (2017). *Life-saving post-ER suicide prevention strategies are cost effective*. Accessed online on 13th Sept at https://www.nih.gov/news-events/news-releases/life-saving-post-er-suicide-prevention-strategies-are-cost-effective.

Orbach, I. (2001). Therapeutic empathy with the suicidal wish: Principles of therapy with suicidal individuals. *American Journal of Psychotherapy, 55*(2), 166–184.

Panagioti, M., Angelakis, I., Tarrier, N., & Gooding, P. (2017). A prospective investigation of the impact of distinct posttraumatic (PTSD) symptom clusters on suicidal ideation. *Cognitive Therapy and Research, 41*(4), 645–653.

Pinheiro, M., Mendes, D., Mendes, T., Pais, J., Cabral, T., Rocha, J. C., et al. (2016). Importance of C-PTSD symptoms and suicide attempt. *European Psychiatry, 33*(Supplement), S215.

Piscopo, K., Lipari, R. N., Cooney, J., & Glasheen, C. (2016). *Suicidal thoughts and behavior among adults: Results from the 2015 National Survey on Drug Use and Health.* NSDUH data review. Accessed online on 24th Feb 2020 at http://www.samhsa.gov/data/sites/default/files/NSDUH-DR-FFR3-2015/NSDUH-DR-FFR3-2015.htm.

Pope, K. S., & Tabachnick, B. G. (1993). Therapists' anger, hate, fear, and sexual feelings: National survey of therapist responses, client characteristics, critical events, formal complaints, and training. *Professional Psychology: Research and Practice, 24*(2), 142–152.

Pope, K. S., & Tabachnick, B. G. (1994). Therapists as patients: A national survey of psychologists' experiences, problems, and beliefs. *Professional Psychology: Research and Practice, 25*, 247–258.

Rimes, K. A., Shivakumar, S., Ussher, G., Baker, D., Rahman, Q., & West, E. (2019). Psychosocial factors associated with suicide attempts, ideation, and future risk in lesbian, gay, and bisexual youth: The youth chances study. *Crisis: The Journal of Crisis Intervention and Suicide Prevention, 40*(2), 83–92.

Simon, R. I. (2006). Suicide risk: Assessing the unpredictable. In R. I. Simon & R. E. Hales (Eds.), *The American Psychiatric Publishing textbook of suicide assessment and management* (pp. 1–32). Arlington: American Psychiatric Publishing, Inc.

Stepp, S. D., Morse, J. Q., Yaggi, K. E., Reynolds, S. K., Reed, L. I., & Pilkonis, P. A. (2008). The role of attachment styles and interpersonal problems in suicide-related behaviors. *Suicide and Life-threatening Behavior, 38*, 592–607.

Stevens, D., Wilcox, H. G., MacKinnon, D. F., Mondimore, F. M., Schweizer, B., Jancic, D., et al. (2013). Post-traumatic stress disorder increases risk for suicide attempt in adults with recurrent major depression. *Depression and Anxiety, 30*(10), 940–946.

Tillman, J. G. (2006). When a patient commits suicide: An empirical study of psychoanalytic clinicians. *International Journal of Psychoanalysis, 87*(1), 159–177.

Turecki, G. (2014). Epigenetics and suicidal behavior research pathways. *American Journal of Preventative Medicine, 47*(3 Supplement 2), S144–S151.

Underwood, M. D., Kassir, S. A., Bakalian, M. J., Galfalvy, H., Dwork, A. J., & Mann, J. J., et al. (2018). Serotonin receptors and suicide, major depression, alcohol use disorder and reported early life adversity. *Translational Psychiatry*, *8*, 279. Accessed online on 12th Oct 2019 at https://www.nature.com/articles/s41398-018-0309-1#Sec7.

Violato, C., & Arato, J. (2004). Childhood attachment and adolescent suicide: A step-wise discriminant analysis in a case-comparison study. *Individual Differences Research, 2*, 162–168.

Watson Coleman, B. (2020). *Ring the alarm: The crisis of black youth suicide in America.* A report to congress from the congressional black caucus emergency taskforce on black youth suicide and mental health. Accessed online on 16th Feb 2020 at https://watsoncoleman.house.gov/uploadedfiles/full_taskforce_report.pdf.

Winnicott, D. W. (1953). Transitional objects and transitional phenomena—A study of the first not-me possession. *International Journal of Psychoanalysis, 34*, 89–97.

Wolford-Clevenger, C., Frantell, P., Smith, P. N., Flores, L. Y., & Stuart, G. L. (2018). Correlates of suicide ideation and behaviors among transgender people: A systematic review guided by ideation-to-action theory. *Clinical Psychology Review, 63*, 93–105.

Woolf, S. H., & Schoomaker, H. (2019). Life expectancy and mortality rates in the United States, 1959–2017. *Journal of the American Medical Association, 322*(20), 1996–2016.

World Health Organization. (2019). *Suicide data.* Accessed 9th Feb 2019 at https://www.who.int/mental_health/prevention/suicide/suicideprevent/en/.

Wright, J., Briggs, S., & Behringer, J. (2005). Attachment and the body in suicidal adolescents: A pilot study. *Clinical Child Psychology and Psychiatry, 10*, 477–491.

Chapter 5
Dissociation: Controversies and Clinical Strategies

Normal vs. Trauma-Related Dissociation

Ideas about dissociation, the causes as well as its role as a result of trauma, are variously and contrarily viewed by clinicians and researchers. Like theoretical camps in psychotherapy approaches, there are strong views on why some people develop extreme dissociation. I will discuss some of these controversies and will speak to a wide variety of research reviewed, interviews with experts, and my own clinical observations regarding this confusing set of clinical phenomena. It is my view that people who have experienced extensive trauma do tend to be troubled by dissociation more than those without these histories. However, mild dissociation is related to normal and frequent experiences in human behavior.

Dissociative phenomena exist on a continuum of normal and common to more maladaptive elements, the latter of which causes disruptions in both functioning and the development of meaning in everyday life. Dissociation is broadly referred to as a loss of access to or control over mental processes that are typically available to conscious awareness, self-attribution, or control under normal circumstances (Cardeña and Carlson 2011).

In regard to trauma reactions, dissociation refers to a defensive mechanism in which we compartmentalize and cleave off memories of things that are traumatic (e.g., Putnam 1991). It's a method designed to promote detachment and keep us from getting overwhelmed. It may also occur when the defensive functions of anxiety fail. I often consider dissociation to be a collapse—when normal modes of coping are unavailable, we simply leave, or to put it more accurately, we narrow our attention and focus, which results in excluding some aspects of experience. An example that comes to mind, from almost 30 years ago, involved a supervisor of mine. There had been severe and unusual flooding in the area in which we lived, and my supervisor had gotten caught in her car in a flash flood. As floods are more common now, many of us may be able to relate. She was trying to get home after work, and she chose to head down a flooded road and found the water up to the windows

T. M. Greenberg, *Treating Complex Trauma*,
https://doi.org/10.1007/978-3-030-45285-8_5

of her car. When she told me about this, she said, "Water was all around me. I knew I made a mistake, but I was trapped. I just told myself, you're in a boat. That's all. Just keep driving, your car is a boat. It was a boat on a pleasant day. I just floated home." Her emotions were flat as she reported this story and she seemed far away. I felt scared for her and wanted to say something, but given the power dynamic, not to mention my relatively young age at the time, I did not want to appear disrespectful. As far as I know, my supervisor did not have a dissociative disorder, but she used the technique of dissociation to keep herself from panicking (not that this was conscious on her part), which could have led to an even worse situation. However, we can also imagine the risk associated with her coping in this way. It's impossible to know if she would have been jolted back to the reality of her situation if she was at serious risk of her car being swept away. In the era before mobile phones, it's unclear what realistic options might have been available to her.

Though trauma histories are associated with an increased tendency to dissociate, people without cPTSD also dissociate, including many people with other psychological problems (van Ijzendoorn and Schuengel 1996; Leavitt 2001). Watson (2003) argues that dissociation is an unstable construct and that the presence of this defense can shift based on when assessment takes place—suggesting that we use it when we need it, though most of the time, not consciously. Indeed, normal dissociation involves the narrowing of attention to keep us from knowing certain facts under stressful situations, suggesting that we all have the capacity to dissociate (Hilgard 1986; Putnam 1997).

Butler (2006) in her review of dissociation emphasizes that it has normal elements and de-emphasizes its defensive function. She notes that absorption in everyday activities, dreaming, daydreaming, and fantasizing all can be considered dissociative but are part of normal, everyday life. For example, many of us daydream, which could have an adaptive element in terms of revisiting what we have done or rehearsing what we might do. In fact, Klinger (1971) postulated that daydreaming might help us to remember things we have forgotten. More recent research suggests that daydreamers might be very smart—they may learn more quickly and efficiently (Godwin et al. 2017).

It's interesting to note that the language of dissociation has made its way into the lexicon of everyday communication, for example, an actress recently referred to being in a different "self-state" when she is acting. A rap song, I happened upon on my car radio, involved a young man speaking about different "versions" of himself. Bromberg (1996) noted that dissociation is common in all of us and that this is related to the shifting nature of consciousness itself: the self is decentered, and the mind is a configuration of shifting, nonlinear, discontinuous states of consciousness in an ongoing clash with the healthy illusion of unitary selfhood. In other words, Bromberg suggests that dissociation can range from everyday shifting states of consciousness to more abrupt shifts to avoid terror.

At the heart of dissociation, whether it's normal or excessive, involves wrestling with the issue of identity. When I have spoken with professional or collegiate athletes, I've seen several aspects of dissociation. These are people who have spent much of their lives training in a particular sport. For some, when unable to compete, they are utterly lost with no sense of who they are. I remember one athlete who got injured and could not play for a period of time, and he said he was not sure if he even *was* himself if he could not play his sport. When I asked him to pay attention to his thoughts so we could get a better sense of what was on his mind, he told me that he literally did not think about anything other than the sport he played. He was three when he started his training, and it's unclear that he was encouraged to think about anything else. I don't know how things turned out for this man, as he eventually got over his injury, went back to his sport, and was transferred to another team. But this case and many others seem to straddle something that is between normal and adaptive dissociation and something that could become more debilitating. It's interesting to note that people with high nonclinical levels of dissociation proneness exhibited less integrity of self-concept and a more polarized and compartmentalized sense of self (Chiu et al. 2017).

Assessing Excessive Dissociation

Despite the fact that dissociation can have normal elements, there are some for whom dissociation becomes a needed and involuntary way of operating in the world. Some people find themselves developing extreme dissociation and symptoms of dissociative disorders. When dissociation becomes a problem, people may unwillingly find that they cannot control their attention in the way they would like. For example, while many of us might find daydreaming a pleasurable experience, people with excessive dissociation experience disconnection and a lack of continuity between thoughts, memories, experiences, actions, and identity. In other words, the narrowing of attention becomes hazardous because of its sheer nature—the exclusion of basic aspects of experience. A client, whom I will call Sheila, described and demonstrated more extreme dissociation when she recounted a rape she had experienced in high school:

I went to their house; I was babysitting, was supposed to babysit for their 5-year-old. I think she was five, maybe older? My mom dropped me off. They were a new family... I got there and only the dad was there? It was...weird. Maybe I don't remember. I did not see the kid. I remember, I think, asking what I was supposed to do. And then, it went dark, I mean in my mind... I was there. I saw the house and I remember talking to the man and then... I don't... I remembered walking home and how much it hurt to walk. It seemed weird and my mom did not ask me why I came home early. I just thought, maybe I made that up, you know, like some kind of dream... But I mean, sometimes, I think, did that really happen? Maybe it didn't....

Sheila indicates the properties of dissociation in sad and tragic detail. She remembers some aspects vividly (she later told me what the décor of the house was like and what she remembered about the details of an air freshener), but the rape only came to her in her bodily memory of the pain at the time and then later in vivid, but disjointed, recurrent dreams about the event. She eventually pieced together her story—she knew she had been raped and eventually could say how the specific event took place. Yet, she wondered if she was crazy, probably more so because she did not have parents who would have been interested in her ordeal. Sheila's speech is important. Clinically, we can suspect the presence of dissociation based on the use of language—the jarring starting and stopping of how she tells the story, as well as what she phrases as questions. Sheila was there, but not there. She protected herself from the violent aspects of her experience, but she knows, nonetheless. And she could not really use language to make sense of her experience until she was in a safe therapeutic relationship, with someone she imagined would be able to think about this event in a neutral way. Though I held in mind the likelihood that she had been raped, I never offered an opinion until she seemed certain about her experience. I noted that it did seem that something bad and frightening happened, but it would have been too risky for me to collude with the part of herself that knew about the assault. I needed to respect her doubt until her story became clearer in her mind.

The American Psychiatric Association (Wang 2018) offers a different typology regarding dissociation than what I have discussed so far and highlights three major types of dissociative disorders. Dissociative identity disorder (DID) is associated with overwhelming experiences, traumatic events, and/or abuse that occurred in childhood and is characterized by different self-states or personality states, and distinct identities are accompanied by changes in behavior, memory, and thinking. Howell (2011) notes that people with DID may tend to refer to themselves with the pronoun "we." This is a phenomenon that I have seen in people who are prone to extreme dissociation and may experience more pronounced different self-states. One young woman I am thinking of was telling me about something she was looking up on the Internet regarding drug use and depression, things she was very familiar with. She said, "We were confused about this and so we looked it up." The idea of "we" suggests multiple states of mind that may be present or possibly that multiple versions of the self coalesce in the service of attempting cohesion.

Dissociative amnesia involves not being able to recall information about oneself that seems beyond normal forgetting. This amnesia is usually related to a traumatic or stressful event. Dissociative amnesia is associated with having experiences of childhood trauma and especially with experiences of emotional abuse and emotional neglect. People may not be aware of their memory loss or may have only limited awareness. And people may minimize the importance of memory loss about a particular event or time. Clinically, I see these phenomena a lot, when clients casually mention, "I don't really remember much about my childhood. I really don't remember much until college." It often does not bother them. While these are people who may have had discrete abusive episodes during childhood, they are often people who were left to their own devices as a young person, such as being left alone a lot at ages in which they were too young to take care of themselves. Equally as important, they had no one to help them manage the overwhelming feelings that take place in childhood in general and more so when being neglected.

Depersonalization/derealization disorder involves a very particular loss of sense of self and identity. Depersonalization involves experiences of unreality or detachment from one's mind, self, or body. People may feel as if they are outside their bodies and watching events happening to them. They may feel as if things and people in the world around them are not real. I've heard people in this state refer to themselves as feeling "dead but alive at the same time." The person is aware of reality and that their experience is unusual. It's often very distressful, even though the person may appear to be numb or dissociated.

Steninberg (1995) describes the five core elements of dissociative disorders in Fig. 5.1.

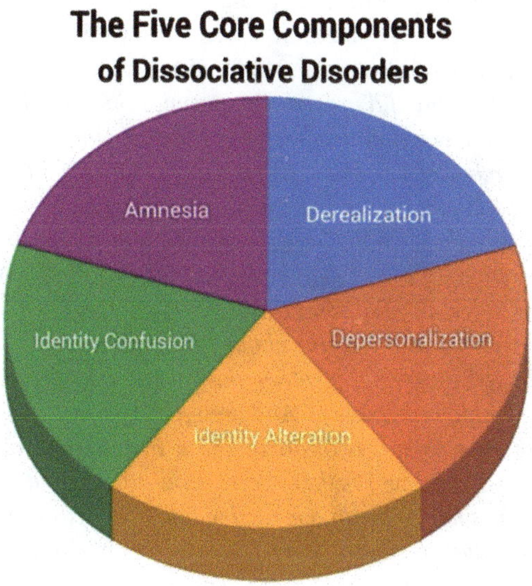

Fig. 5.1 The five core components of dissociative disorders. (Source: *Handbook for the assessment of dissociation: a clinical guide*. Steinberg 1995)

In addition to derealization, depersonalization, and amnesia, Steinberg emphasizes that dissociation impacts identity. Although we may classically think about people who have DID, formerly known as multiple personality disorder, as those who have problems with identity, people who are extremely dissociative, without DID, have problems with self-coherence. For example, a disorganized attachment style (which is also linked with ideas of self-concept) is associated with dissociation (Siegel 1996; Hesse et al. 2003). This makes sense, as people with disorganized attachment styles are unsure of how to attach, and they do so in an almost piecemeal way and based on limited interpersonal data sets. For example, a young man I know with a disorganized attachment style does not really have strong feelings toward anyone he knows. His experience of people changes almost moment to moment, and he has no real recognition of fear that being close to people might involve. Rather, his sense of himself and others is constantly shifting, almost like tectonic plates in constant motion. He has trouble knowing, in a genuine way, when he is with someone with whom he feels comfortable.

Putnam (1992) emphasizes that severe dissociation has a "magical" quality, in that it allows us to transcend difficult circumstances, but it comes with a price. He states the costs of dissociation include "(1) discontinuity of sense of self; (2) a detachment or depersonalization from the physical self that permits or even fosters self-mutilation; (3) An array of amnesias and gaps in the continuity of memory;

(4) inability to transfer basic conceptual information across dissociative states, leading to a failure to learn from experience and erratic access to knowledge and skills; and (5) inner conflicts and self-sabotage" (p. 105).

Putnam adds to the understanding of dissociation by articulating the ways that fragmentation can also be linked with self-destruction. This aspect of thinking about it has been helpful to me, as we will see with Melanie, who has been described in previous chapters of this book. Although I sometimes can pick up on dissociation via the way someone speaks or the fact that clients can appear to be very different from session to session, I was not aware of Melanie's use of this defense, until she worked to sabotage herself and her situation.

Melanie did indeed get a promotion at work, which was a shock to us both, as we both seemed consciously worried about some of her acting out behaviors with a member of her team, as well as her history of "blowing up" various job situations. I had been seeing her for over a year at this point and, yet, felt that I still knew relatively little about her. I began to feel sleepy in sessions with her as she reported seemingly banal details about her job. I found I could not remember or keep track of relevant characters in her life, including her boyfriend, whom I still had little concrete information about and I could barely form a picture of him in my mind, based on anything other than what I might imagine in terms of his basic demographic information. And though she would report fights with her boyfriend, I found there was no emotion in these discussions or really any thoughtful discussion. Regarding work, there were troubles. It sounded like the people reporting to her found her to be an aggressive and dismissive boss, who was at times overly managing and at others frankly neglectful of things she was supposed to keep track of regarding the work of her reports. In other words, while our sessions seemed dead and bland and intolerable, her external world was falling apart. Finally, it occurred to me that there might be something in the realm of dissociation happening. I commented, "I notice that when you talk about these seemingly intense things, I can't quite get a sense of how you are feeling. And I wondered although you can describe some details of what is going on, if maybe something else might be missing?" She said, as though this should have been obvious to me, "Oh yeah, I don't really know sometimes what I am saying. I mean, I do, but I don't. I am outside of myself." I asked her what she meant. She said, "Like, you know, floating." I said, "Like watching yourself?" She said, "Ummm, maybe. I'm not sure." I waited, as I thought she might want to say more. She didn't. So I said, "Is it distressing?" She said, "I think so. I don't know for sure." At that moment, I recalled a dream she had in the beginning of therapy. She was headed to a store to buy something, "something good," as she described it, but as she parked in the parking garage, the sky turned "eerily purple-orange." She was walking into the multistory complex where the store was (my office is in a multistory building), and a giant UFO was hovering over the store. She was not sure if she was going to be abducted. There was so much noise; she "could not think." The dream ended in a state of confusion about what she should do next.

I did not speak then to Melanie about her dream or my recollection of it or what I thought it might mean. I was still trying to piece things together and I was not sure what I should say. After the session, it occurred to me that her dream was about her dissociation. Prior to this moment, I had thought about the dream as a worry about being in therapy, her recent suicide attempt, and her anxiety about attempting to find something good. After it was clear that she had more symptoms of dissociation than I had realized, it occurred to me that she was worried about "alien" aspects of herself, which, in someone who does not have excessive dissociation, could simply be construed as a fear of what is not known in the unconscious. But in this case, "aliens" also represented aspects of her experiences that had been walled off by dissociation and aspects of parts of herself that held on to traumatic events that were terrifying and little known.

To be clear, Melanie did not have clinically diagnosable DID, but as I got to know her, it was clear that under intense anxiety, she became fragmented and dissociated much of her experience. Although there is extensive clinical data that people with DID come to therapy with already formed and named altered states, my experience tends to be both more muted and nuanced. I do see people who present with different personas, though as I have noted, differing self-states have become to be seen as relatively normal by some clinicians and in popular culture. But this is different than the fragmentation caused by trauma. How much fragmentation occurs, how this manifests, and how it's treated seem partly to be based on client- and therapist-dependent narratives. Many of my colleagues and I, in the area in which I practice, tend to deal with "whomever" shows up, knowing that different self-states have a commonality in all of us, though are likely more so among our traumatized clients. And we focus on helping the state of mind that occurs when presenting to us. Noted dissociation expert Chefetz (2015) describes this well when he says, "… although I pay attention to the comings and goings of the dissociated isolated subjectivities in my patients, my main interest in doing so is to track the affect, the emotionality, and the associated cognitive structures that teach me about the mind-body of my patient. I am less interested in the presence of alternate identity for its own sake" (p. 14). Finding emotions is what is most important, no matter the self-state. Accessing affect, in my opinion, is the main tool for truncating fragmentation and limiting dissociation.

Controversies Regarding Dissociation: TM vs. SCM

As a segue to talking about treating dissociative disorders, I'm going to talk about some of the rather significant controversies related to ideas of the causes of dissociation and the two major competing theories. There is some scholarship to these discussions, particularly as it relates to the proposed mechanisms of dissociation. However, it seems that part of the conflict, at least in terms of how it manifests in discussions about the facts of dissociation (including ideas about how real DID is), has to do with beliefs regarding the veracity of "recovered memories" and the "memory wars" of the 1980s and 1990s in the United States, Canada, and Great Britain (Ulatowska and Sawicka 2017). Predating these controversies, however, is a long history of disbelief—professional, as well as cultural dissociation and denial regarding the presence of trauma, particularly in childhood, as well as violence toward vulnerable people in general. This stems back to Freud himself, and I'll address these latter controversies in the next section. My intention in discussing these controversies is not to overtly pick sides, which I think has become an implied expectation when discussing our increasingly polarized therapeutic factions. I think the educated reader can determine for himself or herself what seems to fit based on clinical experience. Also, while it is true that some of the researchers I will discuss (especially those advocating the sociocognitive model) are deemed to be quite controversial by some, I hope the reader will trust that I am laying out arguments for consideration. These research and clinical controversies mirror what survivors of trauma experience all of the time about how real their experience is and, in some cases, how hard it is to find someone who believes them. Like the different schools of psychotherapy, it seems important to understand opposing views and, if possible, to find avenues of consensus.

There are two major theories that attempt to explain dissociation. I've already alluded to one model, the trauma model (TM), which suggests a causal link between trauma and dissociation. The sociocognitive model (SCM) emphasizes social and cognitive variables (e.g., fantasy proneness and suggestibility) as being the primary mechanism of dissociation. It's not quite clear in my mind why these two theories are seen to be so mutually exclusive; however some researchers and clinicians have strong and seemingly disparate views on how extreme dissociation comes about. As I've already suggested, if the idea of recovered memories or beliefs about the reality of DID is in the mix, clinicians and researchers can feel pulled to protect their point of view. Therefore, I would urge the reader to consider that there are interesting arguments on both sides of this debate that can be thought about in a neutral way. In other words, I would like to imagine a way that we can advocate for victims of trauma while still appreciating that trauma has a number of complicated sequelae, many of which we are still trying to understand.

Janet (1889/1973, 1907) is thought to be the parent of the trauma model (TM) by many. He linked dissociation to traumatic hysteria and noted that some traumatized patients experienced more than one state of consciousness (Hart and Rutger 1989). Dalenberg et al. (2012) described dissociation as an "important aspect of the psychobiological response to threat and danger that allows for automatization of behavior, analgesia, depersonalization, and isolation of catastrophic experiences to enhance survival during and in the aftermath of these events" (p. 551). In her and her colleagues' review of the evidence, they note that the association between objectively verified trauma and dissociation was consistent and moderate in strength and remained significant when objective measures of trauma were used, including when fantasy proneness was controlled for in research studies.

As described in Chapter 1, in the DSM-V (APA 2013), the diagnosis of PTSD now involves a subtype that includes dissociation, further reinforcing the link between trauma and dissociation. A study by Stein et al. (2013) sought to corroborate trauma experiences with dissociation and PTSD by surveying over 25,000 people in 16 countries. Symptoms of dissociation in PTSD were associated with reports of re-experiencing symptoms and with male gender, childhood onset of PTSD, high exposure to prior traumatic events and childhood adversities, prior histories of separation anxiety disorder and specific phobia, functional difficulties, and suicidality. A meta-analysis of 31,905 college students found that 11.4% of students met criteria for a dissociative disorder, which is consistent with the prevalence (12%) of experiencing multiple types of trauma during childhood (Kate et al. 2020). This supports the trauma model of dissociation. These authors tested four other hypotheses in this study in an attempt to compare the fantasy model (or SCM) of dissociation to the TM and did not find support for the SCM.

The sociocognitive model (SCM) of dissociation maintains that fantasy proneness, media influences, suggestibility, a tendency to exaggerate symptoms, and memory lapses contribute to self-reports of trauma and dissociative experiences (Lilienfeld et al. 1999; Lynn et al. 2014). Proponents of the SCM note that dissociative people are prone to the construction of fantasies of abuse that are mistaken for memories (Loftus and Ketcham 1994; McNally et al. 2005). Other proponents of the SCM have suggested evidence that fantasy overlaps with dissociation and that variables including fantasy proneness, cognitive distortions, and suggestibility render some individuals vulnerable to the suggestive influences emphasized by the SCM seemingly in the absence of trauma (Merckelbach et al. 2002; Lynn et al. 2012). This includes what some consider to be the tendency of people with dissociation to overreport symptoms of unusual experiences (Merckelbach et al. 2017). Lynn et al. (2012) concede that trauma may sometimes play an etiological role in dissociation, although they view this as less central and specific.

Lilienfeld et al. (1999) question the diagnosis of DID, in a very general sense, with the view that dissociative phenomena are not related to trauma at all. He and his colleagues further conceptualize "DID as a syndrome that consists of rule-governed and goal-directed experiences and displays of multiple role enactments that have been created, legitimized, and maintained by social reinforcement" (p. 507). Lilienfeld et al. go on to note that people with DID may be more prone to therapist suggestion, which may cast doubt on childhood maltreatment in cases in which therapists confirm or suggest the presence of abuse.

Dalenberg et al. (2012) provided a graphical representation of key differences between the trauma model and the fantasy/sociocognitive model in Fig. 5.2.

Dalenberg et al. (2007) noted that the idea of dissociation became conflated with ideas of repressed memories and recovered memories in the early 1990s. This may be one reason for the intense controversy that remains. For example, when I approached people who are proponents of the trauma model, among those who have significant clinical experience with people with DID, some expressed concern that acknowledging any validity of the sociocognitive model meant not accepting the reality of DID. Others expressed concern that the idea of "recovered" memories would be debunked and viewed as fantasy.

Although it may be the case that so-called recovered memories are found to be less factually accurate in some circumstances, it does not mean that there has not been trauma. Memory is complicated and does change. As we will see below in the case discussed by Dalenberg, memories can change even in the presence of objec-

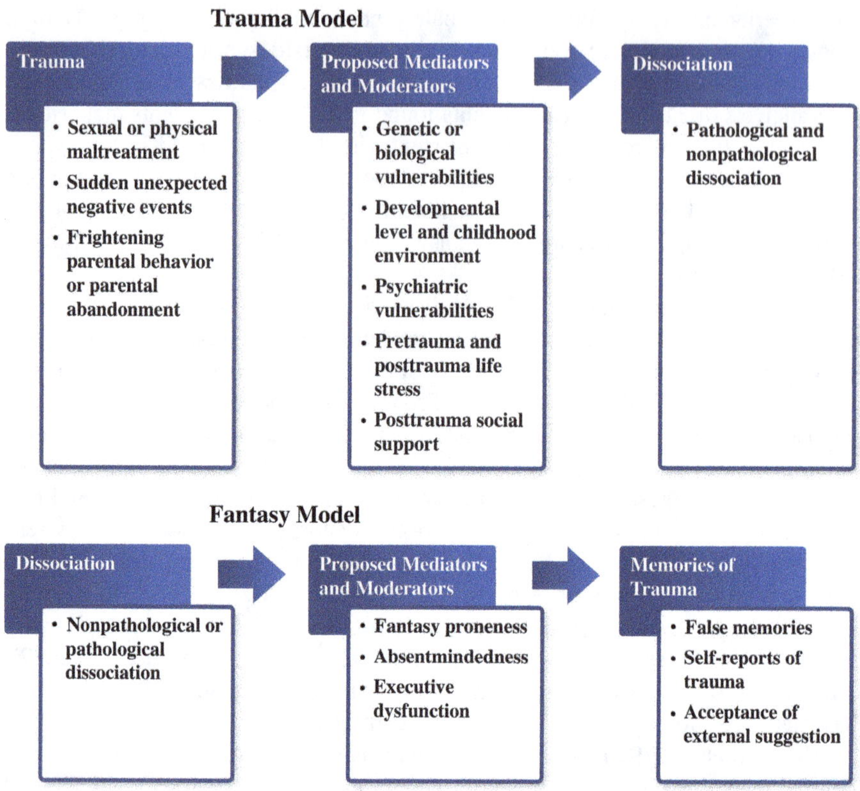

Fig. 5.2 Differences between the trauma model and the fantasy model of dissociation

tively confirmed traumatic events. Further, it's worth noting that psychoanalytic clinicians have long emphasized that trauma is subjective. What matters most is how we evaluate traumatic experiences. In part, this has to do with the extent to which trauma is experienced in isolation or as part of a group that can validate the experience, such as in the World Trade Center attacks in 2001 (Coates et al. 2003). The group experience of trauma can be protective in the development of PTSD. I saw several people who were present at a mass violence event several years ago. Their ability to check facts, to get validation, and to share stories was incredibly healing for all of the people I saw. They all knew that what they experienced was real. This is in stark contrast to when there are only two people in a room where violence takes place.

Proponents of the SCM also note the sticky and complicated history regarding repressed memories, DID, and claims of satanic ritual abuse that swept through the United States in the 1980s and 1990s. Indeed, this history is confusing, as more people reported satanic abuse, witnessing murder, and the experience of sexual assault than law enforcement could account for, though the history of clinical descriptions of DID predates this. It should also be noted that many of the people who claimed to have been abused during this time were in treatment with therapists who used techniques to recover memories that were not empirically validated or the standard of care (Ulatowska and Sawicka 2017).

People who are dissociative and not sure about their histories and identities may be more suggestible as Janet (1907) and Breuer and Freud (1895/1957) stated in various publications. I certainly have heard of cases of clients during the 1980s and 1990s who were explicitly told and then believed they must have experienced satanic abuse; it was a popular way to explain complex symptoms in people who really had no idea what they experienced in childhood. It goes without saying that any therapist who feels confident enough to define the history of a client without appropriate data and clinical material is not the kind of therapy I espouse here. Our work is complicated because trauma and its consequences are confusing and disorienting. To state it even more plainly, our clients have the right to tell us their story; our job is to tolerate not knowing until they can. Dissociation results in confusion. This confusion does not mean that overt traumatic abuse and exploitation did not happen, but it does not mean it did. I have had many clients say to me that they wish they could be hypnotized so they could "go back" and figure out why they have the problems they do, as they imagine something in childhood was not right. These are often people who do not remember much of their childhoods. However, I find that clients eventually can access thoughts and feelings they may not recall at the time they state the wish for hypnosis. Sheila's memory of her rape was not a recovered memory. I gathered earlier and even stressed that she knew something had happened, but she didn't know the details and thinking about it made her emotionally dysregulated. Once she had better control over her emotions, the story began to more fully form in her mind. She could make sense of her flashbacks and nightmares. I witnessed this and thought about it with her. Remaining neutral, curious, caring, and sensitive to emotions is what allows us and our clients to know when and if they are ready to think more about their histories.

It's important to note that severe childhood neglect is associated with dissociative symptoms (Vogel et al. 2009; Vonderlin et al. 2018). As clinicians, we may tend to focus on so-called traumatic events as they can offer clear and defined examples of maltreatment, while neglect has complications that remain relatively less understood. Neglected children have no one to help them with reality testing. In states of fear, all sorts of ideas may come to mind. Think of the normal situation of a child who is convinced there is a monster under her bed. If there is an adult available who can provide comfort (look under the bed and confirm there is, indeed, no monster), she can learn to regulate her fears. She can eventually understand that there are bad thoughts inside of her and that no one will get hurt by them. She can find a sense of safety if the environment is safe and she feels loved. When kids are left alone, particularly in more severe cases in which a child has to find her own food or manage fears about if she will die in the absence of her caretakers, fantasies can take over. This is common and does not mean that trauma is not present, but it may not be in the form of a child molester, a satanic cult, or someone who beats her (though, of course, abuse and neglect do co-occur). Considered in the most neutral light, this may be why proponents of the SCM focus on fantasy, because abuse, neglect, and developmental limitations in children do affect the appraisal of explicit memory. If we consider neglect as a form of trauma, as well as the integration of the fact that dissociation can occur in all of us during fearful situations, we can begin to imagine a way of integrating the sociocognitive models and the trauma models of dissociation.

A Combined Model of Dissociation?

Lynn et al. (2019) have attempted to do this. To be clear, Lynn and several of his colleagues have advocated staunch positions regarding the reality of memories of trauma, and this is rooted in the history of the "memory wars," and their theoretical views are considered controversial if not downright dismissive of the reality of child abuse and maltreatment by some proponents of the trauma model. However, this recent publication seems to allow a bit more room for considering that the trauma model can still be considered valid in the presence of cognitive issues that can occur among some trauma survivors. They suggest ideas that can link both the TM and the SCM of dissociation and speculate that dissociation is linked to "impairments in self-awareness and reflection (i.e., meta-consciousness); cognitive, associational, and affective processes (i.e., "hyperassociation" and shifting cognitive-affective-behavioral sets called "set shifts," emotion regulation); and sleep disruptions." These authors suggest that meta-consciousness relates closely to ideas of mentalization and that people with dissociation struggle to understand themselves and may have symptoms of alexithymia. Sifneos (1973) and Nemiah (1973) in two separate papers characterized alexithymia as occurring in individuals who lack an emotional language to describe internal mental experiences and states. The main qualities in those who are alexithymic include difficulties identifying and describing feelings, differentiating between emotional and physical sensations, and exhibiting a concrete and externally oriented cognitive style (Zackheim 2007). Some authors have described alexithymia as defensive, in which denial, repression, and externalization operate, while others have focused on aspects of limited affective regulation as being primary or woven into character functioning (Glucksman 2000). If we consider any of these definitions of alexithymia, it seems clear to me that this symptom could be associated with trauma.

Regarding hyperassociation, Lynn and his colleagues describe this process as involving a fast-moving mind and the ability to shift quickly in response to stimuli. They state, using clinical examples, that clients responded in a rapid-fire manner with associations to their thoughts, feelings, and behaviors and to external stimuli (e.g., therapist comments, ambient noises). Hyperassociations were often accompanied by strong affect, affect shifts, and avoidance or neglect of the topic at hand, which disrupted the thread of the discussion. They provide an example of a client who was talking with their therapist about being harshly berated by a parent and then quickly associated to an interaction with a beloved pet. Lynn et al. suggest that this behavior represents a failure in meta-consciousness and that emotion was absent from the scenes. This seems to me to be a familiar interaction with clients I see, though I hypothesize that the set-shifting (from the parent to the pet) was an attempt to regulate affect (to keep from getting overwhelmed by thinking about the hostile parent).

Additionally, I view dissociation and set-shifting behaviors from clients as an example of hypervigilance. The astute reader might also note that the above descriptions of a rapidly processing mind (e.g., set-shifting) could be associated with what we often think of as mania or hypomania. It seems to me that at least some people we see whom we might view as having more hypomanic styles or what psychodynamic clinicians refer to as manic defenses might actually be hypervigilance, just in a slightly different presentation. For example, a number of people I have known who seem to possess a manic style to their character also have an exaggerated startle response, problems with aggression, and sleep disturbances. These behaviors are also symptoms in the arousal cluster of PTSD. Hypervigilance, above all, is a kind of cognitive process that attempts to help us keep track of internal and external stimuli. With too much hypervigilance, we can't see the whole picture—not see the forest for the trees, to use a popular idiom. The best reference I have for this explanation comes from the Exner system of interpreting Rorschach ink blots (Exner 2001; Exner and Erdberg 2005). Hypervigilance works well, until physical or psychological processes make it impossible to keep track of everything or the perception that one can keep an eye on all that is needed in the environment. One way to hypothesize about this is that hypervigilance works well until it doesn't and then dissociation takes over. As if the mind behaves in this (admittedly anthropomorphic) way: *I try to keep track of everything, but then too much information comes into my mind, and I must leave.*

Finally, Lynn et al. note that sleep disruption and unusual sleep experiences (e.g., hypnogogic or hypnopompic hallucinations) can also account for symptoms of dissociation. Though they suggest these findings are associated with a non-trauma pathway for dissociation, sleep disturbance is extremely common among those who report trauma, as well as people with various types of psychological disorders, which also have correlates to trauma. Lynn and his colleagues provide a massive amount of data which is only briefly described here, but it seems clear to me that there is room to think of dissociation as linked to both trauma experiences and cognitive problems.

I realize the issue of fantasy proneness is controversial. I understand that for people who practice in forensic settings (which I used to, in juvenile court settings), where the stakes involve appropriate justice for perpetrators of crimes, the idea of suggestibility or other cognitive aspects of dissociation can feel like a lightning rod meant to invalidate victims. However, I think it's a mistake to believe that both cognitive processes and trauma can't be linked to the phenomena of dissociation. For example, Vissia et al. (2016) published a study demonstrating that people with dissociative identity disorder (DID) had experienced trauma and were not more prone to the development of false memories, to challenge the idea that DID was based on fantasies or suggestibility. This issue may be nuanced depending on the chronicity of traumas and the age at which it takes place, but it seems crucial that we recognize that the damage of trauma has multiple sequelae.

Memory is complicated and always shifting to prevent victims from being overwhelmed. Dalenberg (personal communication, 2019) described the following, which clearly elucidates the common problem of so-called accurate memory in those who have been abused:

I recall a child who clearly and cogently describes a rape in childhood. In describing the experience (which was confirmed by confession), she spoke of the sensation of a hot object being thrust inside her, leaving her with a sense of being burned from the inside. This is not an uncommon description, given abrasion and inflammation. Years later, however, the same young woman described the experience as an assault with a hot curling iron, translating a memory of a feeling into a memory of an event. Clearly, her true experience of assault and her false memory of the curling iron are contributing to the memory endpoint here. I juxtapose this example, however, with several dissociative clients who claim to have been attacked with hot objects but show no residual burn evidence. No records of the actual event existed, as is typical, but circumstantial evidence (e.g., contemporary diary evidence or family testimony) supported the possibility of rape. Rather than dismissing these individuals entirely as SCM victims who have been seduced by incompetent therapists, our position is that more evidence would be needed in such a case to disentangle the specifics of the original event. Memory access can be distorted by mood, contaminated by authorities or by nightmare experiences, and made more vivid by repetition. All of these factors should be considered.

Memory shifts based on our developmental level of being able to understand traumatic experiences, as well as to keep us from being overwrought by emotions we can't handle. The physiological experience of being in traumatic situations affects how memories of the event are formed. The secretion of glucocorticoids and norepinephrine disrupts episodic and explicit memory (e.g., LeDoux 1996; Solms and Turnbull 2002), often making it difficult for people to have access to many details of traumatic events, particularly when they are chronic.

Just because cognition is impacted by trauma, it does not mean that trauma has not occurred. I don't see why the TM and the SCM should be mutually exclusive. This seems like more evidence on how tribal and war-like our field has become. And the people who suffer from our infighting are clients. Additionally, despite the scholarship in trying to understand the nuances of memory and what factors contribute to dissociation, the aforementioned controversies may be linked to a long history of trauma survivors not being believed, even by mental health clinicians.

Dissociation of Trauma in the Mental Health Field

If we are to try to find historical ways that people in the mental health field have commonality, it is that many clinicians and researchers have expressed suspicion regarding the prevalence of child abuse. A notable exception to this are the clinicians who developed and treat using the trauma model, as discussed in previous chapters. For them, trauma is common, and they have been advocating for the necessity of believing trauma survivors for about 50 years. While I will discuss the ways that trauma has been negated in general psychology, it's important to begin this discussion with where clinical psychology started, psychoanalysis. While many modern psychodynamic clinicians appreciate the impact of trauma, it has not always been this way. And since psychoanalytic therapy or psychoanalysis has been around longer than any other treatment, it's important to think about how the oldest therapeutic method affected the therapies and research that came after it.

Psychoanalysis or psychoanalytic therapy, which were dominant treatments until the 1960s, when medications and then behavioral methods were developed and flourished, emphasized fantasy. Psychoanalyst Lee Rather (personal communication, 2019) notes that "'fantasy' or 'fantasizing,' are not technical terms about unconscious functions, but rather refer to something very colloquial like consciously day-dreaming or imagining something one wishes could be true. In Freudian theory, unconscious wishes belong to the 'repressed unconscious', that which could be or once was conscious." There is over a century of research and writing on ideas related to unconscious fantasy in psychoanalytic literature. I'm not going to get into details of the volumes of psychoanalytic scholarship related to these points and will refer to unconscious "fantasy," even though it is a general and imprecise term, as Rather notes.

Unconscious fantasy and its influence remain a pillar of psychoanalytic treatment and in today's modern climate, probably even more than dealing with transference for some analytic clinicians. Historically, the emphasis on fantasy presumed that what clients said when they walked in the door was at best a mixture of subjective perceptions and reality. Traumatic childhood experiences were simply not recognized as a priori events. Traditional psychoanalysis has a long and complicated relationship with its valuation of the reality of external circumstances in someone's life, as its theoretical approach has tended to privilege meaning via fantasies over real concerns. Conceptually, the "problem" of reality was never fully resolved within the psychoanalytic school of thought (Renik 1998). Traditional analysts have been concerned that talking about reality in the sense of actual, concrete events and situations diminishes a client's ability to understand their psychic life. Thus, psychoanalysis has historically de-emphasized actual events in favor of the subjective, sometimes distorted perception of those events (Goldschmidt 1986). In contrast, according to psychoanalyst Boulanger, reality matters. Research suggests that regardless of character type and prior psychopathology, a specific set of symptoms arises in many adults in response to life-threatening trauma (Boulanger 2002).

As we can see from the aforementioned authors, there has definitely been a movement among analytic clinicians to weave both reality and subjective perceptions in their understanding of patient experiences. Yet, the emphasis on fantasy has left some patients feeling that they don't know if there is a place for real events and trauma in treatment. To put this idea in concrete clinical perspective, many of us have had the experience as patients of clinicians influenced by psychoanalytic ideas of feeling that we are not believed. A psychoanalyst I saw thought I was being hyperbolic when I described aspects of the home I grew up in, which was a small, rural, not well-maintained, single-family home lacking much insulation. It was cold, both metaphorically and in reality, and in addition to my family, it was host to a number of critters who could easily make their way inside. When I explained this in more detail to the clinician I was seeing, he stated that he assumed that my memories must be influenced by fantasy and its derivative unconscious material. So, the next visit I took to see my family, I took pictures and presented my therapist with a slideshow of my childhood home on my mobile phone. That changed things; he then believed me, but I never quite got over being accused of being overly dramatic. This experience is familiar to many. Several scholars, some who have become quite controversial (e.g., Masson 1984), have described the devastating impact of the abandonment of the "seduction theory" (a very misleading and confusing term) by Freud, which is intricately linked to the emphasis on fantasy. Briefly described, Freud initially thought that his early patients had been physically and sexually abused. As Masson describes the story, Freud presented a paper in 1896 in Vienna on this topic (which would have been timed with his and Breuer's publication of *Studies on Hysteria*) in which he described that his female patients had been sexually abused. His colleagues, all men, derided the findings. At some point, certainly by the time Freud published *The Interpretation of Dreams* (1900), Freud redirected his focus to the wishes of his patients. This was interpreted as something like these female clients had a *conflicted wish* to be seduced by their fathers and negated the possibility that these women actually were abused and exploited by their fathers or other male figures. To be clear, psychoanalytic scholars tend to see this issue as more nuanced, and it may be. But this story illustrates how ideas of fantasy came to be prominent in psychoanalytic theory. In my opinion, as both patient and therapist, fantasies, wishes, and subjective perceptions are just as important as reality. But we need to *start* with the idea that the acknowledgment of reality provides the foundation for healing. When we feel safe enough to tell a story, we need to feel believed. The fact that some people have not felt that their stories would be viewed as real relates, in part, to the backlash against psychoanalysis.

Although behavioral and cognitive behavioral approaches rose to popularity in the 1970s and 1980s because they bypassed the pesky notion of a dynamic unconscious, took much less time, and offered concrete, behavioral symptom reduction, trauma therapists were confronting a whole different set of dilemmas. According to one trauma expert, "Trauma therapy was marginalized, in part, because of the legacy of psychoanalysis's rejection of the reality of much of trauma, particularly childhood sexual abuse, and the pathologizing of people who showed post-traumatic symptoms as being characterologically weak" (Laura Brown, personal communication, 2019). Brown's comments also connect with a dismissive approach to thinking about trauma in the field of psychology in general. Child abuse is rarely mentioned in abnormal psychology textbooks and still receives inadequate and misleading coverage. In an examination of introductory psychology textbooks, there was biased and inaccurate information on childhood maltreatment (Wilgus et al. 2016). Brand et al. (2014) who reviewed the research on the coverage of child abuse in undergraduate textbooks noted the lack of linking childhood maltreatment with psychological disorders, inaccurate discussion of childhood sexual abuse, and biased coverage of false memories and dissociation. Some abnormal psychology texts and graduate school psychopathology volumes present information that recovered memories are false, without presenting research about the accuracy of trauma memories (Brand et al. 2019; Wilgus et al. 2015). Brand and her colleagues (2019) state that, "Despite the lack of empirical support for the fantasy model, it is concerning that the fantasy model perspective was overemphasized, and the role of trauma minimized, in three of the graduate psychology textbooks…" (p. 6).

As I discussed in the previous section, ideas of the fantasy model are deeply steeped in dramatic "recovered memories" of satanic ritual abuse, witness to murder, etc. that occurred in the 1980s and 1990s (e.g., Loftus and Davis 2006). Those specific phenomena involved spurious therapeutic techniques such as hypnosis to "recover" memories (Lynn et al. 2003). These techniques to discover "alters" are not a part of the standard practice of psychology, though many clinicians during this time used these techniques.

Much of the tribalism among therapeutic factions we face today is related in part to how other schools of thought reacted to psychoanalysis, which was a dominant theory for several decades in the twentieth century. In addition the "memory wars" that occurred certainly seem to have caused clinicians on either side of this debate to feel that they have to bunker down and hold steady to their positions. But rigid views risk what's most important—our clients and their ability to tell their own story. My objection to what happened in the 1980s and 1990s regarding claims of abuse is not that such abuse may have been true or not true, it's that people seeking help were prevented from having the time to figure out what their story was. If you tell someone what has happened to them, it is a kind of identity theft. Although our clients may pull for us to describe them and their narrative, our job is to not know and to think with people about what is on their minds, not ours.

Adding to the above developments in psychotherapy, medications, and the ability to truncate or alleviate suffering began the wave of change in offerings of psychotherapeutic approaches to the public, but so did the influence of insurance companies and their hopes that treatment for complex illnesses can be brief. However, treating complex trauma is rarely short term, especially when severe dissociation is involved.

Treating Dissociative Disorders

Dissociation, by definition, indicates how elusive it is. Some researchers have speculated that the presence of dissociation may undermine the seeking of treatment, specifically because "…dissociation may prove especially sensitive to treatment selection bias, given that symptoms such as reduced awareness, fragmented memories, and compartmentalized affects could influence help seeking" (Stein et al. 2013, p. 303). I would add my own less sophisticated reason people with dissociation are hard to both detect and help: Dissociation works to some degree. Losing aspects of this needed way of being is simply terrifying. This returns us to one of my main points in this book: we need to manage and be aware of fear.

Specifically regarding DID diagnoses, most individuals who meet criteria for DID have been treated in the mental health system for 6–12 years before they are correctly diagnosed (Brand et al. 2016). In my clinical experience, these statistics seem about right for dissociative people in general. A nationwide random sample of experienced clinicians found that 53% of clients treated in the community for borderline personality disorder (BPD) had a comorbid dissociative disorder, including 11% meeting criteria for DID (Zittel Conklin and Westen 2005). A study found that up to 8.6% of clients being treated for panic disorder were also diagnosed with a dissociative disorder (Morrison et al. 2003). And in general, people with extreme dissociation present with a number of psychological symptoms and disorders (Brand et al. 2009).

Traumatized clients who use dissociation are difficult to engage in therapy not simply because of the need to not think about aspects of their experience and identity but because of the susceptibility to dissociation. In particular, the discontinuous sense of self that results from dissociation makes it difficult to think and, as Putnam (1992) suggests, to cognitively process information. Thus, for some clients with excessive dissociation, the lack of a cohesive self, required to benefit from some forms of psychotherapy, is simply less available. For example, exposure therapy, which requires clients to tolerate distress and be able to describe feelings related to trauma, seems largely contraindicated in severely dissociative people. This explains why we need to work differently to engage patients in the therapeutic process as well as how people such as Melanie can seem lost and without access to a more nuanced version of emotional thinking and relating. A further complication is that dissociative experiences become an important part of self-experience. As therapists, we threaten to disrupt the very aspects of experience that have helped people survive traumatic events. As Bromberg (1991) puts it, people who use dissociation try to stay the same without changing. This is because the help afforded by psychotherapy results in overwhelming confusion and feelings. Not having a cohesive sense of self, that is, not knowing about confusing and terrifying thoughts and memories, paradoxically serves the purpose of feeling more connected and "whole." Although dissociation can cause confusion, it also serves to ward it off. Not knowing about something too painful to know serves the function of a basic level of protection. Let's return to Melanie's therapy.

Although Melanie did not have clinical DID, she did have mildly different personas that became clear in her second and third years of treatment. For example, when she wore a jean jacket, which seemed a bit too small given her frame, I knew that I would be met with subtle complaints about my work or, at the very least, a more hostile version of herself. I came to think of this version of her as a kind of adolescent. The presence of a baseball hat indicated to me that she had fallen into a very depressed state and she was hopeless and nihilistic. This particular state of mind was reminiscent of when she had tried to kill herself, when she went days without getting out of bed. And there were other, more adjusted states in which she showed up in cute jeans and designer shirts; these were times when she had a sense of confidence about herself and her career. At one point during this time, she developed an intense interest in wine tasting, even though she was not really a drinker. But since a colleague was interested in wine, she became an expert in wine pairings, which varietals she considered best and which regions her preferred wines should come from. And while all of this was going on, her job situation had remained unstable. She was not yet fired though thought she might be. Instead of being able to talk about the reality of her situation, as she became more reliant on me, she asked me endless questions. Did I think a certain person was being hostile toward her? Did I think her new boss was mean? Did I think her boyfriend was using her? These questions were fascinating, as I really had no idea what the answers might be, even if I did feel comfortable enough to answer. However, I did feel incredible pressure to be in her mind, to tell her what to do or even what to think.

I find Boulanger's (2007) discussion of the effects of trauma compelling as they apply to Melanie. Boulanger notes that elements of a core self are likely present among adults who experience overwhelming trauma. However, for children who have experienced complex trauma, it may be more likely that dissociated self-states are woven into psychic experience. I'd add to this by suggesting that for people with cPTSD that involves childhood trauma, if there were some good things in the environment that were able to be gotten hold of, this can form elements of a core self, even if it is somewhat limited. For Melanie, I think her relative resiliency had to do with the fact that she did have access to some good people in her childhood. Teachers often took her under their wing and tried to be emotionally supportive. At least one adult person in her family did care for her without extensive conditions and exploitation (an aunt was particularly loving toward her). The development of self-states was present, though relatively mild. Nevertheless, I was less concerned about the ways Melanie's self-state presentations shifted. I found her demands for me to explain what was on her mind to be much more vexing, frustrating, and clinically meaningful. I realized that more important than the differences in how she appeared and the different affect states that showed up was the fact that she spent most of her time literally "out of her mind." She was good at figuring out who people wanted her to be, more so with men. It was more complicated with women, who were often viewed as enemies. With myself, however, it was another couple of years until she could genuinely tell me, from the most authentic part of herself, actual complaints she had about me and others. It was at this point she had become much more integrated with more coherent stories about some aspects of her life.

Dissociation is an out of mind/out of body experience. In terms of therapeutic technique, I often find that when I can help someone notice how much time they spend outside of themselves, it can initiate a more alive and meaningful avenue of clinical work. Although dissociation involves freezing, being on autopilot, and problems with memories, over time I find that many people who dissociate a lot are very good at figuring out what people want from them. I take questions of me to tell them what they are thinking as a sign that they are starting to realize that they don't know what is on *their* minds, and I point out that it might be useful if they can begin to notice just how much time they spend thinking about what others want from them. I often meet requests from patients for me to tell them what they think, by saying something like, "You are very good at imagining what people want from you. But I wonder if there is a price you pay by doing this. You cheat yourself out of knowing what you want or need." I think this is where there can be some common ground regarding the theories of dissociation (TM and SCM) described earlier in this chapter. I've previously noted links between dissociation and so-called hysteria (Greenberg 2016). The latter term, in this context, emphasizes the intense drive to become who or what others need them to be. Melanie eventually realized this. For example, the wine tasting interest did not last long, as she realized she simply did not like to drink. This resulted in confusion for Melanie (she began to wonder what she wanted in a very general sense), but it was the beginning of me getting to really know her. We started to wonder together which aspects of her being and interests really suited her. It also helped her to slow down and think about more before jumping into situations in which she was "shape-shifting" in who she imagined others wanted her to be.

Kluft (1991) notes that for extremely dissociative persons, treatments need a solid frame and secure boundaries. I agree, but as I have discussed, our work with cPTSD clients does require some flexibility. Therefore with Melanie, I did indulge her questions from time to time while also trying to gently nudge her to get to know her own experience. In general, I don't find self-disclosure useful with extremely dissociated people. In fact, I think it can be very frightening. So I focus on allowing them to have access to my mind so they can have a sense of what I am thinking but without going into detail. I might say something like, "As you were talking, I was reflecting on that story you told me about your boyfriend a couple of months ago when you needed help and he wouldn't provide it. Maybe that's connected with what is on your mind now." Regarding the different personas that were evident from time to time, I did not speak overtly of these. I respect that other clinicians do this; for myself, I worry about promoting fragmentation. Particularly in the beginning of treatment, when the focus is on affect regulation and developing a sense of safety and stabilization, I find it better to communicate with whatever version or self-state that shows up.

Experts in dissociation suggest that early in treatment it's helpful to get clients to notice states of discontinuity and dissociation and relate this to the effects of trauma (e.g., Chefetz 2015; Chu 2011). I do this more judiciously, as many people I see tend to be dismissive of their histories, whether it's adult or childhood trauma. I do find it useful to help people notice states of discontinuous experience but once they feel safe in the therapeutic relationship and using the idea of clinical hypothesis testing. For people who are especially curious as to why they have the symptoms they do, I will often explain something like, "You've had a lot of bad things happen to you and that makes you very aware of your environment at times, but then at others it's like you can't keep track. It's not because you are not smart, but it's more like a way you keep yourself from getting overwhelmed. But the effect is that there are all of these emotions that spring up in unexpected ways, at unexpected times. We see this when people have dissociation. I don't know for sure if that is true for you, but it's something we can think about." If the client wants to talk about it more, we do, but often people need time for that to digest before we talk further about cPTSD in general. I always let the client guide me in terms of what I explain. Though psychoeducation is an important part of therapy with people with cPTSD for some clinicians, I am a bit more measured, and I don't apply the same techniques regarding education to everyone I see. For Melanie, it took years for her to really get curious about her symptoms. When she did, she noticed on her own when she was in a dissociated state. The first time this happened, she came in and said, "I think I was pretty dissociated last week. I don't really remember being here. What do you think?" At that point I could tell her that I agreed and what I thought the external stressor was to explain this.

I do find it helpful for clients to note states of fogginess or disorientation, especially if I imagine that intense anxiety might be an antecedent of dissociation. Often I do this informally, although I find some of the basic mindfulness approaches in dialectical behavior therapy to be helpful, especially those that focus on noticing states of being dissociated (e.g., McKay et al. 2019). My informal approach involves encouraging people to keep track (either mentally or to write it down) what happened internally or externally before they feel foggy or disoriented or have sudden feelings of suicidality or an outburst that seemingly comes out of nowhere. For example, Melanie had "episodes" of suddenly screaming at her boyfriend. She initially presented this data to me by offering more evidence of her "craziness." I encouraged to consider that maybe there was more to it and to notice the next time this happened if there was something going on in her mind or with her boyfriend. She eventually realized that her seemingly random rants had something to do with a kind of "sexual playfulness" her boyfriend and she engaged in but was initiated by him. She had assumed she was fine with this, but it turned out it made her uncomfortable. Since she dissociated during these sexual interactions, she could not link her actions (screaming) with any feelings (fear) about the sexual behavior with her boyfriend. This seemed in part a reenactment of a part of Melanie's sexual trauma history. People who are dissociative can be prone to reenactments of their trauma. I've found the nature of dissociation makes it tough to provide interpretations about reenactments, however. Rather, I focus on the feelings about the behaviors that are frightening once the client becomes more aware of dissociation.

I tend to shy away from urging formal meditation, unless it is guided. For most people I see, meditation can cause too much anxiety or fragmentation. For example, I have seen or heard of a number of clients being told they should attend meditation classes and become quite destabilized if there is too much emphasis on being alone in one's mind. If clients want to meditate, there are excellent resources for this that provide almost constant talking. DBT approaches that encourage recognition of dissociation and associated grounding techniques can also be helpful.

If clinicians want to be especially thorough in diagnosing the severity of dissociation, the Dissociative Experiences Scale (DES) (Bernstein and Putnam 1986) can be used. Since I do not do forensic work and I am aware of the understandable guardedness of many of my clients, I do not use formal instruments. I used to when I was younger but found that people often denied symptoms in formal testing but waited until they felt safe to let me know what was really going on. Therefore, I wait for evidence of dissociation to show up clinically. That said, the DES is one standard instrument in terms of formal evaluation of dissociation.

Treatments with dissociative people can be rocky, often with starts and stops. I have people in my practice who have been seeing me off and on over two decades. They come in for a year or two and then leave but come back when they feel stronger or there is a new crisis. I do not consider these treatments to be failures. In fact, the nature of dissociation requires that people feel in control of their treatments and can go at their own pace. One woman who had returned for a fifth time in therapy announced when she came back that she thought that her mother trying to stab her with a knife (something corroborated by several family witnesses) might have something to do with her difficulties. She said she wanted us to think about that together, but even then, she could not talk about it in detail. The attack and her mother's sadism and envy (that I imagined was present) toward my client was something I needed to keep in my mind. I was able to talk with her about how fearful she was whenever she started to feel close to others or found she needed them; she worried something catastrophic might happen. This was the first time I could have this kind of meaningful conversation with her. I could hold in mind the past while dealing with the here and now.

Horevitz and Loewenstein (1994) note that treatment with people who are extremely dissociative may be punctuated by crises and that what's most helpful is how we manage the unexpected, as opposed to "the outline of a systematic treatment model, which can never fully anticipate the vagaries in the course of treatment…" (p. 291). No matter the level of dissociation, we all have competing aspects of ourselves when going to therapy. We are all afraid of change and getting better. Although psychoanalysis has used the language of resistance to describe this, I think of it as that we are more familiar with what we know, even if it includes suffering. Hope can feel foreboding and terrifying. And although I've argued that many of our clients with cPTSD may never develop a coherent and uninterrupted narrative of one's life and history, getting better does involve the beginning of some stories that have meaning.

Our clients with extreme dissociation need us to provide stabilization, crisis management, a sense of safety, and a slow beginning of the acknowledgment of thoughts and feelings. Feelings need to be titrated, just like a potent medication. Being able to tolerate and know thoughts and feelings is healing but also provides cohesion. Eventually, talking about trauma in detail may be helpful for some. However, we can very often refer vaguely to one's history. For example, when Melanie seemed wary of myself and even her own thoughts, I would say something like, "You never knew what to expect when you were younger; that's probably why it's hard to know if you can trust people or if they are just tantalizing you with the idea of something good that might get ruined or even be a sadistic trick." We can speak to the past more effectively if we have an eye on the present.

Conclusion

The legacy of the cultural dissociation of trauma, as well as neglect of the reality and the ubiquitous nature of trauma in the mental health professions, has led to a complicated valuation of the phenomena of dissociation. Though there are normal aspects of dissociation, there is a great deal of data that excessive dissociation is associated with traumatic events. Yet, it's crucial that we do not define a client's history for them. Our job is to remain neutral, curious, and open to thinking about traumatic events so that clients can, with our support, develop a sense of meaning around what has happened to them, even if the narrative is disjointed. Dissociation already robs people of aspects of their identity because of intense states of discontinuity. In treating clients with excessive dissociation, we need to move slowly and ensure that people feel safe. I'm not an advocate of overly interpreting extreme dissociation until someone becomes more aware of the disruptive aspects of this needed way of being.

For people who are extremely dissociated, our connection with them can be the beginning of them becoming more integrated, but we need to be prepared to shift our approaches quickly. People with extreme dissociation can be hypervigilant and dissociated at different points and time. Even in one session, we can think about affect, but then how to keep from getting overwhelmed and how to take better care of themselves. The ground is always shifting, like a constant earthquake. Our goal is to remain connected and offer all available tools to keep them steady.

Interventions for Working with Dissociative Clients

- Go slow. People who are dissociative can tend to hide from us. This can appear to be suspiciousness, but it's more likely that they are worried about being overwhelmed with emotions, especially in people who are very fragmented.
- If someone presents with more defined self-states, consider interventions that do not reinforce fragmentation, but allow space for full expression of whatever state the client is in.
- Don't rush to label dissociation; it's a needed defense and takes a while for clients to realize its limitations.
- Developing a safe relationship, stabilization, and increasing or maintaining functioning are the key initial goals with people who are extremely dissociative.
- Grounding techniques are so eloquently simple we often overlook their utility. For extreme dissociated states and crises that involve self-harm, grounding is very helpful. Encourage people to notice their external environment and record what they see. Lavender or other essential oils can be used to provide soothing and engagement of olfactory senses.
- When fear and anxiety threaten to overwhelm, consider having the client talk to herself and remind herself that she is safe and no one will hurt her. I suggest that

people literally recite, "I am safe now. No one can hurt me." It's a reminder to the self that any past danger is not present now.

- Some people come to therapy believing they have to tell us every bad thing that has happened to them. Be open to hearing trauma material, but watch for signs of it becoming overwhelming.
- Explain that healing involves dealing with emotions, and these can involve events and relationships in the present.
- Consider that hypomania or manic character styles may involve elements of hypervigilance.
- If a client discusses traumatic events, take these at face value and trust their reality.
- When self-destruction is present, find out if it is troubling. For example, if cutting is present, does it bother them? Would they like to find another way to deal with the need to do this?
- If a client seems "out of his mind" and very focused on what others think of him, try to get him to notice this. We all have more confidence in the world if we can approach situations by knowing what we think and feel. This is the beginning of modeling mentalization.
- Be open to a variety of techniques and to shift approaches as needed. Sometimes dissociative clients need us to stay silent. Sometimes they need us to provide concrete options for coping, such as thinking about how to manage overwhelming feelings and affect.
- Dissociation and trauma rob people of a stable and coherent sense of self. Knowing feelings is the beginning of putting some of the pieces of identity back together.

References

American Psychiatric Association. (2013). *Diagnostic and statistical manual of mental disorders* (5th ed.). Washington, DC: Author.

Bernstein, E. M., & Putnam, F. W. (1986). Development, reliability of a dissociation scale. *Journal of Nervous and Mental Disease, 174*, 727–735.

Boulanger, G. (2002). The cost of survival: Psychoanalysis and adult onset trauma. *Contemporary Psychoanalysis, 38*, 17–44.

Boulanger, G. (2007). *Wounded by reality: Understanding and treating adult onset trauma.* Mahwah: The Analytic Press.

Brand, B., Classen, C., Lanius, R., Loewenstein, R., McNary, S., Pain, C., et al. (2009). A naturalistic study of dissociative identity disorder and dissociative disorder not otherwise specified patients treated by community clinicians. *Psychological Trauma: Theory, Research, Practice, and Policy, 1*(2), 153–171.

Brand, B. L., Loewenstein, R. J., & Spiegel, D. (2014). Dispelling myths about dissociative identity disorder treatment: An empirically based approach. *Psychiatry: Interpersonal and Biological Processes, 77*(2), 169–189. https://doi.org/10.1521/psyc.2014.77.2.169.

Brand, B. L., Sar, V., Stavropoulos, P., Krüger, C., Korzekwa, M., Martínez-Taboas, A., & Middleton, W. (2016). Separating fact from fiction: An empirical examination of six myths about dissociative identity disorder. *Harvard Review of Psychiatry, 24*(4), 257.

Brand, B. L., Kumar, S. A., & McEwen, L. E. (2019). Coverage of child maltreatment and adult trauma in graduate psychopathology textbooks. *Psychological Trauma: Theory, Research, Practice, and Policy, 11*(8), 919–926. https://doi.org/10.1037/tra0000454.

Breuer, J., & Freud, S. (1895/1957). *Studies on hysteria*. New York: Basic Books. (Original work published 1895)

Bromberg, P. (1991). On knowing one's patient inside out: The aesthetics of unconscious communication. *Psychoanalytic Dialogues, 1*, 399–422.

Bromberg, P. M. (1996). Standing in the spaces: The multiplicity of self and the psychoanalytic relationship. *Contemporary Psychoanalysis, 32*, 509–535.

Butler, L. D. (2006). Normative dissociation. *Psychiatric Clinics of North America, 29*, 45–62.

Cardeña, E., & Carlson, E. (2011). Acute stress disorder revisited. *Annual Review of Clinical Psychology, 7*, 245–267.

Chefetz, R. A. (2015). *Intensive psychotherapy for persistent dissociative processes: The fear of feeling real*. New York: W.W. Norton & Company.

Chiu, C. D., Chang, J. H., & Hui, C. M. (2017). Self-concept integration and differentiation in subclinical individuals with dissociation proneness. *Self and Identity, 16*(6), 664–683.

Chu, J. (2011). *Rebuilding shattered lives: Complex PTSD and dissociative disorders* (2nd ed.). Hoboken: Wiley.

Coates, S. W., Rosenthal, J. L., & Schechter, D. S. (2003). *September 11th: Trauma and human bonds*. Hillsdale: The Analytic Press.

Courtois, C. A., & Ford, J. D. (2015). *Treatment of complex trauma: A sequenced, relationship-based approach* (Reprint edition). New York: The Guilford Press.

Dalenberg, C., Loewenstein, R., Spiegel, D., Brewin, C., Lanius, R., Frankel, S., et al. (2007). Scientific study of the dissociative disorders. *Psychotherapy and Psychosomatics, 76*, 400–401.

Dalenberg, C. J., Brand, B. L., Gleaves, D. H., Dorahy, M. J., Loewenstein, R. J., Cardeña, E., et al. (2012). Evaluation of the evidence for the trauma and fantasy models of dissociation. *Psychological Bulletin, 138*(3), 550–588.

Dalenberg, C. J., Brand, B. L., Loewenstein, R. J., Gleaves, D. H., Dorahy, M. J., Cardeña, E., Frewen, P. A., Carlson, E. B., & Spiegel, D. (2014). Reality versus fantasy: Reply to Lynn et al. (2014). *Psychological Bulletin, 140*(3), 911–920. https://doi.org/10.1037/a0036685. Hooboken: Wiley.

Exner, J. E. (2001). *A Rorschach workbook for the comprehensive system* (5th ed.). Asheville: Rorschach Workshops.

Exner, J. E., & Erdberg, P. (2005). *The Rorschach: Advanced interpretation* (Vol. 2). Hooboken: Wiley.

Freud, S. (1900/1913/2010). *The interpretation of dreams* (A. A. Brill, Trans.) (3rd ed.). New York: Macmillan (1913). Bartleby.com (2010).

Glucksman, M. L. (2000). Affect dysregulation: Defense or deficit? *Journal of the American Academy of Psychoanalysis, 28*, 263–273.

Godwin, C. A., Hunter, M. A., Bezdek, M. A., Lieberman, G., Elkin-Frankston, S., Romero, V. L., et al. (2017). Functional connectivity within and between intrinsic brain networks correlates with trait mind wandering. *Neuropsychologia, 103*, 140. https://doi.org/10.1016/j.neuropsychologia.2017.07.006.

Goldschmidt, O. (1986). A contribution of the subject of "psychic trauma" based on a course of a psychoanalytic short therapy. *International Review of Psychoanalysis, 13*, 181–199.

Greenberg, T. M. (2016). *Psychodynamic perspectives on aging and illness* (2nd ed.) New York: Springer.

Hart, O., & Rutger, H. (1989). The dissociation theory of Pierre Janet. *Journal of Traumatic Stress, 2*, 397–412.

Hesse, E., Main, M., Abrams, K. Y., & Rifkin, A. (2003). Unresolved states regarding loss or abuse can have "second-generation" effects: Disorganization, role inversion, and frightening ideation in the offspring of traumatized non-maltreating parents. In M. F. Solomon & D. J. Siegel (Eds.), *Healing trauma: Attachment, mind, body and brain*. New York: W.W. Norton & Company, Inc.

Hilgard, E. R. (1986). *Divided consciousness: Multiple controls in human thought and action*. New York: Wiley.

Horevitz, R., & Loewenstein, R. J. (1994). The rational treatment of multiple personality disorder. In S. J. Lynn & J. W. Rhue (Eds.), *Dissociation: Clinical and theoretical perspectives*. New York: The Guilford Press.
Howell, E. (2011). *Understanding and treating dissociative identity disorder*. New York: Routledge.
Janet, P. (1907). *The major symptoms of hysteria: Fifteen lectures given in the Medical School of Harvard University*. New York: Macmillan.
Janet, P. (1973). *L'automatisme psychologique*. Paris: Société Pierre Janet. (Original work published 1889)
Kate, M.-A., Hopwood, T., & Jamieson, G. (2020). The prevalence of dissociative disorders and dissociative experiences in college populations: A meta-analysis of 98 studies. *Journal of Trauma & Dissociation, 21*(1), 16–61.
Klinger, E. (1971). *Structure and function of fantasy*. New York: Wiley.
Kluft, R. P. (1991). Multiple personality disorder. In A. Tasman & S. M. Goldfinger (Eds.), *American Psychiatric Press review of psychiatry* (Vol. 10, pp. 161–188). Washington, DC: American Psychiatric Press.
Leavitt, F. (2001). MMPI profile characteristics of women with varying levels of normal dissociation. *Journal of Clinical Psychology, 57*(12), 1469–1477.
LeDoux, J. (1996). *The emotional brain: The mysterious underpinnings of emotional life*. New York: Touchstone.
Lilienfeld, S. O., Lynn, S. J., Kirsch, I., Chaves, J., Sarbin, T., Ganaway, G., & Powell, R. (1999). Dissociative identity disorder and the sociocognitive model: Recalling the lessons of the past. *Psychological Bulletin, 125*, 507–523.
Loftus, E. F., & Davis, D. (2006). Recovered memories. *Annual Review of Clinical Psychology, 2*, 469–498.
Loftus, E., & Ketcham, K. (1994). *The myth of repressed memory: False memories and allegations of sexual abuse*. New York: St. Martin's Press.
Lynn, S. J., Lock, T., Loftus, E. F., Krackow, E., & Lilienfeld, S. O. (2003). The remembrance of things past: Problematic memory recovery techniques in psychotherapy. In S. O. Lilienfeld, S. J. Lynn, & J. M. Lohr (Eds.), *Science and pseudoscience in clinical psychology* (pp. 205–239). New York: Guilford Press.
Lynn, S. J., Lilienfeld, S. O., Merckelbach, H., Giesbrecht, T., McNally, R., Loftus, E., & Malaktaris, A. (2012). The trauma model of dissociation: Inconvenient truths and stubborn fictions: Comment on Dalenberg et al. (2012). *Psychological Bulletin, 140*, 896–910.
Lynn, S. J., Berg, J., Lilienfeld, S. O., Merckelbach, H., Giesbrecht, T., Accardi, M., & Cleere, C. (2014). Dissociative disorders. In D. Beidel, B. C. Frueh, & M. Hersen (Eds.), *Adult psychopathology and diagnosis* (7th ed., pp. 497–538). New York: Wiley.
Lynn, S.J., Maxwell, R., Merckelbach, H., Lilienfeld, S.O., van Heugten-van der Kloet, D., & Miskovic, V. (2019). Dissociation and its disorders: Competing models, future directions, and a way forward. *Clinical Psychology Review, 73*, 101755.
Masson, J. M. (1984). *Assault on truth: Freud's suppression of the seduction theory*. New York: Farrar Straus & Giroux.
McKay, M., Wood, J. C., & Brantley, J. (2019). *The dialectical behavior therapy skills workbook: Practical DBT exercises for learning mindfulness, interpersonal effectiveness, emotion regulation & distress tolerance*. Oakland: New Harbinger.
McNally, R. J., Clancy, S. A., Barrett, H. M., & Parker, H. A. (2005). Reality monitoring in adults reporting repressed, recovered, or continuous memories of childhood sexual abuse. *Journal of Abnormal Psychology, 114*, 147–152.
Merckelbach, H., Horselenberg, R., & Schmidt, H. (2002). Modeling the connection between self-reported trauma and dissociation in a student sample. *Personality and Individual Differences, 32*, 695–705.
Merckelbach, H., Boskovic, I., Pesy, D., Dalsklev, M., & Lynn, S. J. (2017). Symptom overreporting and dissociative experiences: A qualitative review. *Consciousness and Cognition, 49*, 132–144.

Morrison, K. H., Bradley, R., & Westen, D. (2003). The external validity of controlled clinical trials of psychotherapy for depression and anxiety: A naturalistic study. *Psychology and Psychotherapy: Theory, Research and Practice, 76*, 109–132.

Nemiah, J. C. (1973). Psychology and psychosomatic illness: Reflections on theory and research methodology. *Psychotherapy and Psychosomatics, 22*, 106–111.

Putnam, F. W. (1991). Dissociative phenomena. In A. Tasman & S. M. Goldfinger (Eds.), *American Psychiatric Press review of psychiatry* (Vol. 10, pp. 145–160). Washington, DC: American Psychiatric Press.

Putnam, F. W. (1992). Discussion: Are alter personalities fragments or figments? *Psychoanalytic Inquiry, 12*(1), 95–111.

Putnam, F. W. (1997). *Dissociation in children and adolescents*. New York: Guilford.

Renik, O. (1998). Getting real in analysis. *Psychoanalytic Quarterly, 67*, 566–593.

Siegel, D. J. (1996). Cognition, memory, and dissociation. *Child and Adolescent Psychiatric Clinics of North America, 5*(2), 509–536.

Sifneos, P. E. (1973). The prevalence of "alexithymic" characteristics in psychosomatic patients. *Psychotherapy and Psychosomatics, 22*(2), 255–262.

Solms, M., & Turnbull, O. (2002). *The brain and the inner world: An introduction to the neuroscience of subjective experience*. New York: Other Press.

Stein, D. J., Koenen, K. C., Friedman, M. J., Hill, E. D., McLaughlin, K. A., Petukhova, M. V., et al. (2013). Dissociation in posttraumatic stress disorder: Evidence from the world mental health surveys. *Biological Psychiatry, 73*(4), 302–312.

Steinberg, M. (1995). *Handbook for the assessment of dissociation: A clinical guide*. Washington, DC: American Psychiatric Press.

Ulatowska, J., & Sawicka, M. (2017). Recovered memories in clinical practice—A research review. *Psychiatria Polska, 51*(4), 609–618. https://doi.org/10.12740/PP/62770.

van Ijzendoorn, M. H., & Schuengel, C. (1996). The measurement of dissociation in normal and clinical populations: Meta-analytic validation of the Dissociative Experiences Scale (DES). *Clinical Psychology Review, 16*(5), 365–382.

Vissia, E. M., Giesen, M. E., Chalavi S., et al. (2016). Is it trauma- or fantasy-based? Comparing dissociative identity disorder, post-traumatic stress disorder, simulators, and controls. *Acta Psychiatr Scand, 134*(2):111–128. https://doi.org/10.1111/acps.12590.

Vogel, M., Spitzer, C., Kuwert, P., Möller, B., Freyberger, H. J., & Grabe, H. J. (2009). Association of Childhood Neglect with adult dissociation in schizophrenic inpatients. *Psychopathology, 42*, 124–130.

Vonderlin, R., Kleindienst, N., Alpers, G., Bohus, M., Lyssenko, L., & Schmahl, C. (2018). Dissociation in victims of childhood abuse or neglect: A meta-analytic review. *Psychological Medicine, 48*(15), 2467–2476.

Wang, P. (2018). *What are dissociative disorders?* American Psychiatric Association. Accessed online on 4th Nov 2019 at https://www.psychiatry.org/patients-families/dissociative-disorders/what-are-dissociative-disorders.

Watson, D. (2003). Investigating the construct validity of the dissociative taxon: Stability analyses of normal and pathological dissociation. *Journal of Abnormal Psychology, 112*(2), 298–305.

Wilgus, S. J., Packer, M. M., Lile-King, R., Miller-Perrin, C. L., & Brand, B. L. (2015, May 25). *Coverage of child maltreatment in abnormal psychology textbooks: Reviewing the adequacy of the content. Psychological trauma: Theory, research, practice, and policy*. Advance online publication. https://doi.org/10.1037/tra0000049.

Wilgus, S. J., Packer, M. M., Lile-King, R., Miller-Perrin, C. L., & Brand, B. L. (2016). Coverage of child maltreatment in abnormal psychology textbooks: Reviewing the adequacy of the content. *Psychological Trauma: Theory, Research, Practice, and Policy, 8*(2), 188–197. https://doi.org/10.1037/tra0000049.

Zackheim, L. (2007). Alexithymia: Expanding the realm of research. *Journal of Psychosomatic Research, 63*, 345–347.

Zittel Conklin, C., & Westen, D. (2005). Borderline personality disorder in clinical practice. *American Journal of Psychiatry, 162*, 867–875.

Chapter 6
The Need to Numb: Substance Use and Therapeutic Management

Substance Use Problems: Evolving Social Perceptions and Reality

People have long used substances for pleasure, self-medication, and experimentation or due to pressure from friends and families, to enhance concentration, advance creativity, decrease social anxiety, and/or decrease inhibition, to name just a few common reasons. Thinking about this topic is complicated and risks inherent judgments and perilous speculation. For example, in the United States, there is a long tradition of moralistic condemnation of intoxication with all types of psychoactive drugs (Des Jarlais 2017).

In just my career, I have witnessed extremes regarding how we view people who use opiates. For example, in the 1990s I worked in an inpatient chronic pain clinic in which the goal of treatment was for clients to not take any narcotics for pain, no matter the condition and no matter how responsibly they used them. Also during that time, any hospitalized patient who requested narcotics was viewed with a sense of deep suspicion and with the often-unspoken assumption that they might be an addict. This shifted about a decade later, when it was clear we were undertreating pain. Then there was a very relaxed approach to prescribing, with little thought to the potentials or dangers of doing so. And now, with enhanced regulations and the opiate crisis, doctors are wary in prescribing many types of prescription medications for fear of people becoming addicted. A less severe example of shifting views on use of substances is when I was in training, caffeine was viewed as negative. In my education as a health and behavioral psychologist, our goal was to essentially get people to stop using any product with this supposedly dangerous substance! Of course, we now know that certain caffeinated drinks (tea and coffee) and food (dark chocolate) are thought to have antioxidant qualities and nutritional benefits. Admittedly, too much caffeine can worsen anxiety, but my experience of my training was that it involved messages to clients that at least hinted of value judgments.

T. M. Greenberg, *Treating Complex Trauma*,
https://doi.org/10.1007/978-3-030-45285-8_6

In the wider culture, there was a time when a two-martini lunch and a half a pack of cigarettes seemed normal (especially for certain white-collar professionals) and a time when smoking an occasional joint seemed criminal. I mention all of this as a way of pointing out just how much social and cultural values impact our view of people who take substances. These views not only shift over time but are also very dependent on the countries we live in, not to mention our socioeconomic status and racial and ethnic identities.

As a clinician, I respect people's need or interest in using substances of all kinds, and when thinking about client's use of substances, I take a curious and neutral stance. I always have a dialogue with them about how they view their use and whether or not they consider it a problem or an obstacle to functioning. These ways of dealing with clients seem important, as people who use or abuse substances, particularly if they have histories of trauma, can feel a great deal of shame. Further, excessive use of drugs and alcohol can be a factor influencing further victimization, highlighting the need for compassion and sensitivity when dealing with substance use issues.

Substance use is complicated and difficult to treat for both psychological and neurological reasons. Many reward centers in the brain are triggered when we take certain substances. Additionally, using substances can seem to make dealing with emotions easier. Stimulating drugs promote activation and distraction; sedating drugs can quiet the mind. Since people with cPTSD are often constantly at risk of being overwhelmed by thoughts and feelings that they feel may harm them, my view is we need to treat substance use like any other symptom. What do our clients want to do about their use, if anything? It's not our call to make. We can, however, weave this issue into our treatments, and like a lot of the things we try to help our clients with, it may take a long time and a bit a creativity to influence different coping mechanisms.

Many of us, as mental health clinicians, have had little formal training on dealing with substance use disorders, and the worlds of drug and alcohol treatment are often very separate from the work of other kinds of therapists (Najavits and Hien 2013). I hope this chapter can offer some ideas of how to think about treating trauma survivors who are over-reliant on substances for coping or who have become dependent.

The Increase in Problematic Substance Use

We are living in a time of extreme use of drugs and alcohol and deaths of despair, which are related. Woolf and Schoomaker (2019) analyzed life expectancy data collected by the Centers for Disease Control and Prevention and all-cause mortality rates listed in the US Mortality Database from 1959 to 2017. These authors note that although life expectancy had been steadily rising, it decreased after 2014 related to an increase in mortality from specific causes (drug overdose, suicides, organ system diseases) among young- and middle-aged adults of all racial groups, with an onset as early as the 1990s and with the largest relative increases occurring in the Ohio

Valley and New England. But in many places in the United States, midlife mortality increased, caused by drug overdoses, alcohol abuse, suicides, and a diverse list of organ system diseases, related to substance use. Of course, it makes sense to partially blame the opioid epidemic, which has been plaguing the United States and Canada for a number of years. And while substance abuse and dependency are complicated, there is strong evidence that these afflictions are linked with trauma histories, PTSD, and cPTSD.

Links Between Trauma and Substance Use

Below I will highlight some of the data that suggests links between substance use and trauma. I should note that many of the studies I will describe use DSM criteria for PTSD, not cPTSD (which is not included in the DSM-V). This is due, in part, to the relative newness of cPTSD diagnostic criteria, and cPTSD has not been explicitly described in many of the studies I will mention. However, many of the participants described in the following studies would likely meet criteria for cPTSD. For example, the study by Lee et al. (2019) (described below) involved one cohort of street-entrenched youth under the age of 25. I additionally discuss research regarding veterans who have had multiple deployments, which is associated with cPTSD. Regarding veterans, recent data suggest that many, if not most, people who enter the military have trauma histories before enlisting, enhancing the burden of military service (Kesling 2019). Therefore, there seems to be a case to be made that the study participants mentioned below are not suffering from so-called simple PTSD.

Trauma is a risk factor for substance abuse, and substance abuse is also a risk factor for trauma (Najavits et al. 1997). For example, among people who were dependent on cocaine and seeking treatment, the most common traumatic events reported were witnessing someone's death or serious injury, experiencing a disaster, physical assault, accident, and/or sexual assault (Back et al. 2000).

Up to 65% of people with PTSD have been found to have a comorbid substance use disorder (Pietrzak et al. 2011). Lee et al. (2019) found that a provisional PTSD diagnosis using DSM-V diagnostic criteria nearly doubled the risk of nonfatal overdose among people who used illicit drugs, including opiates. PTSD is also associated with cannabis use (Kevorkian et al. 2015), though overall associations between cannabis consumption and trauma are not as strong as other drugs. PTSD is also associated with cigarette smoking, and one study found emotional numbing to be particularly linked with the likelihood of lifetime smoking (Greenberg et al. 2012).

About one-third of people with PTSD have comorbid alcohol dependence and are more likely to have experienced childhood adversity (Blanco et al. 2013; Kessler et al. 1997), with the latter study finding a higher likelihood of using substances to relieve PTSD symptoms and higher rates of other psychiatric disorders. Among individuals with PTSD, heavy alcohol use is associated with a greater number and more severe PTSD symptoms (Behar 1987; Saladin et al. 1995). The odds of having an alcohol use disorder increase with the number of PTSD criteria (Pietrzak et al. 2011).

Although substance abuse and PTSD are concurrent in a large number of civilian populations, veterans are even more likely to have both PTSD and substance use disorders. For example, in a large national cohort of Vietnam veterans, 73% of male Vietnam veterans met diagnostic criteria for comorbid PTSD and a lifetime diagnosis of alcohol use disorder (Kulka et al. 1990). In a study looking at more than 400,000 Iraq and Afghanistan veterans who sought care at Veterans Affairs medical centers from 2001 to 2010, veterans who had both drug and alcohol use disorders had a threefold increase in having a diagnosis of PTSD (Seal et al. 2011). Among more recent veterans, polysubstance use is associated with increased severity of PTSD symptoms (Bhalla et al. 2018).

Combined Vulnerability: Psychological and Biological Models

Like all psychiatric disorders that have labels, substance use diagnoses are thought to impact people who have biological/genetic vulnerabilities and those who experienced environmental stress. Considering any one of these factors in isolation risks oversimplifying the complexities of problematic substance use. With that caveat, I will describe some of the ideas regarding the reasons for the high association between trauma and substance use or misuse.

Khantzian (1997) suggested the self-medication hypothesis of substance use, an idea that is familiar to many clinicians:

> Traumatized individuals with limited capacities to psychologically dissociate may attempt to produce similar soothing or numbing effects by using psychoactive substances … These substances are used to enter and maintain dissociative-like states. (p. 197)

Stewart and Conrod (2003) also suggest that continued PTSD symptoms could promote and maintain substance misuse through peoples' attempts to control PTSD symptoms. Substance misuse could maintain, prolong, or exacerbate PTSD symptoms, which in turn could serve to promote further substance misuse and so on. Figure 6.1 presents a graphic by the aforementioned authors on the vicious cycle of substance use and PTSD.

There is a lot of support for the self-medication hypothesis, with Flanagan et al. (2016) arguing that it has the most empirical support to date and that ideas about self-medication have been garnered by studies demonstrating that PTSD typically emerges before co-occurring substance use disorders. According to a recent study, people with features of borderline personality disorder (who are more likely to have histories of trauma, as I've described) were more likely to use alcohol, cannabis, and prescription opioids as a method of coping with symptoms (Vest and Tragesser 2019).

Roesler and Dafler (1993) used the term "chemical dissociation" to ward off PTSD symptoms. Indeed, some studies have suggested that dissociation is more common among people who abuse substances (Najavits and Walsh 2012). In this

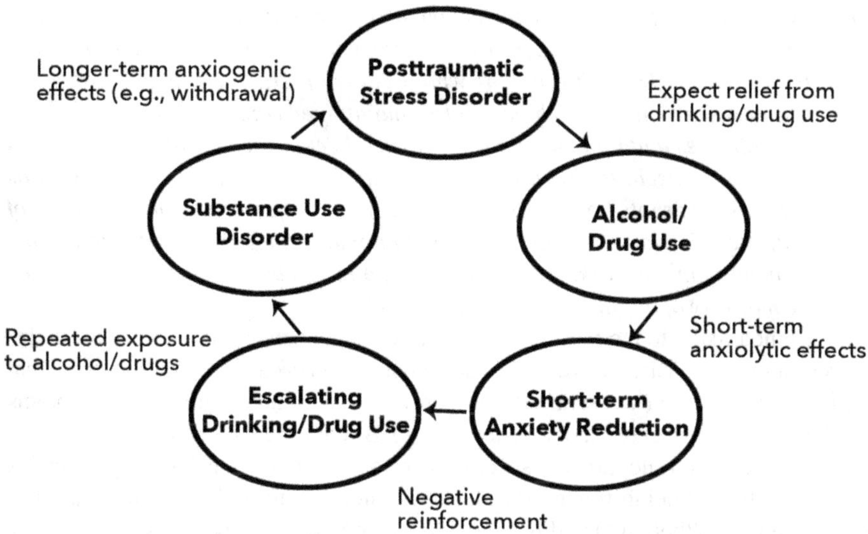

Fig. 6.1 Proposed cycle of substance use and PTSD. (Stewart and Conrod 2003)

latter study, people with high levels of dissociation had more trauma-related symptoms and childhood histories of emotional abuse and physical neglect and held beliefs that substances could help manage psychological symptoms. An experimental study found that among people with cocaine or alcohol dependence and PTSD, exposure to trauma cues or reminders increased substance cravings, and severity of PTSD symptoms predicted the intensity of the cravings (Coffey et al. 2002). Sexual assault survivors with PTSD, who believed that substance use would reduce distress, were more likely to have problematic alcohol use (Ullman et al. 2006). Additionally, several studies have suggested that people with substance use disorders, without PTSD, tend to relapse in *tempting* situations, whereas people with PTSD and substance use disorder report using substances in response to *negative* situations (Kramer et al. 2014).

However, Najavits (2002) also notes that some people use substances to access negative feelings as opposed to escaping from them. An example of this is someone who likes to drink alcohol in order to cry or to be able to tolerate thinking about negative things. Although I have witnessed this, it's been more my experience to see people with cPTSD who use substances do so with a hope of reducing PTSD symptoms. Let's consider the example of David:

David, who I saw many years ago, was 61 years old and served in-country in Vietnam after he was drafted. He told me little about his experiences there, except once to joke he had been a POW. What he talked about most was how he didn't want to go into the Army, including thinking at one point about moving to Canada. He had few resources though, having grown up in a small Midwestern town with poor and disinterested parents. He appeared to adjust after the war. After a stint of using heroin, he started a successful import/export business. After he quit heroin, which he did with the assistance of a detox center, he began to drink daily. He was also a heavy smoker, smoking up to two packs a day. He met criteria for PTSD but shrugged this off by stating, "Doesn't everyone who was over there?" He married once but then divorced. Only one of his three children maintained contact with him. He noted he had nightmares and told me that when he had been asleep for about 90 minutes (when most of us begin to dream), he'd wake up and smoke a cigarette as well as drink "a couple of shots" of vodka. He continued in this fashion throughout most of the night, literally waking up about every 90 minutes, though denied it interfered with his functioning at work. However, at that point, his business partner had taken over the majority of day-to-day responsibilities.

It seemed likely to me that David had started using substances to ward off nightmares, at the very least. However, his dependency had escalated to such a point that he likely needed near-constant alcohol consumption so he did not have symptoms of alcohol withdrawal (e.g., delirium tremens). At the time I knew him, he had been very dependent on alcohol for several years and had little insight regarding his drinking. He was being treated for alcohol-related health problems but refused to stop drinking. Although David is an extreme example, many people spontaneously articulate using substances for help with PTSD symptoms. For example, a young woman I worked with who had survived being hit by a car but was left with significant injuries (she also had a history of sexual assault) told me she drank 8–10 drinks in the evening, just to manage her anxiety, which involved severe hypervigilance. She said she loved how when she drank she didn't feel she had to "pay attention" to anything, plus it helped her get to sleep. In her case she had also seemed to use just enough to sleep several hours, which, she also told me, reduced her nightmares.

Related to substance dependence, heritability estimates for nicotine, alcohol, and drug addiction are in the range of 50–60% (Heath et al. 1997; Kendler et al. 2003; Li 2006; Tsuang et al. 1998). Research suggests that environmental factors have a stronger effect on the behavior of initiating substance use, whereas genetic factors play a larger role in the transition from occasional use to the development of addiction (Bierut 2011). A shared genetic association has been observed between substance use and PTSD. McLeod et al. (2001) described the "shared vulnerability hypothesis," in that combat exposure, PTSD symptoms, and alcohol use are associated because some portion of the genes that influence vulnerability to combat (measured by volunteering for service) also influence vulnerability to alcohol consumption and to PTSD symptoms. Another study found that PTSD, alcohol dependence, and drug dependence have common additive genetic influences suggesting a significant contribution for PTSD (Xian et al. 2000).

Both PTSD and substance use disorders have been associated with abnormal hypothalamic–pituitary–adrenal axis (HPA-axis) levels and specifically low cortisol levels (Hruska and Delahanty 2014). The HPA-axis is a hormonal response system in which cortisol levels are impacted via neurological responses to stress. It's the complicated version of what most of us think of as the fight/flight response. Over 20 years of research suggests that altered HPA-axis functioning is associated with problematic alcohol use and dependence and that the nature of this dysregulation varies with respect to the stages of progression toward alcohol dependence (Stephens and Wand 2012). Brady et al. (2009) note that the HPA-axis, including extrahypothalamic corticotrophin-releasing factor (CRF), and the noradrenergic system are all intimately involved in the stress response, PTSD, and pathophysiology of substance use disorders. Both PTSD and substance use disorders are found to have abnormalities in the prefrontal cortex and in the anterior cingulate cortex suggesting that this brain region may represent a common pathway between the two disorders (Hruska and Delahanty 2014).

Assessing Substance Use

In terms of actual definitions, it's worth mentioning the ranges and types of use described in this chapter. I'll be describing excessive use, that is, use of a substance that is determined to be more than what a client wants and may be associated with negative consequences. More severe use is described by the DSM-V (APA 2013) as substance abuse disorder. Substance use disorder is more akin to what was described as substance dependence when I was in training. It involves using more of a substance over an extended period of time, persistent efforts to cut down, cravings, tolerance, withdrawal, and negative physical or environmental consequences, and the use also interferes with functioning. In the middle of this range would be something like problematic use, such as a heavy drinker who drinks a lot (such as five or more drinks) in the evenings but still manages to go to work the next day and may not meet all criteria for substance use disorder but who still may be aware of the excessive or even compulsive nature of the drinking and where there may be negative physical and/or psychological effects. An example of the former might be liver damage, and an example of the latter might be not being available to take care of children in an attentive way. The lines between all of these criteria may become blurry, in part because my emphasis is client-centered, meaning that they control the narrative about their use. While this approach does not fit neatly with exacting diagnostic criteria, it has a more real-world applicability for dealing with clients in the outpatient setting in which I practice.

As I stated in Chapter 2, it's important that any kind of assessment with people who have cPTSD should be as non-intrusive as possible. I see assessment of substance use as an ongoing part of treatment as described by harm reduction clinicians (Tatarsky and Kellogg 2010). I find that if people are concerned about their use of a particular substance, they let me know within the first couple of sessions. If they are not concerned, it comes up in other contexts. Let's consider the case with a young woman I will call Sabrina:

Sabrina, who was 23 and just starting grad school, said she was coming to therapy because of anxiety. She was from the East Coast, with parents she described as "very liberal," one of whom was a daily and heavy drinker and the other who used to "smoke weed" with her brothers. Sabrina was never involved in these activities, which mirrored her feelings about her childhood. Her older brothers were viewed as much more interesting and got a lot more attention from her parents. Particularly when her parents were using substances, Sabrina was treated to a host of complaints about everything from her looks to her level of intelligence. She told me later in her therapy that she realized from very young age that she was "born into the wrong family."

She was isolated throughout much of high school and described herself as "mostly out of it," but when she relocated to the West Coast for college, she lived with 5–6 different roommates in a large home, all of whom were enthusiasts of using substances of all kinds. Sabrina favored lysergic acid diethylamide (LSD or acid) but used literally any hallucinogenic she could get her hands on. She also enjoyed 3,4-methylenedioxy-methamphetamine (MDMA or Molly/Ecstasy) in addition to her daily diet of beer, marijuana, and cigarettes. Perhaps even more mind-boggling than her polysubstance use was that she used a variety of "experimental" drugs, which, from what I could tell, could literally have been any kind of tablet someone could buy from the various drug purveyors she and her housemates had contact with. Adding to that, she admitted that sometimes she took two "tabs" of LSD or Molly when she was partying. She did wonder at times whether the latter use might be linked with occasional "symptoms of depression" and I assured her this was very possible, though this did not change her behavior. As she was entering into what I imagined to be a more demanding grad school curriculum (she had found college "easy and boring" and got straight As), I asked if she wondered if she'd be able to keep up her partying pace. She said it wasn't a problem.

As we'll see with Sabrina in the next section, I dealt with her substance use by allowing her to tell me when it became a problem. As with most diagnostic issues, our clients need to feel that their symptoms are an issue before we can address them. That said, I think we can weave in ways to encourage people to think about their substance use, and I'll discuss that below.

As far as formal assessment, the National Institute on Drug Abuse has a comprehensive list of assessment devices for drugs and alcohol and can be accessed at https://www.drugabuse.gov/nidamed-medical-health-professionals/screening-tools-prevention. My approach when evaluating and thinking about substance abuse with clients is to simply ask a lot of questions about it, assuming the client wants to discuss it. I listen for ambivalence, as identifying this is a window into really considering the possibility of change (Miller and Rollnick 2002). While these authors are advocates of motivational interviewing, a related idea was suggested to me many years ago by psychoanalyst Lee Rather. Rather (personal communication) emphasized the importance of asking and exploring in some depth what the client likes about the psychological, emotional, and physical effects of using their preferred substance(s). I've found this suggestion highly useful, even in situations in which substance abuse has resulted in problems. For example, a young man with a severe marijuana addition that impacted his standing at his job was able to think more about the impact of his use when I simply asked what he liked about being stoned. This was soothing to him, as he had heard from everyone else in his life that he should simply quit. But these demands (as he experienced them) negated the importance and meaning of the pot smoking for him. If you think about it, this is common sense. We have historically lived in a culture that encourages abstinence—

a kind of all or nothing approach. And while I do think that abstinence approaches can be helpful, many people need space and time to thinking about their use and what it means. And some people really do not want to be abstinent. Fortunately there are a variety of ways to help people think about and moderate their use of substances, if this is something they are interested in.

It's worth noting that some schools of therapy, particularly psychoanalytic approaches, have a history of suggesting to clients that therapy cannot be useful if they are involved in excessive substance use. I'm not sure if this remains the case, as many clinicians have become more flexible. But the old teaching was that if someone was using substances they could not benefit from treatment, presumably because it could interfere with the development of transference. I find this tradition curious, as analysts have long prided themselves on being neutral observers of human behavior. Whatever the reasoning, my experience is that people who want to tell me about their taking of substances are mentioning it because they are concerned about it and want us to think about it with them. It seems important we welcome any kind of discussion about any behavior with a curious stance, even if it makes us worried or uncomfortable.

I also think it's important we think of one's use of substances as an important, albeit, complicated relationship. For example, a friend referred to her "addiction" to diet soda. I laughed this off as a cute joke. She corrected me and said, "No, I'm serious. I think about it, I imagine how good it will taste. It gives me so much pleasure! But I only allow myself to have two a day as I know it's not the best thing for me. But I can't stop." Substances, no matter how seemingly innocuous, may have many meanings. It is vital that we explore that relationship—what it provides and what it does not and its pleasures and consequences. This is a vital part of an ongoing assessment of substance use. For people with cPTSD, it's important to evaluate any connection the client is aware of regarding use and PTSD or other mood symptoms, as this helps with deciding what approaches to take. My approach to assessment is to let someone's use of substances unfold throughout the treatment, unless people bring the issue in as a something that requires help right away. In those cases, there are a number of options for helping people.

Treatment Approaches for cPTSD and Substance Use

Seeking Safety

People with combined substance use disorder (SUD) and PTSD have worse outcomes in addiction treatment and higher rates of relapse (Jacobsen et al. 2001; Najavits 2007). Seeking Safety has been widely adopted for treating people with both SUD and PTSD. Concurrent Treatment of PTSD and Substance Use Disorders Using Prolonged Exposure (COPE) is a newer model that is used primarily within the Veterans Affairs system.

Seeking Safety (SS), developed by Lisa Najavits, PhD, is a present-focused, coping skills approach. It was designed to address both PTSD and SUD at the same time but without having clients delve into their trauma narratives in detail. Najavits developed Seeking Safety as a first-stage approach that could be used with any client and by any provider. Seeking Safety research and clinical implementation include the most vulnerable cPTSD clients, who are often excluded from classic PTSD treatments: people with drug disorders, psychosis, criminal justice involvement, current domestic violence, suicidality and self-harm behaviors, low cognitive ability, personality disorders, severe and chronic childhood trauma, etc. According to Najavits, SS "addresses PTSD without requiring clients to move into their trauma narrative, which can be too intense when they are still actively addicted or have other major current vulnerabilities" (personal communication, 2019). "Seeking Safety was designed to be optimistic, flexible, and engaging," she says, in part to offset the fear some clients have about starting PTSD treatment and the high dropout of models such as prolonged exposure. (These are concerns I also noted in Chapter 1.) A meta-analysis by Lenz et al. (2016) that included complex PTSD clients found that SS showed a moderate effect size for PTSD and modest effect for SUD, across 12 randomized controlled trials with 1997 patients.

When I first read about Seeking Safety, it struck me as the kind of therapy I imagined many clinicians might intuitively conduct if they and their clients wanted to address trauma while staying focused on the present. Another potential advantage to SS is that it does not need to be conducted by licensed mental health professionals. Peers and paraprofessionals can conduct the model, which has public health implications regarding its scope, especially in community settings. The main goal of SS is to help clients attain safety in their relationships, thinking, behavior, and emotions. The treatment encompasses the following (accessed from https://www.treatment-innovations.org/ss-description.html, December 22, 2019):

- Interpersonal topics: Honesty, Asking for Help, Setting Boundaries in Relationships, Getting Others to Support Recovery, Healthy Relationships, Community Resources
- Cognitive topics: PTSD: Taking Back Your Power, Compassion, When Substances Control You, Creating Meaning, Discovery, Integrating the Split Self, Recovery Thinking
- Behavioral topics: Taking Good Care of Yourself, Commitment, Respecting Your Time, Coping with Triggers, Self-Nurturing, Red and Green Flags, Detaching from Emotional Pain (Grounding)
- Combination topics: Introduction/Case Management, Safety, Life Choices, Termination

Seeking Safety is flexible and emphasizes empowering clients to choose coping that can work for them. It allows for harm reduction or abstinence approaches and encourages but does not require 12-step and other self-help groups.

COPE

The other new approach, Concurrent Treatment of PTSD and Substance Use Disorders Using Prolonged Exposure (COPE), is a treatment originally developed for use with veterans (Back et al. 2012, 2015). A recent randomized clinical trial with veterans directly compared COPE and Seeking Safety and found that COPE was associated with greater PTSD symptom reduction and greater likelihood of PTSD remission than Seeking Safety (Norman et al. 2019). This fits with what I heard from clinicians at the VA, that there is a preference for exposure treatments. It's also consistent with a managed care model; COPE is conducted in 12 sessions, and SS allows for more meetings (Najavits and Hien 2013). Among civilians with PTSD and substance dependence, the combined use of COPE plus usual treatment (substance dependence treatment), compared with usual treatment alone, resulted in improvement in PTSD symptom severity without an increase in severity of substance dependence (Mills et al. 2012).

COPE involves 12 individual, 60–90 minute therapy sessions, and the program includes several components (adapted from Back et al. 2015):

- Education about the relationship between PTSD and substance use disorders
- Education about common reactions to trauma
- Cognitive behavioral techniques to help patients manage cravings and high-risk thoughts about using alcohol or drugs
- Coping skills to help prevent relapse to substances
- Breathing retraining relaxation exercise
- In vivo (real-life) exposures and imaginal exposures

Seeking Safety and COPE are two popular treatments for treating complex PTSD combined with substance abuse. They were developed with the acuity of veterans in mind (though they can be applied to civilian populations), and both may serve valuable functions. However, as COPE involves exposure, it should be considered if it is deemed that exposure therapy is safe and preferred by the client. Given the data I discussed in Chapter 1 on drop-out rates in exposure therapy as well as the fact that exposure therapies can cause a great deal of distress, my approach is more similar to what is described in the Seeking Safety model, unless I am seeing someone with a straightforward case of PTSD that involved one acute event in adulthood. I have done exposure therapy in cases of simple PTSD, but this is a very small fraction of the people I see. Many of my clients obliquely mention their complex trauma backgrounds in the first few sessions. They do so often by asking if I feel it's important to talk about them. I emphasize that if thoughts about their trauma histories come up in a spontaneous and authentic way, I'd be happy to discuss it and think with them about how they understand and feel about these events. I go on to say that since trauma always is in the background (by this I am implying the presence of the unconscious and that, even in small ways, we often find the past repeats itself in the present), we can focus on the here and now. Healing can be linked with thinking, in particular, about current relationship functioning. And while it is true that I eventually do more intense processing of trauma with some of the people I see, this takes place after a year or more of therapy. People with cPTSD simply need more time to feel safe, as I've emphasized throughout this book. This is even more true for people who use substances, as in order to stop using, many of them need other coping mechanisms in place in order to deal with potentially overwhelming thoughts and feelings. Perhaps this is why longer-term treatments have symptom improvements that last longer than short-term treatments (e.g., Shedler 2012). Let's return to Sabrina's treatment:

In the first year of her therapy, Sabrina's use was always in the background. We discussed a number of topics common in younger women, problems with roommates, an argument with her boyfriend, sexuality, etc. As she had some medical knowledge, she might fact-check certain ideas about the dangers of her substance use, and I always answered matter-of-factly with what I understood to be the risks. However, whenever her drug use came up, I also asked her what she liked about it. She was explicit that she loved being "out of her mind" and in the "universe of a different kind of life with different possibilities." I noted how desperate she seemed in chasing a kind of feeling in which there were no worries and everyone could seem happy together. I was also thinking about her desire for a real family, one in which her parents might recognize Sabrina's talents and abilities or, as I thought of it, that she was a really "good kid" in many respects. I also spotted how much she felt that her friends who used with her were her family. This reinforced my clinical decision to tread lightly regarding her substance use. After about a year, Sabrina mentioned that she had begun having hallucinations. She had never had these symptoms before, and I wondered out loud if they may be due to her use of hallucinogens and/or the massive amounts of pot she was consuming. I suggested she consider experimenting with using drugs less to see if this helped, and it did. This was in addition to some other harm reduction techniques that helped her consider her risks and motivations regarding her relationship with drugs. The hallucinations disappeared, and she realized the danger she was putting herself in. Following that, she started having more arguments with her roommates. After 2 years of therapy, she had moved into a new apartment with roommates who did not use drugs, and eventually her use declined to marijuana and alcohol only on weekends.

I treated Sabrina using a variety of approaches for cPTSD including some CBT (such as keeping track of anxiety and when it manifested and noticing coexisting thoughts) assertiveness training and psychodynamic techniques (though focusing on here-and-now family relationships) and addressing normal developmental concerns that are common in young adults (such as feeling independent, normalizing sexual issues and concerns, deciding what kinds of friends she wanted to have, etc.). Her substance abuse remained very much on my mind, and I think hers too, but I didn't push her. I did worry about her use a lot, which I think, from a mentalizing stance, offered a kind of relationship she had never had before. Additionally, Sabrina had many dissociative symptoms, which I suspected, but could not be sure of until she started using fewer drugs. It seemed to me that her drug use was just as she said, a way to be "out of her mind." Although when she stopped the majority of her use, it was clear that her dissociation would be a clinical issue, but she felt safer in therapy at that point and could tell me more about aspects of her dissociation.

What I also want to highlight here with Sabrina is that she is one of many people I have seen with a substance use problem who eventually decides on her own to reduce or stop harmful substance use. The oldest person I have seen with a similar trajectory was 67 years of age, supporting the idea that Sabrina's young age was not the only factor in her making a life changing decision. I think since Sabrina felt so unseen in her childhood, invisible really, it was important that I could know about her substance abuse and be able to think about it with her in a non-judgmental and curious way. At times I felt like a mother of a teenager, worried if she might flunk out of school, worried if she might get arrested for having too many drugs in her possession (as she took several trips across state lines with considerable amounts of drugs in her car), and worried she was hanging out with the wrong kinds of friends. But holding and containing of these issues, much like you see in psychodynamic work and in mentalizing treatments (as discussed in Chapter 3), served the function of a kind of loving and concerned parenting she desperately needed.

While one may assume based on the research I discussed that substance abuse is partly related to self-medication, I have found commenting on this to carry limited therapeutic traction. Most people I see know on some level that the use of substances makes them feel better or helps to avoid difficult symptoms. When I've mentioned their use serves a purpose for them, maybe even to ward off difficult feelings, I've sometimes been met with a stare that indicates that this is obvious! This was certainly the case with Sabrina and she knew using made her feel less anxious. As the therapy progressed, she became less anxious, which also likely helped her consider the benefits of reducing her consumption of substances.

Treatment Approaches Specifically for Substance Use

As I've described, an overwhelming majority of people who use substances excessively have histories of trauma. Therefore, especially outpatient clinicians have a few good options for combining substance abuse treatment approaches into psychotherapy treatments (in addition to Seeking Safety and COPE) that can be combined with virtually any kind of therapy. This latter point is important, as the historical split between psychotherapy and substance abuse treatments often implies we have to send our clients away for *that kind* of treatment while we wait for them to get their substance use under control so they can come back for what we do. Of course, some people do need and want intensive inpatient treatment for severe substance use disorders, and I am not suggesting as outpatient therapists we can do it all. But I am making the point that there has been such shame and moral judgment about substance use that it's imperative that we allow a space to think with clients about how and if they want to address substance use and how we may be helpful, in addition to the engagement of other forms of support and treatment.

I'll describe three commonly used techniques for people who are interested in substance use treatment. People who use, abuse, or become dependent on substances are very diverse. It's important to think with clients about what avenues of treatment interest them.

Twelve-Step Programs

Twelve-step programs were adapted from the 1939 book, *Alcoholics Anonymous: The Story of How More Than One Hundred Men Have Recovered from Alcoholism* (Alcoholics Anonymous World Services 2001). The current title of the Big Book, as it is affectionately called by proponents, is *Alcoholics Anonymous* (AA). There are now over twenty-five 12-step groups that help "addicts" (this term is part of 12-step culture) involving everything from drugs and alcohol to gambling, food, sex, and even workaholics. It's an abstinence model of treatment, meaning the goal is to refrain from any substance or behavior that's deemed an addiction. Groups are peer led and use a sponsor system that encourages or requires a senior person in the program to offer support and mentoring. For example, one person I work with in one of the food addict-related programs speaks with a sponsor every day. Their conversations are not just related to food; they often sound like mini-counseling sessions. However, different 12-step programs have different levels of flexibility regarding sponsor contact. The other unique thing about 12-step programs is that they are global and relatively consistent. People can find an AA meeting, for example, in many parts of the world. Each group has a different culture, and participants are encouraged to find meetings that seem like a good fit.

Critics of 12-step programs suggest that it is a white male model that encourages the belief in a monotheistic god. For example, "surrendering to a higher power" is involved in 12-step work (AA World Services, 2001). Indeed, spirituality and religiosity are associated with better coping while involved in 12-step programs (Carrico et al. 2007). In general, empirical support for 12-step programs is widely inconsistent and depends on which reviews or individual studies are viewed. A Cochrane review (often viewed as the gold standard of unbiased research reviews) concluded that people involved in 12-step programs (particularly Alcoholics Anonymous) should be made aware that there is a lack of experimental evidence regarding efficacy (Ferri et al. 2006). A 1999 meta-analysis found that attendance of AA was worse than no treatment (Kownacki and Shadish 1999). However, another analysis found that support for rates of abstinence is about twice as high among those who attend AA and that higher levels of attendance are related to higher rates of abstinence and prior AA attendance is predictive of subsequent abstinence (Kaskutas 2009).

Engagement in the 12-steps is important and associated with abstinence outcomes. For example, participants with both drug and alcohol dependency who had a sponsor had read 12-step literature, were involved with service work, called other members for help, and were almost three times more likely than those less involved to maintain abstinence at 2 years (Majer et al. 2013).

Clinically, I have found people who benefit from 12-step programs are those who do seem to have an all or nothing approach to their use as well as an associated increase in risk-taking behaviors when taking their preferred substance. Although these folks may have some sense of the self-medication benefit of drugs, they also tend to be people, in my experience, who seem to literally change behaviors based on even minor use and for whom use seems particularly compulsive. For example, I recall a friend from college who seemed to become a different person as soon as she started drinking. Further, I remember when we would go to a bar to have a drink, I'd have given my beer minor attention (meaning I'd taken a couple of sips) and she was already on to ordering a second and then third and fourth while I was still finishing my first glass. My friend changed from the first drink, and drinking led her to engage in all kinds of risk-taking behaviors. Though I had grown up in a culture of drinking in rural Minnesota, this behavior was surprising to me. I couldn't imagine having the literal physical capability of drinking alcohol in that way. Since that time, I have noticed that clients who have benefited from 12-step programs have similar patterns. In addition, it's been my clinical observation that people who benefit from 12-step programs are more likely to be alexithymic. Sifneos (1973) and Nemiah (1973) characterized alexithymia as occurring in individuals who lack an emotional language to describe internal mental experiences and states. The main qualities in those who are alexithymic include difficulties identifying and describing feelings, differentiating between emotional and physical sensations, and exhibiting a concrete and externally oriented cognitive style (Zackheim 2007). For people who have traits of alexithymia, what I have found helpful about 12-step programs is that they are particularly good for people who really don't know a lot about their motivations and for whom using their preferred substance is their primary drive. The steps involved, as well as the jargon people learn, strike me as a very good introduction to a psychological language. Many of my clients over the years have participated in 12-step programs while seeing me for in-depth psychotherapy. For clinicians in this position, however, I'd suggest acquainting yourself with the language of 12-step programs or even to attend a 12-step meeting. At the time I got licensed to practice in the state of California, it was a requirement that we attend two 12-step meetings as part of a substance abuse training requirement. This is really an invaluable education that I can't recommend highly enough. For clients involved in 12-step programs, it has been helpful to integrate their cultural language into psychotherapy. For example, one client with a long history of involvement in 12-step programs uses the term "stay in my lane." We use this phrase when he is tempted to externalize his behaviors and minimize his part in his problematic situations.

Harm Reduction

Harm reduction is a framework for addressing substance use and other potentially risky behaviors and aims to reduce the consequences of these behaviors without requiring abstinence. It is an alternative to traditional treatments that require no substance use and extends the reach of treatment to substance users who are unwilling or unable to embrace abstinence (Tatarsky and Marlatt 2010).

Harm reduction was born out of activism in the United States and linked to the criminalization of drug use behaviors which remain differentially enforced among disenfranchised and discriminated groups (Moore and Clear 2012). Methadone maintenance and needle exchange programs were early forms of harm reduction as many of the problems from drug use were related to lifestyle-associated behaviors as well as the route of administration (i.e., needles). Methadone offered a safer form of medication for treating intravenous heroin use (Courtwright et al. 1989). Needle exchange programs were met initially with considerable resistance in the 1980s but have been found to reduce HIV and hepatitis B transmission.

Harm reduction approaches have now been expanded for clinical use with many different substance-using populations. Tatarsky and Marlatt (2010) described the clinical principles of harm reduction, which are as follows (pp. 120–121):

1. Substance use problems are best understood and addressed in the context of the whole person in her social environment.
2. Meet the client as an individual.
3. The client has strengths that can be supported.
4. Challenge stigmatization.
5. Substances are used for adaptive reasons.
6. Drug use falls on a continuum of harmful consequences.
7. Not holding abstinence (or any other preconceived notions) as a precondition of the therapy before really getting to know the individual.
8. Engagement in treatment is the primary goal.
9. Start where the patient is.
10. Look for and mobilize the client's strengths in service of change.
11. Develop a collaborative, empowering relationship with the client.
12. Goals and strategies emerge from the therapeutic process.

As you can see, harm reduction is a flexible and comprehensive approach designed for therapists and emphasizes a connection with the client. In fact, harm reduction may be especially suited for therapies that emphasize the therapeutic relationship. For example, Rothschild (2010) described using harm reduction in modern relational psychoanalytic treatments and notes that "…both harm reduction and relational psychoanalysis are utilized as underlying principles rather than techniques or methods of treatment" (p. 137).

Tatarsky and Kellogg (2010) describe a model of harm reduction psychotherapy that integrates biological, psychoanalytic, cognitive behavioral, and humanistic therapies. They emphasize a negotiated, collaborative therapeutic relationship and a focus on how healing aspects of the therapeutic relationship are. Once clients are willing to change their use behavior, they set goals on what they would like their use to look like (e.g., drinking alcohol only on weekends and no more than three drinks a day on drinking days). With an experimental attitude, clients are encouraged to try different ways to change, while the therapist helps with the teaching of techniques such as urge-surfing, which is a strategy for reflecting on urges and not acting from impulse (Marlatt 1994), reflection, managing triggers, and other behavioral methods. In addition there are a number of workbooks that one can use with clients or that people can buy on their own in order to deal with substance use.

In terms of demonstrated efficacy, it's interesting to note that harm reduction is still relatively new, and the approach is as much philosophy as it is technique. A number of research articles I reviewed address topics regarding its acceptance in the wider chemical dependency treatment community as opposed to clinical trials regarding efficacy. The other difficulty in studying harm reduction is that it is frequently implemented as part of public health programs as part of wider interventions. Additionally, any non-manualized treatment is difficult to study and often conducted in the course of long-term therapies, which are rarely the subject of research. The theory is also not without critics. For example, some believe that harm reduction misleads the substance user who may be addicted and allows for denial of the seriousness of the problem (Dimeff et al. 1999).

Harm reduction does have some demonstrated efficacy in a number of populations, including persons with general illicit drug use (Ritter and Cameron 2006); those who use stimulants and engage in high-risk sexual behavior (Carrico et al. 2014); among college-aged people with self-reported heavy alcohol use (Logan and Marlatt 2010); and among employees when integrated into treatment in employee assistance programs (Osilla et al. 2008).

Motivational Interviewing

It's likely obvious to some that harm reduction involves aspects of motivational interviewing (Logan and Marlatt 2010), which is another popular way of engaging clients in thinking about changing substance use behavior. Motivational interviewing is different in that it is typically supplied as a brief intervention. It also has a wide application, with adaptations of it being used for not only substance abuse and other behaviors that can become problematic (such as gambling) but physical behaviors of all kinds. It has been defined as a client-centered and directive method for enhancing motivation to change by exploring and resolving client ambivalence (Miller and Rollnick 2002).

Motivational interviewing is very focused on the desires and interests of clients and uses aspects of reflective listening and developing discrepancy, which is essentially raising the client's awareness of the negative aspects of substance use. In an adapted version of motivational interviewing, clients are given feedback on their substance use based on assessment and then encouraged to discuss the problem in a nonthreatening manner.

Motivational interviewing has some good success rates for addressing problematic drug and alcohol use. For example, an analysis of 30 studies found reduced excessive drinking by 56% and also reduced drug abuse (Burke et al. 2003). Another review found similar results for people abusing alcohol, though motivational interviewing was less helpful for drinkers diagnosed with alcohol dependence (Vasilaki et al. 2006). A more recent review, however, strikes a more cautious tone. Frost et al. (2018), utilizing strict criteria, including risk of bias, reported that 8 out of 13 studies showed a moderate reduction in excessive drinking and limited data for reduction of other substances.

It's important to note that substance use, specifically when use escalates to dependency, is very difficult to treat. Again for severe substance use disorder, inpatient programs are ideal but even those have relatively limited outcomes. That said, let me describe a case of someone without complex trauma but for whom a combination of motivational interviewing and harm reduction was effective:

Alex was born into a family of successful immigrant parents, and he went to a prestigious college and had a career in finance. He married in his thirties, which was a little later than his parents would have liked, and described his wife as "caring but busy" as they had a 2-year-old son. He admitted that he "partied hard" in college and noted his grades could have been better. He really could not tell me much about his life, other than he came to therapy because his wife was threatening to divorce him over his drinking. He said that he drank daily, and his wife did not seem to mind that. Where things went awry, however, was when he went out with his college buddies. He reported that he would drink 12–15 drinks and that the evenings began with beer but then moved on to the ordering of shots of alcohol in quick succession. On these evenings, he would come home nearly incoherent. He would stumble around and break things and, on a few occasions, urinated in the closet, as he mistook this for the toilet. He approached the therapy in a pragmatic way and said he was open to ideas for addressing his problem. We discussed whether or not he wanted to stop his drinking, and initially he said he was not sure. I asked him what he thought were the downsides of his drinking were. In addition to noting his wife's dissatisfaction, he wondered out loud what some of the physical effects of heavy drinking might be, and we talked about this. As far as what he thought was positive about his drinking, he actually did not describe positive sensations of being drunk. Rather, his excessive drinking seemed very much about connecting with his friends and a fairly concrete idea that drinking was "just what they did." I questioned this in a curious way. I wondered if there were guys in his group that drank as much as he did. He noted that one man also had a young child and he had reduced his drinking. This allowed him to think about whether or not it might be possible to cut down. Therefore, we started by developing ways he could manage his drinking when out with his friends. I suggested he integrate water with his alcohol consumption. Many professionals suggest one glass of water for every drink. He did not want to do that, as it seemed "too obvious," but he agreed to try having at least a couple of glasses of water when he was out with his friends. The other thing I encouraged was that he limit or stop drinking shots at the end of the night, as he identified that this was what really put him "over the edge." Again, he was hesitant, as he did not want to be viewed as different than his friends. I noted that he could talk with the one friend who had begun drinking less and see if he would spend more time with him at that point in the evening—the two of them could stick together. This worked. And he reported that he could go out with his friends without losing control. He decided to continue his daily drinking, though decided it might be helpful to limit this to three drinks a day. This seemed to appease his wife and he left therapy, feeling satisfied.

Alex was not aware of any other reasons to stay in therapy, though I imagined there were many things about his internal life he either was not aware of or had not told me, or both. Nevertheless, it was helpful to use motivational interviewing and harm reduction as tools that could help him get his drinking to a place where it felt more under control.

Conclusion

Treating people with combined cPTSD and substance use requires a great deal of compassion and patience, as well as knowledge of the different models for helping people address their relationships with alcohol and drugs. There is a lot of data that PTSD and substance use overlap and that many people use substances to numb and dissociate. It's important that we let our clients be in control of discussions about their use, and my approach advocates curiosity and neutrality about use.

Interventions for Helping People with Excessive Substance Use

- Evaluate substance use in a casual way and consider assessment as part of treatment. Like all issues for clients with cPTSD, it takes a great deal of time to develop trust and to discuss the extent of problems.
- Discuss what the client likes about their use. Consider if use is designed to promote dissociation.
- For clients who are fine with their use, allow problems with it to come up in a spontaneous way.
- As the client is more able to talk about substance use, ask if they think about what's negative about their use.
- As substance use is often related to anxiety/PTSD, encourage other behaviors that can help, such as exercise, distraction and mindfulness, and social support.
- Motivational interviewing and harm reduction can be easily integrated into any kind of therapy, but it's also worth mentioning the idea of 12-steps programs. I often suggest to clients they simply go to a meeting and see if they like the idea of it.
- Think with clients about triggers for using, as PTSD symptoms are often antecedents, but so are issues in relationships or negative feelings in general. Encourage them to talk about instances in which other people are disappointing or when interactions result in fear.

- Seeking Safety and COPE are newer treatments for both cPTSD and substance use disorders.
- Clinicians can integrate substance use treatment with a variety of different therapeutic approaches by integrating 12-step principles, motivational interviewing, or harm reduction.

References

American Psychiatric Association. (2013). *Diagnostic and statistical manual of mental disorders* (5th ed.). Washington, DC: Author.

Back, S., Dansky, B. S., Coffey, S. F., Saladin, M. E., Sonne, S., & Brady, K. T. (2000). Cocaine dependence with and without post-traumatic stress disorder: A comparison of substance use, trauma history and psychiatric comorbidity. *American Journal on Addictions, 9*(1), 51–62.

Back, S. E., Killeen, T. K., Foa, E. B., Santa Ana, E. J., Gros, D. F., & Brady, K. T. (2012). Use of an integrated therapy with prolonged exposure to treat PTSD and comorbid alcohol dependence in an Iraq veteran. *American Journal of Psychiatry, 169*(7), 688–697.

Back, S. E., Foa, E. B. T. K., Mills, K., Teesson, M., & Carroll, K. (2015). *Concurrent treatment of PTSD and substance use disorders using prolonged exposure (COPE)* (Therapist manual. Treatments that work). New York: Oxford University Press.

Behar, D. (1987). Flashbacks and posttraumatic stress symptoms in combat veterans. *Comprehensive Psychiatry, 28*, 459–466.

Bhalla, I. P., Stefanovics, E. A., & Rosenheck, R. A. (2018). Polysubstance use among veterans in intensive PTSD programs: Association with symptoms and outcomes following treatment. *Journal of Dual Diagnosis, 15*, 36. https://doi.org/10.1080/15504263.2018.1535150. Advance online publication.

Bierut, L. J. (2011). Genetic vulnerability and susceptibility to substance dependence. *Neuron, 69*(4), 618–627.

Bill, W. (2001). *Alcoholics anonymous* (4th ed.). Alcoholics Anonymous World Services. ISBN 1-893007-16-2. OCLC 32014950, United States.

Blanco, C., Xu, Y., Brady, K., Pérez-Fuentesa, G., Okudaa, M., & Wang, S. (2013). Comorbidity of posttraumatic stress disorder with alcohol dependence among US adults: Results from National Epidemiological Survey on alcohol and related conditions. *Drug and Alcohol Dependence, 132*(2013), 630–638.

Brady, K. T., Tuerk, P., Back, S. E., Saladin, M. E., Waldrop, A. E., & Myrick, H. (2009). Combat posttraumatic stress disorder, substance use disorders, and traumatic brain injury. *Journal of Addiction Medicine, 3*(4), 179–188.

Burke, B. L., Arkowitz, H., & Menchola, M. (2003). The efficacy of motivational interviewing: A meta-analysis of controlled clinical trials. *Journal of Consulting and Clinical Psychology, 71*(5), 843–861.

Carrico, A. W., Gifford, E. V., & Moos, R. H. (2007). Spirituality/religiosity promotes acceptance-based responding and 12-step involvement. *Drug and Alcohol Dependence, 89*(1), 66–73.

Carrico, A., Carrico, A. W., Flentje, A., Gruber, V. A., Woods, W. J., Discepola, M. V., et al. (2014). *Community-based harm reduction substance abuse treatment with methamphetamine-using men who have sex with men*. UCSF. Retrieved from https://escholarship.org/uc/item/3r04g63v. Accessed online on 22 Dec 2019.

Coffey, S. F., Saladin, M., Drobes, D. J., Brady, K. T., Dansky, B. S., & Kilpatrick, D. G. (2002). Trauma and substance cue reactivity in individuals with comorbid posttraumatic stress disorder and cocaine or alcohol dependence. *Drug and Alcohol Dependence, 65*(2), 115–127.

Courtwright, D., Joseph, H., & Des Jarlais, D. C. (1989). *Addicts who survived: An oral history of narcotic use in America 1923–1965*. Knoxville: University of Tennessee Press.

Des Jarlais, D. C. (2017). Harm reduction in the USA: The research perspective and an archive to David Purchase. *Harm Reduction Journal, 14*, Article 51.

Dimeff, L. A., Baer, J. S., Kivlahan, D. R., & Marlatt, G. A. (1999). *Brief Alcohol Screening and Intervention for College Students (BASICS): A harm reduction approach*. New York: The Guilford Press.

Ferri, M., Amato, L., Davoli, M. (2006). Alcoholics anonymous and other 12-step programmes for alcohol dependence. *Cochrane Database of Systematic Reviews, 3*. Art. No.: CD005032. https://doi.org/10.1002/14651858.CD005032.pub2.

Flanagan, J. C., Korte, K. J., Killeen, T. K., et al. (2016). *Current Psychiatry Reports 18*, 70. https://doi-org.ucsf.idm.oclc.org/10.1007/s11920-016-0709-y. Accessed online on 22 Dec 2019.

Frost, H., Campbell, P., Maxwell, M., O'Carroll, R. E., Dombrowski, S. U., Williams, B., et al. (2018). Effectiveness of motivational interviewing on adult behaviour change in health and social care settings: A systematic review of reviews. *PLoS One, 13*(10), e0204890. https://doi.org/10.1371/journal.pone.0204890.

Greenberg, J. B., Ameringer, K. J., Trujillo, M. A., Sun, P., Sussman, S., Brightman, M., Pitts, S. R., & Leventhal, A. M. (2012). Associations between posttraumatic stress disorder symptom clusters and cigarette smoking. *Psychology of Addictive Behaviors, 26*(1), 89–98.

Heath, A. C., Bucholz, K. K., Madden, P. A., Dinwiddie, S. H., Slutske, W. S., Bierut, L. J., Statham, D. J., Dunne, M. P., Whitfield, J. B., & Martin, N. G. (1997). Genetic and environmental contributions to alcohol dependence risk in a national twin sample: Consistency of findings in women and men. *Psychological Medicine, 27*, 1381–1396.

Hruska, B., & Delahanty, D. L. (2014). PTSD-SUD biological mechanisms: Self-medication and beyond. In P. Ouimette & J. P. Read (Eds.), *Trauma and substance abuse: Causes, consequences, and treatment of comorbid disorders* (pp. 35–52). Washington, DC: American Psychological Association.

Jacobsen, L. K., Southwick, S. M., Kosten, T. R. (2001). Substance use disorders in patients with posttraumatic stress disorder: A review of the literature. *American Journal of Psychiatry, 158*(8):1184–1190. https://doi.org/10.1176/appi.ajp.158.8.1184.

Kaskutas, L. A. (2009). Alcoholics anonymous effectiveness: Faith meets science. *Journal of Addictive Diseases, 28*(2), 145–157.

Kendler, K. S., Prescott, C. A., Myers, J., & Neale, M. C. (2003). The structure of genetic and environmental risk factors for common psychiatric and substance use disorders in men and women. *Archives of General Psychiatry, 60*, 929–937.

Kesling, B. (2019, December 5). For many soldiers, mental-health issues start before enlistment. *Wall Street Journal*. Accessed online at https://www.wsj.com/articles/for-many-soldiers-mental.

Kessler, R. C., Crum, R. M., Warner, L. A., Nelson, C. B., Schulenberg, J., & Anthony, J. C. (1997). Lifetime co-occurrence of DSM-III-R alcohol abuse and dependence with other psychiatric disorders in the national comorbidity survey. *Archives of General Psychiatry, 54*, 313–321.

Kevorkian, S., Bonn-Miller, M. O., Belendiuk, K., Carney, D. M., Roberson-Nay, R., & Berenz, E. C. (2015). Associations among trauma, posttraumatic stress disorder, cannabis use, and cannabis use disorder in a nationally representative epidemiologic sample. *Psychology of Addictive Behaviors, 29*(3), 633–638.

Khantzian, E. J. (1997). The self-medication hypothesis of substance use disorders: A reconsideration and recent applications. *Harvard Review of Psychiatry, 4*, 231–244.

Kownacki, R. J., & Shadish, W. R. (1999). Does alcoholics anonymous work? The results from a meta-analysis of controlled experiments. *Substance Use & Misuse, 34*(13), 1897–1916.

Kramer, M. D., Polusny, M. A., Arbisi, P. A., & Krueger, R. F. (2014). Comorbidity of PTSD and SUDs: Toward an etiologic understanding. In P. Ouimette & J. P. Read (Eds.), *Trauma and substance abuse: Causes, consequences, and treatment of comorbid disorders* (pp. 53–75). Washington, DC: American Psychological Association.

Kulka, R. A., Schlenger, W. E., Fairbank, J. A., Hough, R. L., Jordan, B. K., Marmar, C. R., & Weiss, D. S. (1990). *Trauma and the Vietnam War generation: Report of findings from the National Vietnam Veterans Readjustment Study*. New York: Brunner/Mazel.

Lee, W. K., Hayashi, K., DeBeck, K., Milloy, M. J. S., Grant, C., et al. (2019). Association between posttraumatic stress disorder and nonfatal drug overdose. *Psychological Trauma: Theory, Research, Practice, and Policy*. Advance online publication. Accessed on 6th Dec 2019 at https://doi.org/10.1037/tra0000511.

Lenz, S. A., Henesy, R., & Callender, K. (2016). Effectiveness of seeking safety for co-occurring posttraumatic stress disorder and substance use. *Journal of Counseling and Development*. Accessed online on 18th Dec 2019 at https://doi.org/10.1002/jcad.12061.

Li, M. D. (2006). The genetics of nicotine dependence. *Current Psychiatry Reports, 8*, 158–164.

Logan, D. E., & Marlatt, G. A. (2010). Harm reduction therapy: A practice-friendly review of research. *Journal of Clinical Psychology, 66*(2), 201–214.

Majer, J. M., Jason, L. A., Aase, D. M., Droege, J. R., & Ferrari, J. R. (2013). Categorical 12-step involvement and continuous abstinence at 2 years. *Journal of Substance Abuse Treatment, 44*(1), 46–51.

Marlatt, G. A. (1994). Addiction, mindfulness, and acceptance. In S. C. Hayes, N. S. Jacobson, V. M. Follette, & M. J. Dougher (Eds.), *Acceptance and change: Content and context in psychotherapy* (pp. 175–197). Reno: Context Press.

McLeod, D. S., Koenen, K. C., Meyer, J. M., Lyons, M. J., Eisen, S., True, W., et al. (2001). Genetic and environmental influences on the relationship among combat exposure, posttraumatic stress disorder symptoms, and alcohol use. *Journal of Traumatic Stress, 14*, 259–275.

Miller, W. R., & Rollnick, S. (2002). Motivational interviewing. In *Preparing people to change* (2nd ed.). New York: The Guilford Press.

Mills, K. L., Teesson, M., Back, S. E., et al. (2012). Integrated exposure-based therapy for co-occurring posttraumatic stress disorder and substance dependence: A randomized controlled trial. *Journal of the American Medical Association, 308*(7), 690–699.

Moore, L., & Clear, A. (2012). History and context of harm reduction in the United States. In R. Pates & D. Riley (Eds.), *Harm reduction in substance use and high-risk behaviour: International policy and practice* (pp. 370–381). Chichester: Wiley-Blackwell.

Najavits, L. M. (2002). *Guilford substance abuse series. Seeking safety: A treatment manual for PTSD and substance abuse*. New York: Guilford Press.

Najavits, L. M. (2007). Seeking safety: An evidence-based model for substance abuse and trauma/PTSD. In K. A. Witkiewitz & G. A. Marlatt (Eds.), *Practical resources for the mental health professional. Therapist's guide to evidence-based relapse prevention* (pp. 141–167). San Diego: Elsevier Academic Press. https://doi.org/10.1016/B978-012369429-4/50037-9.

Najavits, L. M., & Hien, D. (2013). Helping vulnerable populations: A comprehensive review of the treatment outcome literature on substance use disorder and PTSD. *Journal of Clinical Psychology, 69*(5), 433–479.

Najavits, L. M., & Walsh, M. (2012). Dissociation, PTSD, and substance abuse: An empirical study. *Journal of Trauma & Dissociation, 13*(1), 115–126.

Najavits, L. M., Weiss, R. D., & Shaw, S. R. (1997). The link between substance abuse and posttraumatic stress disorder in women: A research review. *American Journal on Addictions, 6*, 273–283.

Nemiah, J. C. (1973). Psychology and psychosomatic illness: Reflections on theory and research methodology. *Psychotherapy and Psychosomatics, 22*, 106–111.

Norman, S. B., Trim, R., Haller, M., Davis, B. C., Myers, U. S., Colvonen, P. J., Blanes, E., Lyons, R., Siegel, E. Y., Angkaw, A. C., Norman, G. J., & Mayes, T. (2019). Efficacy of integrated exposure therapy vs integrated coping skills therapy for comorbid posttraumatic stress disorder and alcohol use disorder: A randomized clinical trial. *JAMA Psychiatry, 76*(8), 791–799. https://doi.org/10.1001/jamapsychiatry.2019.0638.

Osilla, K. C., Zellmer, M. S., Larimer, M. E., Neighbors, C., & Marlatt, G. A. (2008). A brief intervention for at-risk drinking in an employee assistance program. *Journal of Studies on Alcohol and Drugs, 69*, 14–20.

Pietrzak, R. H., Goldstein, R. B., Southwick, S. M., & Grant, B. F. (2011). Prevalence and Axis I comorbidity of full and partial posttraumatic stress disorder in the United States: Results from

Wave 2 of the National Epidemiologic Survey on Alcohol and Related Conditions. *Journal of Anxiety Disorders, 25*, 456–465.

Ritter, A., & Cameron, J. (2006). A review of the efficacy and effectiveness of harm reduction strategies for alcohol, tobacco and illicit drugs. *Drug and Alcohol Review, 25*(6), 611–624.

Roesler, T. A., & Dafler, C. E. (1993). Chemical dissociation in adults sexually victimized as children: Alcohol and drug use in adult survivors. *Journal of Substance Abuse Treatment, 10*, 537–543.

Rothschild, D. (2010). Partners in treatment: Relational psychoanalysis and harm reduction therapy. *Journal of Clinical Psychology, 66*(2), 136–149.

Saladin, M. E., Brady, K. T., Dansky, B. S., & Kilpatrick, D. G. (1995). Understanding comorbidity between PTSD and substance use disorders: Two preliminary investigations. *Addictive Behaviors, 20*, 643–655.

Seal, K. H., Cohen, G., Waldrop, A., Cohen, B. E., Maguen, S., & Ren, L. (2011). Substance use disorders in Iraq and Afghanistan veterans in VA healthcare, 2001–2010: Implications for screening, diagnosis and treatment. *Drug and Alcohol Dependence, 116*(1–3), 93–101.

Shedler, J. (2012). The efficacy of psychodynamic psychotherapy. In R. A. Levy, J. S. Ablon, & H. Kächele (Eds.), *Psychodynamic psychotherapy research: Evidence-based practice and practice-based evidence* (pp. 9–25). Totowa: Humana Press/Springer.

Sifneos, P. E. (1973). The prevalence of "alexithymic" characteristics in psychosomatic patients. *Psychotherapy and Psychosomatics, 22*(2), 255–262.

Stephens, M. A., & Wand, G. (2012). Stress and the HPA axis: Role of glucocorticoids in alcohol dependence. *Alcohol Research: Current Reviews, 34*(4), 468–483.

Stewart, S. H., & Conrod, P. J. (2003). Psychosocial models of functional associations between posttraumatic stress disorder and substance use disorder. In *Trauma and substance abuse: Causes, consequences, and treatment of comorbid disorders*. Washington, DC: American Psychological Association.

Tatarsky, A., & Kellogg, S. (2010). Integrative harm reduction psychotherapy: A case of substance use, multiple trauma, and suicidality. *Journal of Clinical Psychology, 66*(2), 123–135.

Tatarsky, A., & Marlatt, G. A. (2010). State of the art in harm reduction psychotherapy: An emerging treatment for substance misuse. *Journal of Clinical Psychology, 66*(2), 117–122.

Tsuang, M. T., Lyons, M. J., Meyer, J. M., Doyle, T., Eisen, S. A., Goldberg, J., True, W., Lin, N., Toomey, R., & Eaves, L. (1998). Co-occurrence of abuse of different drugs in men: The role of drug-specific and shared vulnerabilities. *Archives of General Psychiatry, 55*, 967–972.

Ullman, S. E., Filipas, H. H., Townsend, S. M., & Starzynski, L. L. (2006). Correlates of comorbid PTSD and drinking problems among sexual assault survivors. *Addictive Behaviors, 31*(1), 128–132.

Vasilaki, E. I., Hosier, S. G., & Cox, W. M. (2006). The efficacy of motivational interviewing as a brief intervention for excessive drinking: A meta-analytic review. *Alcohol and Alcoholism, 41*(3), 328–335.

Vest, N. A., & Tragesser, S. (2019). Coping motives mediate the relationship between borderline personality features and alcohol, cannabis, and prescription opioid use disorder symptomatology in a substance use disorder treatment sample. *Personality Disorders: Theory, Research, and Treatment*. https://doi.org/10.1037/per0000385. Advance online publication.

Woolf, S. H., & Schoomaker, H. (2019). Life expectancy and mortality rates in the United States, 1959-2017. *Journal of the American Medical Association, 322*(20), 1996–2016.

Xian, H., Chantarujikapong, S. I., Scherrer, J. F., Eisen, S. A., Lyons, M. J., Goldberg, J., et al. (2000). Genetic and environmental influences on posttraumatic stress disorder, alcohol and drug dependence in twin pairs. *Drug and Alcohol Dependence, 61*, 95–102.

Zackheim, L. (2007). Alexithymia: Expanding the realm of research. *Journal of Psychosomatic Research, 63*, 345–347.

Chapter 7
When Trauma Is in the Body: Managing Physical Concerns

Effects of Trauma on the Body

Many people who have histories of complex trauma have the chaos of their childhoods living in their bodies in that they are more likely to have or develop a number of physical problems. Historically, some clinicians have left the body out of treatment or worse, labeled people with illnesses that are hard to explain as "psychosomatic." We now know that a number of psychological states as well as adverse child events impact the body in a number of physiological ways. I'll discuss this research as it makes it clear that both the mind and the body are injured as a result of chronic trauma. Because of this, some of our clients are harder to reach because they are plagued by physical concerns. Such clients come to therapy either reluctantly or with some aim to feel better, but not necessarily curious about how their psychology could be exacerbating their symptoms. As therapists, we can feel overwhelmed and unclear if we can help. Consider the case of Lisa as an introduction:

Lisa entered an inpatient chronic pain program where I saw her as part of her multidisciplinary treatment. She had just turned 30 and had unrelenting back pain for the last 2 years, which kept her from working. She had lost her mother approximately 2 years ago due to breast cancer and also became engaged around that time. Lisa cared for her mother in the last 6 months of her life. Lisa had no history of health problems, but by the time I met her, she was debilitated by low back pain (though an organic finding regarding her pain had not been found), a possible diagnosis of fibromyalgia, and a fair amount of narcotic use, which was deemed to be excessive. Lisa described a curious story of the onset of her pain. She reported that after the death of her mother and after she had become engaged, she had taken a road trip to see her fiancé, who resided in another state at the time. It was during this trip she reported she had been on a "rough road" and "went over several bumps." Ultimately, something "snapped" in her back. She said despite multiple procedures and medications, nothing helped. It sounded as if she spent the last 2 years feeling miserable. Despite this, she resented being in the chronic pain program and had

T. M. Greenberg, *Treating Complex Trauma*,
https://doi.org/10.1007/978-3-030-45285-8_7

nothing to say to anyone on the multidisciplinary team, except the physician. When I met with her, she was not overtly resentful but rather very physically oriented in her remarks, almost as if she had no access to her mind at all. As she told her story of the onset of her illness, her comments begged for a symbolic and metaphorical understanding of possible feelings and anxieties, and she remained convinced that a psychological understanding of any kind was not useful to her.

Anyone who has worked in multidisciplinary treatment settings recognizes Lisa as someone who is forced to meet with a mental health professional but genuinely sees the encounter as obligatory. It can be hard to reach people like Lisa, but one approach that I try (and is a common method in chronic pain programs) is to acknowledge that symptoms are real even if psychological interventions help. Additionally, providing factual information regarding the autonomic nervous system or the "fight/flight" response can sometimes help make people less wary of psychological services. This kind of education is also the foundation of cognitive behavioral (CBT) treatments for some physical illnesses and chronic pain and warrants brief explanation. The term "fight or flight" was coined by Walter Bradford Cannon in the early twentieth century and has served as a foundation of understanding how our basic evolution leads us to be primed not only to appraise stress as a bodily threat but also to react in a physical way that may interfere with homeostasis (Cannon 1915; Fink 2009). It has been long known that anxiety, or fear, in particular, can cause a number of changes in the body—including increased heart rate, acid production in the stomach, and increased muscle tension. And the latter amplifies the sensation of pain. In the 1930s, Hans Selye described the condition of general adaptation syndrome and noticed how a number of people presented with common nonspecific physical symptoms in response to stress (Chrousos and Gold 1992; Selye 1936/1998). Again, thinking in this way about how stress can physically exacerbate physical symptoms is the foundation of treatments developed primarily by health psychology researchers over the last 60 years.

And though this basic understanding of how the mind and the body interact has been known to researchers for decades, current data (described below) provide a more clear understanding of how the mind and the body are connected and how chronic stress can alter basic responses of the neuroendocrine system and render people vulnerable to a variety of illnesses, particularly those that are often cast in the light of having more psychological influence.

A number of illnesses that had been previously referred to as being caused by one's mind are actually highly influenced by physical susceptibilities and early stress related to abuse, neglect, and other adverse events. Several physical problems are now understood to be a result of a complicated interplay of psychology, neurophysiology, altered gene expression, and the havoc stress hormones bring to bear on the body in those that seem biologically vulnerable. This research is daunting, and it can be hard not to feel that there is little we can do to help the beleaguered bodies of some of our clients. However, there are some symptoms and illnesses that do seem to be especially helped with psychological treatment and thus imply (though we can never really know for sure) the primary influence of stress and emotional factors. It's reasonable to assume that in all matters involving physical complaints, there is a complex feedback loop in which the body and emotions activate each other. It may be the case that some illnesses are particularly sensitive to stress and that some people are biologically vulnerable to become ill when faced with emotional challenges. However, no matter the disease, there is a preponderance of evidence that psychological intervention helps to reduce healthcare visits and procedures and that some people actually do feel better, with a reduction in physical symptoms, when involved in psychotherapy. However, as we'll see later in this chapter, no matter the therapeutic modality used, longer-term approaches work much better than short-term approaches. Although we can't undo what has resulted from trauma, relationships can be soothing and regulating and can teach people they don't have to live in fear or be alone with negative emotions. A primary goal in all therapies is to help people find others in their lives who make them feel safe. In addition, psychotherapy is an important relationship and, particularly when it is long term, can provide an important reparative emotional experience. As we'll see, people in healthy relationships may be protected from the development or worsening of some illnesses. In contrast, conflictual relationships are associated with the development of or exacerbation of some medical illnesses.

Links Between Childhood Adversity and Physical Illness

As I've stated, people who experience child abuse, neglect, and stressful life circumstances in childhood are more likely to have a number of physical problems. There are a few ways to consider this research and the mechanisms associated with the findings. First, early childhood adversity results in changes to the immune system via the hypothalamic–pituitary–adrenal axis as I've described in previous chapters. Second is the pathway linked with health behaviors. As we saw in the chapter on substance abuse, people with trauma histories are more likely to use substances that can cause physical problems. Third, there are changes in the expression of genes related to environmental stress as I discussed in Chapter 2. Finally, trauma and subsequent stress (via enhanced arousal and negative emotions) appear to impact telomere length, which may be associated with illness (Glei et al. 2016).

The most well-known study on child maltreatment and medical illness was conducted by Felitti et al. (1998) and was based on survey responses from 9508 people from Kaiser Permanente's San Diego Health Appraisal Clinic. This was a groundbreaking study not only because of the results; its novel approach to evaluating trauma and adverse childhood experiences seemed to open the door for research on trauma and physical health. The adverse childhood experience questionnaire, known now by the acronym, ACE-Q, developed by Felitti and his colleagues is now widely used in research that studies the effects of childhood maltreatment in adults. The advantage of this scale is that it covers a wide range of difficulties children may experience beyond neglect and physical and sexual abuse. Felitti (1998) and his colleagues found in a large sample of adults that adverse childhood experiences or ACEs (which included physical, psychological, sexual abuse, violence in the home, a mentally ill or suicidal family member, or someone in the household abusing substances) were associated with not only an increase in psychological problems but also increased health risk behaviors and medical illness. The more adverse events respondents reported, the more likely they were to have medical problems that included heart disease, cancer, chronic bronchitis, chronic obstructive pulmonary disease, liver disease, and skeletal fractures. Regarding the relationship between increased incidence of liver disease and adverse childhood experiences, a follow-up publication to the Felitti et al. study found that high-risk behaviors (such as substance use, intravenous drug use, over 50 sexual partners, and other high-risk sexual behaviors) were associated with an increase in illnesses affecting the liver. Again the more adverse childhood experiences reported, the more likely were people to engage in high-risk behaviors (Dong et al. 2003). This data has since been replicated and expanded beyond just liver disease. For example, Campbell et al. (2016) found that four or more ACEs increased the likelihood of binge or heavy drinking, smoking, risky HIV behavior, diabetes, heart attack, coronary heart disease, stroke, depression, disability caused by health problems, and use of special equipment because of disability. The data described in the last chapter on substance use and trauma fits neatly with the health behavior part of the trauma and illness link.

It's not only risky behaviors that explain these findings. In another follow-up study to the Felitti et al. data, it was found that health behaviors, depression, and anger were associated with the development of heart disease (Dong et al. 2004). This is consistent with data from the last 25 years—depression and anger (especially hostility and cynical mistrust) are linked with heart disease and this has been demonstrated in multiple studies (e.g., Frasure-Smith et al. 1993; Barefoot et al. 2000; Rutledge et al. 2006; Myrtek 2001; Smith et al. 2004).

And though depression and anger are commonly seen in people with trauma histories, again, these factors don't tell the whole story. Researchers at Yale University found that women who reported abuse or neglect as children had an almost ninefold increase in cardiovascular disease; however, depression did not explain the increased prevalence of heart disease in these women (Batten et al. 2004). Additionally, a more recent study that looked at older adults found that childhood adversity was associated with an increased risk of cardiovascular disease, lung disease, asthma, as well as a number of psychiatric disorders (McCrory et al. 2015). Both socioeconomic factors and health behaviors did not explain these findings.

Though research has demonstrated inconsistent findings, a review found physical and psychological victimization were associated with risk of any cancer in five studies and significant associations with regard to sexual abuse victimization in two studies (Holman et al. 2016).

Regarding studies of people diagnosed with PTSD or likely cPTSD, there is a very high incidence of chronic pain (Fishbain et al. 2017). A study of over 4000 Vietnam veterans (who often have repetitive complex trauma histories) found that those who met diagnostic criteria for PTSD were twice as likely to die from heart disease as those without PTSD (Boscarino 2008). Additionally, veterans with PTSD were more likely to have metabolic syndrome, which is a risk factor for heart disease and diabetes (Heppner et al. 2009). A study that specifically looked at the presence of traumatic events and subsequent PTSD in women found that both a history of traumatic events and the presence of four or more PTSD symptoms predicted cardiovascular disease (Sumner et al. 2015).

Proposed Mechanisms Explaining the Trauma-Illness Connection

Although the possibilities are numerous as to what might further explain the relationship of child abuse and disease, a study found that childhood maltreatment predicts adult multi-organ inflammation, which is thought to be connected to a variety of maladies, including heart disease, and many chronic diseases (Danese et al. 2007; Pahwa et al. 2019). Another study found links between child abuse and biological markers of increased inflammation, in particular, C-reactive protein (Baumeister et al. 2015).

In a review article by Lohr et al. (2015) on the physical effects of PTSD, it was reported that people with PTSD had reduced telomere length and, thus, accelerated aging. Telomeres are protective caps on the end of DNA strands on chromosomes and become shorter as people age. These authors also reported a link between PTSD and higher inflammation markers and that people in the study had higher rates of aging-related conditions such as heart disease, type 2 diabetes, dementia, and ulcers. They also found a mild-to-moderate association between PTSD and premature death.

Complex PTSD and all of the intense emotional states that are part of it are just bad for the body. As I've described in previous chapters, HPA-axis dysfunction is implicated in neurological and other physical changes in response to trauma. It is thought that the susceptibility to HPA-axis stress is in part related to heredity (Nicolaides et al. 2015). Yet, it does seem that our childhoods and the level of safety provided at this crucial time may be related to how resilient our ability to manage stress is and how robust our individual HPA-axis systems are (Kalmakis et al. 2015). In the study conducted by the aforementioned authors, chronic adverse childhood experiences led to HPA-axis dysfunction in the form of reduced cortisol levels, which may make us susceptible to illness later in life. For example, low cortisol is implicated in the development of chronic fatigue syndrome (Papadopoulos and Cleare 2012), endometriosis, and chronic pelvic pain (Petrelluzzi et al. 2008). Dysfunctional reactions of the glucocorticoid system (though not necessarily low cortisol) are thought to be associated with fibromyalgia (Geiss et al. 2012). Additionally, the effects of HPA-axis dysfunction are also thought to predispose people to asthma, eczema, migraines, and a number of gastrointestinal symptoms (Nicolaides et al. 2015). Kempke et al. (2015) found that people with chronic fatigue syndrome and histories of emotional neglect were more likely to have disrupted cortisol and HPA-axis functioning. Whether it is too low or high, cortisol seems to be an important endpoint in an overworked HPA-axis system.

Relationships and the Buffer Against Illness

Although the above research is daunting, it's important to remember that good relationships can provide a protective buffer against the psychological and physical hits from traumatic experiences. Before I describe some of the research that supports this, let's consider a case example of someone I'll call Ruth.

Ruth was in her mid-50s and saw me 2 years after she had been diagnosed and treated for breast cancer. She had a very mild case and needed only a lumpectomy. Yet, she was very disturbed about her diagnosis, and she worried that her occasional martinis with friends might have contributed to her illness. What really pulled her to seek therapy, however, was that she had developed a number of physical symptoms 6 months after her surgery. She had become achy all over and felt tired all of the time. She also had frequent headaches and this was new for her as well. She was really worried she had another malignancy, but her doctors assured her she was fine. Eventually, she sought the help of a rheumatologist who told her she had fibromyalgia. When we met she was unable to tell me much about her history. She had been married for over two decades and had teenage daughters but assured me that her life was fine outside of her medical issues. She and her husband also had very successful careers. They were also very wealthy, which she felt the need to tell me right away and often. As far as her background, she alluded to a very difficult childhood, and a rape in college, but again said there was nothing really that "important or interesting" about her history. She wanted to talk about how to manage her symptoms and said she hoped her time with me would be short term.

From health psychology and pain management standpoint, it's important to assess social relationships as they are an extremely important part of helping clients cope. At least that's what the teaching says. Yet, many clients like Ruth see no point in talking about relationships, other than a matter-of-fact agreement that they have "social support." This concept is not foreign to them, as physicians have learned to ask patients with pain about their social support as a way of coping. To them, at least in the beginning of therapy, nothing really matters that is outside of their body. I'll describe how I work with clients like Ruth when I discuss treatment, but thinking about current relationships for people who have medical conditions can help us understand situations that might contribute to stress that exacerbates illness symptoms. And with the right initial interventions, we can eventually talk about them and make them a focus of therapy. This is because while some CBT interventions can help people who are troubled by their bodies, the most robust data on coping has to do with the kinds of meaningful relational support clients like Ruth receive.

The data on relationships and health can be summed up as such: good relationships are protective and can improve health; negative and conflictual relationships are bad for the body. When I was in training in the early 1990s, I was taught to emphasize social support as a main intervention to improve coping for people with physical symptoms. Yet, it wasn't until several years later that research began to focus and expand on the quality of social support. Before there was much data on this, I remember being in hospital rooms and seeing people who clearly had unhappy relationships with spouses or other family members. I recall thinking that I was not sure how to emphasize support; at times it was clear patients did not want to be anywhere near their families! In some cases people had many more symptoms when so-called close support persons were around. I learned then the importance of helping people choose whom they wanted around them when they were ill and to set limits and boundaries with those that seemed to make them feel worse. While there are health risks associated with social isolation, negative relationships appear to be literally toxic in some cases.

Marital cohesion is associated with lower systolic blood pressure (Tobe et al. 2007). In general, marriage is protective against heart disease, especially for men. Even in men who are anxious (which is a risk factor for heart disease), marriage has been found to serve as a protective factor against heart attacks (Shen et al. 2008). Though this latter finding is encouraging, women are more sensitive to the effects of romantic relationships as women may be more attuned to emotional quality in relationships than men (Gerson and Gerson 2012; Wanic and Kulik 2011). In a study of women who had been maltreated as children and thus at risk for both mental and physical health problems, researchers found that having safe and nurturing romantic relationships in adulthood was associated with reductions in rates of depression and better overall health and lower rates of sleep problems when compared with women who had histories of abuse but did not report safe romantic relationships at the time of the study (Jaffee et al. 2017). This study demonstrates what researches refer to as the "buffering" effect of social relationships. The buffering hypothesis suggests that social relationships may provide concrete or emotional resources that promote more positive health behaviors or more adaptive neuroendocrine responses to stressful events via the HPA-axis. The support from social relationships moderates or buffers the deleterious influence of stressors on health and relates to both real and perceived support (Cohen 2004). Again, the right kind of support matters. People need to feel safe in order to benefit from social support. In another study that looked at research involving 308,849 individuals, followed for an average of 7.5 years, people with adequate social relationships had a 50% greater likelihood of survival (lower risk of death) compared to those with poor or insufficient social relationships, and the results were stronger the more enhanced and socially integrated the relationships were (Holt-Lunstad et al. 2010). An example of socially integrated support might be someone who volunteers, but instead of showing up and not having much contact with others where they are volunteering, they have relationships and connections with people who care about how they are. In other words, they have relationships that are not just superficial. In people with irritable bowel syndrome (IBS), relationships with partners and family that were supportive were associated with fewer symptoms (Gerson et al. 2006). Additionally, a major finding in regard to pain research found that the presence of close attachment figures not only reduced the sensation of pain but activated a neural region of the brain that is associated with a sense of safety (Eisenberger et al. 2011).

And while good relationships provide a buffer against illness, negative and conflictual relationships increase health risks. Research has found that poor-quality or unhappy relationships have a higher negative influence on physical health, particularly cardiovascular disease (Robles et al. 2014). Another study found that conflictual marital relationships were associated with an increase in heart disease, especially among men and women in lower socioeconomic groups (De Vogli et al. 2007). Persons in poor marriages have an increased risk of periodontal disease, which is thought to increase the risk of heart disease (Amabile et al. 2008; Kiecolt-Glaser and Newton 2001). These latter researchers also found that people who reported poor marital quality also had increases in reports of pain. Hostile romantic partnerships are associated with reports of being less healthy overall as well as increased symptoms in those with rheumatoid arthritis (Kiecolt-Glaser and Newton 2001; Zautra et al. 1998).

Research on the Decrease of Physical Symptoms in Therapy

Much (though not all) of the research looking at a decrease in symptoms from psychotherapy has taken place among people who have physical symptoms without demonstrated medical findings. In more severe cases, this used to be referred to as somatoform disorder and more generally in clinical jargon as somatization. The DSM-V (APA 2013) refers to an excessive preoccupation with physical symptoms that interferes with functioning as somatic symptom disorder.

In a study by Altmann et al. (2018) that took place in Germany, patients who were in either cognitive behavioral therapy (CBT), psychodynamic therapy, or psychoanalytic therapy showed reduced symptoms of depression, anxiety, stress, and what the authors termed as somatization—defined as physical complaints including back pain, headaches, stomach pain, dizziness, generalized pain, shortness of breath, and gastrointestinal distress. All groups showed improvement in physical symptoms and had fewer missed days of work. It should be noted that CBT in Germany usually involves 45–80 sessions; while psychodynamic therapy, considered shorter term than psychoanalytic therapy, is about 80 sessions, psychoanalytic therapy is up to 240 sessions. This is obviously a very different model than we have in the United States but supports that longer-term therapy reduces physical complaints and emotional symptoms. It also bolsters what I described in Chapter 1; all therapies have roughly the same efficacy rates, and the relationship with the therapist is the most important outcome variable. Certainly in the case of the German study, people in all three groups developed longer-term relationships with their therapists. In contrast, in a review of studies using very strict criteria and involving a very limited number of sessions (up to 13), CBT was found to have a small effect on the reduction of symptoms among people who have somatoform disorders (van Dessel et al. 2014). Similar results have been found in other reviews (e.g., Kleinstäuber et al. 2011). In fact, according to three reviews published in the Cochrane database, which has very strict methods and criteria, there was no evidence that short-term CBT treatments provide reduced pain complaints among people with neuropathic pain (Eccleston et al. 2015) and evidence for just small amounts of symptom reduction in people who have multiple sclerosis or fibromyalgia (Young and Khan 2018; Theadom et al. 2015)

Abbass et al. (2009) looked at 23 studies of over 1800 medically ill patients with illnesses as diverse as heart disease, musculoskeletal illnesses, and even dermatological diseases. The study found psychodynamic therapy to be effective not only for psychological symptoms but for physical symptoms as well. Incredibly, in studies that reported data on healthcare utilization, there was a 77.8% reduction in medical visits among those who had been in a psychodynamic therapy. Since psychodynamic treatments provide longer-term therapies, this may account in part for the reduction in symptoms.

There also may be a connection between expressing trauma-related events through writing and health. Researchers found that healthy college students who write about traumatic events have stronger immune functioning, visit university health clinics less frequently, and experience greater subjective well-being compared with a control group that were instructed to write about superficial topics (Pennebaker et al. 1988). In people with asthma or rheumatoid arthritis, about half of people who wrote about traumatic events had significant improvement in lung function among asthma patients and improvement in illness as blindly rated by a physician in the case of the patients with rheumatoid arthritis (Smyth et al. 1999).

Treating People Who Are Somatically Focused

I think many of us in the field are appropriately nervous about labeling any illness as purely psychosomatic. It seems prudent to try to hold the idea in mind that every illness has both psychological and physical contributions. What matters most is not the cause but what works to alleviate symptoms. Additionally, as I've already suggested, it's crucial that we treat all symptoms as real. This is not only a therapeutic strategy to encourage engagement in therapy. I've seen many people throughout my career who have been told by many doctors that symptoms are "all in their heads" only to find that they have a physical illness that can be treated. I recall one man I treated who developed severe depression because of vision problems. He saw several specialists across the country who told him there was nothing wrong with his eyes. He felt crazy, thought he was *going crazy* until he saw a vestibular physical therapist who correctly diagnosed his problem and literally cured him within a couple of months. Such situations have been humbling for me. However, this does lead to a major clinical issue among our clients who have physical problems and are still looking for concrete fixes. For every client I have seen who has found an answer to their physical dilemmas and been able to get treated, I have seen as many who go down the rabbit hole of questionable or even dubious treatment methods that have no effect or, worse, cause a great deal of physical harm. Therefore, it is important that we can think with clients about how much they want to spend (in time, money, and iatrogenic medical risks) looking for a solution. I try to think with people about the risks and benefits of various treatments and encourage them to really consider what they are putting their body through. Additionally, I explain that at some point, most people (particularly those with chronic pain) decide they need to function on coping and healing with tools they can learn through therapy and managing stress associated with relationships. As I've described previously (Greenberg 2012), it can be disempowering and even debilitating to expect that physicians have all of the answers. Dealing with people who have complicated and not well-understood medical problems requires us to proceed with a sense of balance and the recognition that we, as well as our clients, may not ever really understand the complex interplay of the mind and the body. That said, there are some people who respond to stress with various physical complaints, but even in these situations, I always keep in mind that certain people likely have a biological predisposition to manifest stress in a physical way.

In older health psychology research, pessimism, passivity, and learned helplessness were thought to be associated with increased likelihood of illness of all kinds (Peterson and Seligman 1987). These authors note that passivity might be linked with not caring about one's health or feeling that seeing a doctor, for example, could do little to improve health. Therefore, a main goal in therapy for people who are somatically focused is to help people see where they do have control over their symptoms. To be clear, this is not meant as an indirect way of suggesting that symptoms are psychosomatic. I tend to stay away from that discussion, and I always emphasize that the mind and the body are impacted by one another. In fact, I emphasize that stress and anxiety are physical symptoms. This tends to be helpful as people aware of stress or anxiety often feel ashamed about this and worry they are causing their symptoms.

In the majority of cases, I begin treatment with people who are somatically focused by starting with more directive and concrete interventions and education about the body. This is usually in the form of modified CBT techniques, with an emphasis on behavioral approaches to reduce physical symptoms. Although I described earlier that there is not an overwhelming amount of evidence that short-term CBT approaches help with some medical symptoms, I use them in the context of developing a relationship with the client, and I explain that treating issues related to physical functioning can take a long time. I suggest CBT approaches using a framework that these ideas may help with some aspects of their symptoms and that it can be helpful to start with concrete interventions, especially if they work and can offer some quick relief. However, before doing any kind of CBT work with clients, it's important to evaluate the extent to which they feel that they are willing to try to see if they can get some control over symptoms. Further, it's extremely important to find out if clients link stress of any kind with their symptoms. If not, the buy-in regarding CBT can be limited. That said, if I can, I explain the fight/flight response and note that physical symptoms, especially pain, can cause a reaction that can seem just like anxiety. Additionally, pain is worse if the body is tense. If someone is willing, I teach them diaphragmatic breathing with an emphasis that it's a natural tool to help with physical symptoms because muscle tension makes pain worse. Another key approach that can work for people in pain is the idea of pacing. Pacing is essentially a strategy to moderate activities and to know when to slow down. People with chronic illnesses often try to do too much when they are feeling well (having a "good day") only to feel worse, often with increased pain or symptoms the next day.

I rarely encourage (and definitely never require) formal homework, unless someone asks for it. Some people who tend to be more focused on their bodies are generally less aware of what is going on in their minds. I don't mean this in a critical sense at all. In fact, the reason I originally became interested in health psychology is that early in my career I noticed that people who sought therapy for medical problems had never been in therapy before. Most felt they simply had never needed it. I didn't assume that they must have needed therapy before and did not receive it; instead I surmised that whatever they were doing before worked for them. In many cases, as we will see with Ruth, they simply kept themselves busy. I've described this in previous writing as a kind of "manic" defense (Greenberg 2012, 2016). However, I don't think of this as clinical mania. Rather, it's a process or style of functioning geared toward keeping oneself distracted from painful emotional material. Avoiding therapy and not thinking about past traumatic events can work when one is not inhibited from using the body as a distraction. This is often adaptive and leads to success in many cultures. However, when the body stops working, there is a need for increased reliance on the mind in part because people cannot sustain constant activity. I'll describe how this impacted Ruth.

In the first several sessions with Ruth, she wanted to know what to "do" about her pain and discomfort. She wanted the focus to be just on her body. The paradox of this was that she wasn't sure therapy could help at all but came at the urging of her doctor. Therefore in the first few sessions, we discussed behavioral ways she could manage her symptoms. I explained to her that although she can't control some aspects of her body, it helps to focus on factors she can control. We discussed exercise, mindfulness approaches, and strategies for sleeping better. When I suggested pacing, she clearly got anxious and was hesitant. Ruth did not know how to slow down, and she certainly did not want to, no matter the price her body paid. It was at that point I was able to ask what her life was like before she got cancer, as she felt "everything had fallen apart"(though she consciously meant physically) since her cancer diagnosis. She said that she was thinking about leaving her husband as she had met someone else with whom she had begun an affair. When she was diagnosed with cancer, she assumed this was her "punishment," and she broke things off with this other man. The next session she came in telling me that her affair was not that big of a deal and that she and her husband were fine. She also said she had read about catastrophizing online and said she wanted to talk about that. We then did discuss how people in pain can assume from the moment something starts to hurt that the pain may ruin their day or assume that they will have a pain flair that will keep them from functioning. Ruth became extremely anxious and said, "Yeah, I know I do that." "I think it's better if you just tell me what to do." At that point, I tried to check in on how she was managing some of her behaviors we had talked about, and then she became frustrated and said, "I'm not stupid. I already know all of this stuff." I felt both flustered and annoyed. I then said, "You're right. Some of these strategies do seem straightforward, particularly for people who read a lot and are highly educated. So the dilemma for me is that you are obviously super smart and I can try to tell you things you may already know, but also there is a great deal of research on how relationships can impact people with pain and medical problems, and while I don't know a ton about your situation, it does seem like you may have some things that might be good to talk about. I've certainly never met anyone who has teens at home and not had any stress or difficulty associated with that." She paused and looked at the floor. I thought it was possible she might walk out the door any second. Instead she said, "My husband has been seeing other women for years. We both want out, but we stay just for the kids. But the kids know we are miserable and they barely talk to me. They think the fact that our marriage is bad is my fault."

Ruth illustrates the different modalities required with someone who has more of a bodily focus and who doesn't want to talk about things related to emotions or relationships. People like Ruth seem to move in and out of their mind and body (meaning focusing on thoughts or emotions only to switch back to a more concrete focus on their bodily symptoms) in just moments and it's important we try to keep up. This behavior seems to be a kind of dissociation in which the body is a vessel for the mind and emotions. When thoughts and feelings become too much, they disappear into their body. People like Ruth also illustrate the limitations of CBT for some people and the related binds we therapists can find ourselves in. There are many ways CBT can help people cope with physical illnesses, yet, especially cognitive approaches do require some awareness and relationship with one's mind. For people like Ruth, who have spent their whole lives being externally focused, by marking success with how much money they have, how they look, or how well their kids turn out, even so-called straightforward cognitive strategies may not be helpful. This is why I start with behavioral interventions and limit discussions regarding catastrophizing and other "cognitive distortions." For people with more active defenses, they often can handle being told what to do by someone they perceive as an expert. But when there is underlying trauma or current relationship stress, people often (though out of awareness) say they want something concrete from us but then get frustrated when we provide it, because it seems too simple. It also goes without saying that such people have more narcissistic defenses than most. In situations like Ruth's, they are often waiting to see when and if they can talk about other aspects of their lives that have the potential to offer more healing. To do this, though, they have to tolerate a great deal of shame about needing help. Therefore often with physically oriented clients, treatment involves talking about the body, with occasional forays into emotional material, only then to return to a focus on somatic symptoms. In Ruth's case, however, I was able to weather the back and forth between discussions about her body and her mind. Eventually, in this treatment which lasted over 2 years, her health began to be in the background.

Ruth had been coming to see me for about 6 months when she stopped talking about her physical symptoms as much. She also no longer needed me to "tell her what to do" about her physical discomfort. She did begin an exercise program, which she acknowledged helped her pain, in part, she thought because it helped her sleep better. Although she initially denied any symptoms of depression, she did have a number of depressive symptoms that she told me about after she settled into therapy and as she found talking about her mind a little more tolerable. She agreed to talk with her physician about an antidepressant that could also help with pain. She began to talk about her marriage and her children as those relationships were fraught with conflict that resulted in part from passivity on her part. Although she had a prominent leadership role at work, she seemed unable to set even the most basic limits with her children. This became a major focus of her treatment. She and her husband decided to try couples therapy, but they ultimately decided to end the marriage, as her husband had decided to leave the marriage for another woman he had recently been seeing. Although this was difficult and destabilizing, as the endings of all long-term marriages are, Ruth ultimately felt she should have taken better care of herself years ago, when she knew of her husband's pattern of being with other women. She wondered if this relationship, which felt toxic to her, might have led to her illnesses.

Although Ruth's situation ended up being emotionally painful, she left therapy feeling that she could have more control over her life. Ruth never discussed past traumas. I don't think this was a failure in terms of her therapy. Given her level of emotional functioning, specifically her sense of grandiosity in some aspects of her life, thinking about her vulnerability in her childhood might have been too destabilizing, especially given the ending of her marriage. She did leave therapy with her medical symptoms well under control and with an increased understanding of how her mind worked and how she felt about people in her present life.

Although people such as Ruth can be challenging, another common scenario are people who tend to seem good natured, with relatively few personality issues or pathology. They may or may not have a formal diagnosis but have a number of physical symptoms that fit with somatization. These tend to be people who are more open to CBT approaches for managing physical symptoms and may get physically better relatively quickly. I see this more often in young adults. Yet once symptoms get better (or plateau), they keep coming to therapy. They no longer seem interested in talking about their bodily symptoms, but they are not sure what to talk about. In such cases, I often have the feeling that I am not being useful, and sometimes I wonder why they keep seeing me! And sometimes people in this situation can become "chatty" in the therapy, with bland updates about work or physical symptoms. If I was a clinician who just used CBT approaches, these are the kinds of clients who might be simply graduated from therapy. But since they keep coming, I often wonder with them what else might be on their minds. Again, these are people who are mostly naïve to the therapy process, and I find some education is needed about how to use therapy. This is often the case for people with trauma histories that they had been able to successfully compartmentalize. They know they need something more, but they are not sure how to get it.

In moving beyond CBT approaches with clients, one of the things I find most helpful with clients who have bodily concerns, particularly if their disease(s) seems to be especially impacted by stress, is to get them to notice if they ever find themselves nervous. I find with most of my clients, even those that do not describe physical complaints, that I need to nudge them to consider if they feel anxious or nervous. I see this as a consequence of our increasingly manic culture and the propensity to focus more on external aspects of being rather than developing a rich internal life. For example, one woman in her late 20s, who saw me for severe depression and a managed autoimmune disease, joked with me after her first year of therapy, saying, "Until I met you, I had no idea that I was anxious." This woman had seen several therapists before myself. Later, she wondered if her previous therapies focused too much on her depression and her family. Although we eventually concentrated a great deal on her family and her childhood, which was fairly traumatic, I feel that I gained traction in helping her because she could see how nearly every relationship she had made her anxious. She had never been aware of this. She was fairly dissociative, and so interactions with others were mostly geared around her figuring out what they needed from her. She had little access to her mind and could not really relate to people in a way that involved her subjectivity, as psychoanalytic clinicians would describe it. So she did what she knew best, she focused on others. This is a common behavior among both people with dissociation and physical problems. Anxiety is important as it is often the beginning of an emotional language. As is the case with people who present to me with only bodily symptoms, I see it as my job to help people develop the foundation of an emotional language. This often starts with anxiety or a milder version of a sense of being nervous.

Conclusion

When trauma lands in the body, we need to utilize a number of creative and flexible treatment methods in order to help. Clients who are focused on physical problems need to feel safe before other issues can be discussed. Historically clinicians have felt they have little to offer clients with medical problems because of the idea that symptoms are "psychosomatic." But if we think of the body as the living story of trauma, we can become more patient and understand that the mind and body have been injured. We are limited in ways we can discuss this however, as many of our clients need us to be physically and practically focused in the beginning of therapy. Positive relationships can provide a buffer to help people manage their physical symptoms and may help strengthen the body and the immune system in preventing an exacerbation of current illness or the development of new medical problems.

Interventions for Helping People Who Are Physically Focused

- Assume all physical symptoms are real but explain that real symptoms can be helped with therapy because of the ways the mind and body interact.
- Evaluate the extent to which clients have some awareness on the impact of stress on their symptoms. If not, then focus more on behaviors than cognitions in therapy.
- Try to get a sense of relationships in the present, if possible.

- Provide education about how therapy can help, both behaviorally and by thinking about relationships.
- Provide education about the fight/flight response.
- Emphasize that stress and anxiety are physical and that pain, in particular, can cause anxiety.
- Teach diaphragmatic breathing as a quick easy-to-learn technique for managing illness-related distress. One resource is here: https://www.health.harvard.edu/lung-health-and-disease/learning-diaphragmatic-breathing.
- Encourage exercise. Even if uncomfortable at first, it reduces pain in the long run.
- Address sleep; if someone is not sleeping well, it makes everything in the mind and the body worse.
- Allow time for emotional discussions to develop.
- If possible, get client to notice things they become anxious about, particularly in relationships.
- If physical symptoms improve, don't assume it's the end of treatment; it could be just the beginning.
- People with medical issues often take much longer to discuss or disclose trauma histories. Therefore, focus on the here-and-now symptom relief approaches (if tolerated) and watch for the presence of anxiety, especially in relationships.

References

Abbass, A., Kisely, S., & Kroenke, K. (2009). Short-term psychodynamic psychotherapy for somatic disorders: Systematic review and meta-analysis of clinical trials. *Psychotherapy and Psychosomatics, 78*(5), 265–274.

Altmann, U., Thielemann, D., Zimmermann, A., Steffanowski, A., Bruckmeier, E., Pfaffinger, I., et al. (2018). Outpatient psychotherapy improves symptoms and reduces health care costs in regularly and prematurely terminated therapies. *Frontiers in Psychology, 9*, 748. Accessed online on 27 Dec 2019 at https://www.frontiersin.org/article/10.3389/fpsyg.2018.00748. https://doi.org/10.3389/fpsyg.2018.00748.

Amabile, N., Susini, G., Pettenati-Soubayroux, I., Bonello, L., Gil, J. M., Argues, S., et al. (2008). Severity of periodontal disease correlates to inflammatory systemic status and independently predicts the presence and angiographic extent of stable coronary artery disease. *Journal of Internal Medicine, 263*(6), 644–652.

American Psychiatric Association. (2013). *Diagnostic and statistical manual of mental disorders* (5th ed.). Washington, DC: Author.

Barefoot, J. C., Brummett, B. H., Helms, M. J., Mark, D. M., Siegler, I. C., & Williams, R. B. (2000). Depressive symptoms and survival of patients with coronary artery disease. *Psychosomatic Medicine, 62*, 790–795.

Batten, S. V., Aslan, M., Maciejewski, P. K., & Mazure, C. M. (2004). Childhood maltreatment as a risk factor for cardiovascular disease and depression. *Journal of Clinical Psychiatry, 65*(2), 249–254.

Baumeister, D., Akhtar, R., Ciufolini, S., Pariante, C. M., & Mondelli, V. (2015). Childhood trauma and adulthood inflammation: A meta-analysis of peripheral C-reactive protein, interleukin-6 and tumour necrosis factor-α. *Molecular Psychiatry, 21*(5), 642–649. https://doi.org/10.1038/mp.2015.67. Epub ahead of print.

Boscarino, J. A. (2008). A prospective study of PTSD and early age mortality among Vietnam veterans: Implications for surveillance and prevention. *Psychosomatic Medicine, 70*(6), 668–676.
Campbell, J. A., Walker, R. J., & Egede, L. E. (2016). Associations between adverse childhood experiences, high-risk behaviors, and morbidity in adulthood. *American Journal of Preventive Medicine, 50*(3), 344–352.
Cannon, W. B. (1915). *Bodily changes in pain, hunger, fear and rage*. New York: D. Appleton.
Chrousos, G. P., & Gold, P. W. (1992). The concepts of stress and stress system disorders: Overview of physical and behavioral homeostasis. *Journal of the American Medical Association, 267*(9), 1244–1252.
Cohen, S. (2004). Social relationships and health. *American Psychologist, 59*(8), 676–684.
Danese, A., Pariante, C. M., Caspi, A., Taylor, A., & Poulton, R. (2007). Childhood maltreatment predicts adult inflammation in a life course study. *Proceedings of the National Academy of Sciences of the United States of America, 104*(4), 1319–1324.
De Vogli, R., Chandola, T., & Marmot, M. G. (2007). Negative aspects of close relationships and heart disease. *Archives of Internal Medicine, 167*(18), 1951–1957.
Dong, M., Dube, S. R., Felitti, V. J., Giles, W. H., & Anda, R. F. (2003). Adverse childhood experience and self-reported liver disease: New insights into the causal pathway. *Archives of Internal Medicine, 163*, 1949–1956.
Dong, M., Giles, W. H., Felitti, V. J., Dube, S. R., Williams, J. E., Chapman, D. P., et al. (2004). Insights into causal pathways for ischemic heart disease: Adverse childhood experiences study. *Circulation, 110*, 1761–1766.
Eccleston, C., Hearn, L., & Williams, A. C. D. C. (2015). Psychological therapies for the management of chronic neuropathic pain in adults. *Cochrane Database of Systematic Reviews, 10*, CD011259. https://doi.org/10.1002/14651858.CD011259.pub2.
Eisenberger, N. I., Master, S. L., Ingaki, T. K., Taylor, S. E., Shirinyan, D., Lieberman, M. D., et al. (2011). Attachment figures activate a safety signal-related neural region and reduce pain experience. *Proceedings of the National Academy of Sciences of the United States of America, 108*(28), 11721–11726.
Felitti, V. J., Anda, R. F., Nordenberg, D., Williamson, D. F., Spitz, A. M., Edwards, V., et al. (1998). Relationship of child abuse and household dysfunction to many leading causes of death in adults. *American Journal of Preventive Medicine, 14*(4), 245–258.
Fink, G. (2009). Stress: Definition and history. In L. R. Squire (Ed.), *Encyclopedia of neurological sciences* (pp. 549–555). Oxford: Academic.
Fishbain, D. A., Pulikal, A., Lewis, J. E., & Gao, J. (2017). Chronic pain types differ in their reported prevalence of Post-Traumatic Stress Disorder (PTSD) and there is consistent evidence that chronic pain is associated with PTSD: An evidence-based structured systematic review. *Pain Medicine, 18*(4), 711–735.
Frasure-Smith, N., Lesperance, F., & Talajic, M. (1993). Depression following myocardial infarction: Impact on 6-month survival. *Journal of the American Medical Association, 270*, 1819–1824.
Geiss, A., Rohleder, N., & Anton, F. (2012). Evidence for an association between an enhanced reactivity of interleukin-6 levels and reduced glucocorticoid sensitivity in patients with fibromyalgia. *Psychoneuroendocrinology, 37*(5), 671–684.
Gerson, M. J., & Gerson, C. D. (2012). The importance of relationships in patients with irritable bowel syndrome: A review. *Gastroenterology Research and Practice, 2012*, 157340. https://doi.org/10.1155/2012/157340. Published online December 1, 2011.
Gerson, M. J., Gerson, C. D., Awad, R. A., Dancey, C., Poitras, P., Porcelli, P., et al. (2006). An international study of irritable bowel syndrome: Family relationships and mind-body attributions. *Social Science and Medicine, 62*, 2838–2847.
Glei, D. A., Goldman, N., Risques, R. A., Rehkopf, D. H., Dow, W. H., Rosero-Bixby, L., et al. (2016). Predicting survival from telomere length versus conventional predictors: A multinational population-based cohort study. *PLoS One, 11*(4), e0152486. Accessed online on 29 Dec 2019 at https://doi.org/10.1371/journal.pone.0152486.

Greenberg, T. M. (2012). *When someone you love has a chronic illness*. Springville: UT. Plainsight Publishing.

Greenberg, T. M. (2016). *Psychodynamic perspectives on aging and illness* (2nd ed.). New York: Springer.

Heppner, P. F., Crawford, E. F., Haji, U. A., Afari, N., Hauger, R. L., Dashevsky, B., et al. (2009). The association of posttraumatic stress disorder and metabolic syndrome: A study of increased health risk in veterans. *BMC Medicine, 7*, 1.

Holman, D. M., Ports, K. A., Buchanan, N. D., Hawkins, N. A., Merrick, M. T., Metzler, M., & Trivers, K. F. (2016). The association between adverse childhood experiences and risk of cancer in adulthood: A systematic review of the literature. *Pediatrics, 138*(Suppl 1), S81–S91. https://doi.org/10.1542/peds.2015-4268L.

Holt-Lunstad, J., Smith, T. B., & Layton, J. B. (2010). Social relationships and mortality risk: A meta-analytic review. *PLoS Medicine, 7*(7), e1000316. https://doi.org/10.1371/journal.pmed.1000316.

Jaffee, S. R., Takizawa, R., & Arseneault, L. (2017). Buffering effects of safe, supportive, and nurturing relationships among women with childhood histories of maltreatment. *Psychological Medicine, 47*(15), 2628–2639.

Kalmakis, K. A., Meyer, J. S., Chiodo, L., & Leung, K. (2015). Adverse childhood experiences and chronic hypothalamic–pituitary–adrenal activity. *Stress: The International Journal on the Biology of Stress, 18*(4), 446–450. https://doi.org/10.3109/10253890.2015.1023791.

Kempke, S., Luyten, P., De Coninck, S., Van Houdenhove, B., Mayes, L. C., & Claes, S. (2015). Effects of early childhood trauma on hypothalamic–pituitary–adrenal (HPA) axis function in patients with Chronic Fatigue Syndrome. *Psychoneuroendocrinology, 52*, 14–21.

Kiecolt-Glaser, J. K., & Newton, T. L. (2001). Marriage and health: His and hers. *Psychological Bulletin, 127*, 472–503.

Kleinstäuber, M., Witthöft, M., & Hiller, W. (2011). Efficacy of short-term psychotherapy for multiple medically unexplained physical symptoms: A meta-analysis. *Clinical Psychology Review, 31*(1), 146–160.

Lohr, J. B., Palmer, B. W., Eidt, C. A., Aailaboyina, S., Mausbach, B. T., Wolkowitz, O. M., et al. (2015). Is post-traumatic stress disorder associated with premature senescence? A review of the literature. *The American Journal of Geriatric Psychiatry, 23*(7), 709–725.

McCrory, C., Dooley, C., Layte, R., & Kenny, R. A. (2015). The lasting legacy of childhood adversity for disease risk in later life. *Health Psychology, 34*(7), 687–696.

Myrtek, M. (2001). Meta-analyses of prospective studies on coronary heart disease, type A personality, and hostility. *International Journal of Cardiology, 79*(2–3), 245–251.

Nicolaides, N. C., Kyratzi, E., Lamprokostopoulou, A., Chrousos, G. P., & Charmandari, E. (2015). Stress, the stress system and the role of glucocorticoids. *Neuroimmunomodulation, 22*, 6–19.

Pahwa, R., Singh, A., & Jialal, I. (2019). Chronic inflammation. In: StatPearls [Internet] Treasure Island (FL): StatPearls Publishing. Accessed online on 29 Dec 2019 at https://www.ncbi.nlm.nih.gov/books/NBK493173/.

Papadopoulos, A., & Cleare, A. (2012). Hypothalamic–pituitary–adrenal axis dysfunction in chronic fatigue syndrome. *Nature Reviews Endocrinology, 8*, 22–32.

Pennebaker, J. W., Kiecolt-Glaser, J. K., & Glaser, R. (1988). Disclosure of traumas and immune function: Health implications for psychotherapy. *Journal of Consulting and Clinical Psychology, 56*(2), 239–245.

Peterson, C., & Seligman, M. E. P. (1987). Explanatory style and illness. *Journal of Personality, 55*, 237–265.

Petrelluzzi, K. F. S., Garcia, M. C., Petta, C. A., Grassi-Kassisse, D. M., & Spadari-Bratfisch, R. C. (2008). Salivary cortisol concentrations, stress and quality of life in women with endometriosis and chronic pelvic pain. *Stress: The International Journal on the Biology of Stress, 11*(5), 390–397.

Robles, T. F., Slatcher, R. B., Trombello, J. M., & McGinn, M. M. (2014). Marital quality and health: A meta-analytic review. *Psychological Bulletin, 140*(1), 140–187.

Rutledge, T., Reis, S. E., Olson, M., Owens, J., Kelsey, S. E., Pepine, C. J., et al. (2006). Depression is associated with cardiac symptoms and hospitalization among women with suspected coronary heart disease: The NHLBI-sponsored WISE study. *Psychosomatic Medicine, 68*, 217–223.

Selye, H. (1998). A syndrome produced by diverse nocuous agents. *The Journal of Neuropsychiatry and Clinical Neurosciences, 10*(2), 230–231. (Original work published 1936).

Shen, B. J., Avivi, Y. E., Todaro, J. F., Spiro, A., Laurenceau, J. P., Ward, K. D., et al. (2008). Anxiety characteristics independently and prospectively predict myocardial infarction in men: The unique contribution of anxiety among psychologic factors. *Journal of the American College of Cardiology, 51*(2), 113–119.

Smith, T. W., Glaser, K., Ruiz, J. M., & Gallo, L. C. (2004). Hostility, anger, aggressiveness, and coronary heart disease: An interpersonal perspective in personality, emotion, and health. *Journal of Personality, 72*(6), 1217–1270.

Smyth, J. M., Stone, A. A., Hurewitz, A., & Kaell, A. (1999). Effects of writing about stressful experiences on symptom reduction in patients with asthma or rheumatoid arthritis: A randomized trial. *Journal of the American Medical Association, 281*, 1304–1309.

Sumner, J. A., Kubzansky, L. D., Elkind, M. S. V., Roberts, A. L., Agnew-Blais, J., Chen, Q., et al. (2015). Trauma exposure and posttraumatic stress disorder symptoms predict onset of cardiovascular events in women. *Circulation, 132*(4), 251–259. https://doi.org/10.1161/CIRCULATIONAHA.114.014492.

Theadom, A., Cropley, M., Smith, H. E., Feigin, V. L., & McPherson, K. (2015). Mind and body therapy for fibromyalgia. *Cochrane Database of Systematic Reviews, 4*, CD001980. https://doi.org/10.1002/14651858.CD001980.pub3.

Tobe, S. W., Kiss, A., Sainsbury, S., Jeslin, M., Geerts, R., & Baker, B. (2007). The impact of job strain and marital cohesion on ambulatory blood pressure during 1 year: The double exposure study. *American Journal of Hypertension, 20*, 148–153.

van Dessel, N., den Boeft, M., van der Wouden, J. C., Kleinstäuber, M., Leone, S. S., Terluin, B., et al. (2014). Non-pharmacological interventions for somatoform disorders and medically unexplained physical symptoms (MUPS) in adults. *Cochrane Database of Systematic Reviews, 11*, CD011142. https://doi.org/10.1002/14651858.CD011142.pub2.

Wanic, R. A., & Kulik, J. (2011). Toward an understanding of gender differences in the impact of marital conflict on health. *Sex Roles, 65*, 297–312.

Young, A. B., & Khan, J. (2018). Non-pharmacological interventions for chronic pain in multiple sclerosis. *Cochrane Database of Systematic Reviews, 12*, CD012622. https://doi.org/10.1002/14651858.CD012622.pub2.

Zautra, A. J., Hoffman, K. S., Matt, K. S., Yocum, D., Potter, P. T., Castro, W. L., et al. (1998). An examination of individual differences in the relationship between interpersonal stress and disease activity among women with rheumatoid arthritis. *Arthritis Care and Research, 11*(4), 271–279.

Chapter 8
When Fight Impulses Dominate: Managing Aggression and Anger

Anger and Clinical Avoidance

I have described how we can help people with trauma histories deal with anger by slowly encouraging them to notice how fearful they are because anger is one part of the fight/flight response and linked to surviving trauma. Some people with cPTSD, however, are entrenched in angry states of mind, and the only response to real or perceived threats is aggression. Such people simply cannot tolerate ideas or feelings related to being afraid. In fact, it's often an intense fear of vulnerability, helplessness, and a sense of over-responsibility that keeps people clinging to anger. Anger can make us feel powerful, as if we can protect ourselves from getting hurt again. Attachment to one's anger can also be connected to the idea of revenge and the belief that someone should pay for one's suffering. Traumatized people may also feel an excessive need to control their surroundings, which can make them inflexible because change in their environment elicits an internal sense of chaos and overstimulation, which must be immediately stopped by attacking the source of their frustration. Let's consider the case of Darlene.

Darlene was in her 50s and came to therapy after her previous therapist had retired. She had been in and out of some form of therapy for much of her life and reported she was an "angry child" though she was not able to provide more detail about her anger, other than, "I was just difficult." She described cruel and sadistic caretakers. For example, it was not uncommon to be locked in a closet for even a minor infraction. She married quite young and had three children, one of whom died by suicide. One of her children did not speak to Darlene and moved out of the country for college and never came back to the United States. Her third adult child still lived in the area and did maintain contact, but Darlene rarely had any good things to say about her daughter. She criticized most every aspect of her daughter's being, though, from what I could tell, her daughter created a nice and successful life for herself, which I imagined must have been difficult given Darlene's disposition. Darlene was in no romantic relationship and had been on disability for many years

T. M. Greenberg, *Treating Complex Trauma*,
https://doi.org/10.1007/978-3-030-45285-8_8

because of bipolar disorder which was currently controlled through psychiatric medications. As I got to know Darlene, her diagnosis of bipolar disorder seemed to be just the tip of the iceberg in terms of her symptoms. She was mean to literally everyone in her wake. She fought with bus drivers, customer service agents, and even other clients in my waiting room. With me, she tended to vacillate between being obsequious (e.g., repeatedly apologizing for being even a minute late) or being very condescending (e.g., commenting once that I wore an outfit that "made me look fat"). If there was lint on the fabric of a chair in my office, she wouldn't sit there because it was "disgusting," and while she exercised the option of sitting on my leather sofa, she clearly resented choosing to move. Just being in her presence was a strain and I always felt on edge.

Although anger and related expressions of it are common reactions to trauma, it's not especially adaptive in terms of cultivating or maintaining relationships. Traumatized individuals who devalue others and project their anger often have difficulty in therapy. In extreme cases, they can treat us poorly and/or assume that since we're getting paid, we're required to tolerate their abuse. I'll discuss this issue further, as it's especially important with really aggressive clients that we set limits and do not tolerate verbal assaults. In this chapter, I'll describe the research on manifestations of anger among both civilian and veteran clients. However, first I want to consider the paucity of research and writing on clients who present with a lot of anger, because anger and aggression are often difficult for us to think about.

Despite the fact that many people with PTSD or cPTSD have issues with aggression, this topic has barely been covered in the literature. Between 1987 and 2011, McHugh et al. (2012) noted that only about 1.4–1.5% of research articles on PTSD looked at the role of anger and hostility. Researchers have also argued that anger is unique to PTSD because of its inclusion in the diagnostic criteria for PTSD. Anger critically differentiates PTSD from other anxiety disorders (Olatunji et al. 2010). Interestingly, although many of us assume the emotion of anger and aggression are related (that anger often precedes aggression), aggression can occur without awareness of anger (Miles et al. 2019).

Anger is a "fuzzy" concept that encompasses a number of different emotions (Russell and Fehr 1994). We're often uncomfortable with how we deal with aggression in clinical settings; anger and hostility are uneasy and confusing, and because of this, we shy away from thinking about these emotions both in ourselves and in our clients. In addition, anger can be wrapped up in a number of feelings, such as disappointment. It can be viewed as secondary, as when I suggest it can be a mask for fear or sadness. Anger and/or aggression can also encompass irritation, frustration, rage, hostility, outrage, and even boredom. Anger can be experienced as a short-term state of mind or can live on as an entire aspect of someone's personality functioning. And then there is the fact that gender, race, and ethnicity play a role in how aggression is expressed, perceived, and tolerated.

And yet, anger disrupts relationships. I tend to have a fairly high tolerance for generalized anger—it often does not bother me—but I'm certainly not at my best as a therapist when I feel that clients such as Darlene are belittling or mocking toward me. The variety of anger people such as Darlene express makes it difficult for us to mentalize or be empathic, in part because the very things we have to offer (a supportive relationship) are foreign and also potentially enraging to them. Clients who have a lot of narcissistic vulnerabilities hate the idea of dependency and needing help from others. They can also be envious of our capacity for helping them, because they do not possess such a skill within themselves. These versions of anger can seem more destructive. When anger is at the forefront, establishing a solid therapeutic relationship is tricky, since a sturdy alliance is the needed ingredient for therapeutic change.

It goes without saying that it's better if clients begin therapy with a feeling that we are helpful. In fact, Kohut suggested that successful therapies often begin with clients who idealize their therapists, as this is a needed part of early development (Kohut 1971). Idealization can be problematic in the long term because we need to realize that no one is without fault and people we love will inevitably disappoint us. But given therapy can be frightening, clients who start out seeing us through an idealized lens can create the beginning of a sense of safety. Clients who have experienced repetitive childhood trauma may have never had a situation in which they could bask (even temporarily) in the warmth of a caregiver. With angry and more narcissistic clients, however, they may only engage with us if we validate the ways they have been mistreated, which means agreeing with the belief that the world is a horrible place and everyone is awful. Though I don't suggest the latter approach, it can happen a lot with therapists who feel overwhelmed by a client's anger. It's simply just difficult to figure out how to connect with people who are really angry.

Historically it's been challenging to incorporate theories of aggression into psychotherapy. The most comprehensive models come from within psychodynamic thinking. For example, Freud's ideas of slips of the tongue, in which we unconsciously expose an aggressive wish, have made their way into popular culture. Other psychoanalytic theories of aggression have failed to land in non-analytic therapies or in psychodynamic communities in the United States. Melanie Klein has one of the most prolific and comprehensive theories regarding aggression, but her view of infantile sadism is a tough sell for many therapists and patients alike (e.g., Mills 2006). Despite the paucity of useful theories regarding aggression, there is also a practical aspect to the dilemmas posed by this state of mind and behavior, particularly when anger is woven into one's personality. Most clients shy away from owning their aggression and being told they come across as angry. It's very hard to talk about because it can promote shame and sometimes more anger. And sometimes when clients hear us remark about their anger, it's often met with a comment such as "Of course I am!" In other words, many people do not see their anger as a problem to be addressed, but merely a fact of life. That is, unless it gets them in trouble. When addressed with care, this can be an entry point into dealing with people who have anger woven into their characters.

Even more common are clients who are not sure how useful it is to talk about and explore their anger. While they may acknowledge their anger, they may feel stuck and say, "What do I do with that?" And this is where I can't help but wonder if maybe theories of psychology don't know how to fully address anger. In many therapeutic methods, the idea has mainly been about bypassing anger to get to the "good parts" where we get along and can focus on common goals. Even in anger management, a focal part of treatment is to help people manage the expression of their anger by teaching them do so in a more appropriate way. While this is useful for certain clients, it occurs to me that the culture of psychology orbits around the avoidance of this prickly emotion. Certain exceptions exist, such as when Arthur Janov's Primal Scream therapy was popular in the 1970s. While this treatment never really took off, it strikes me as an attempt to deal with the very issues I'm describing. Anger is frightening or at the very least unsettling for many of us in the mental health field. I think it is fairly common for us to avoid thoughts and feelings of our own anger, especially around our professional peers. For instance, when we compare people in the mental health field to those who practice in law and medicine, we often see different models of comfort with anger and aggression. This may also be due to temperament/personality type. For instance, many therapists are people pleasers and feeling-oriented individuals who shy away from anger, even outside of their professional lives. Class components contribute to how we cope with anger, too. I grew up in a lower-class background where anger was expressed much more directly. If I'm honest, there is a certain comfort I feel with people who grew up similarly—clients who can just tell me I said something perceived as wrong—or that I did something offensive. That said, I think most of us go into the mental health field with ideas that we are good people who want to help others. For many people in the field, "good" equals not seeming even remotely aggressive.

Anger may be frightening to many of us, but it's also ubiquitous in our culture. Consider the rise in aggression on social media. Because aggression can be linked with negative consequences, it's easier to be hostile or even vitriolic when we are not face to face with the object of our anger. In my experience on social media (which I now intentionally limit my involvement in), I remember a neighbor who seemed lovely in person, a good mother with nice kids, only to find on social media she espoused wildly racist views and rants of all kinds which seemed quite unhinged. If we think about conflicting presentations of anger like this through the lens of fight/flight reactions we humans have evolved with, there was a time (more regularly) when "fight" meant to literally kill someone. Most of us are terrified by this. The fact that social media is an outlet for such rage provides a window into how much some people hold in aggressive thoughts because of fear or even just awareness that there's something wrong with being too belligerent.

We do need outlets for our aggressive instincts however. Think of the wide interest in the hundreds of crime dramas on television that start with a murder and then the hunt for the villain. Such shows represent a search for justice, but there's also a deep fascination of who kills and why. In nearly every one of these programs, the murderer is the person you least expect, like the nice neighbor introduced in the first 10 minutes of the show. We watch and wait to find out the identity of yet another person whose aggression led them to commit a crime. This detour in thinking about cultural aggression and the normative, yet hidden nature of it, is a way of saying that anger is everywhere, even in ourselves. And it may have to do with the wider practice of avoiding research and discussion about anger and aggression in the mental health field. Many of us have been taught to sublimate our anger by finding socially acceptable ways of dealing with it. For example, a colleague I once knew who appeared to have a great deal of aggressive feelings developed an interest in hockey later in her life. She told me that the fighting was her favorite part of going to games. Yet, for people with cPTSD, especially those with childhood and adult trauma experiences, it's not so easy to find socially sanctioned outlets. And as we will see, people with cPTSD and anger seem to endure more suffering, possibly because they cannot tolerate just how angry and aggressive they feel.

Links Between Anger and Trauma

The lack of research regarding anger and PTSD is surprising, given how important it is in understanding and treating people who are bearing intense feelings. For example, the arousal symptom cluster of PTSD, which includes anger among its criteria, predicts severity of PTSD symptoms and it's also related with intrusive PTSD symptoms (Schell et al. 2004). Further, anger and hostility predict worse treatment outcomes in people with PTSD and cPTSD (e.g., Burns et al. 1999; Rao et al. 2004).

Among veterans seeking therapy for PTSD, approximately 75% of males and 45% of females reported clinically significant anger symptoms (Hoge et al. 2006; Wilk et al. 2015; Mackintosh et al. 2015). Anger, including thoughts of harming others, is intensified among veterans who have both PTSD and major depression (Gonzalez et al. 2016). Veterans and active duty military members have higher rates of intimate partner aggression than civilians (Love et al. 2015). One theory suggests that combat veterans with PTSD have difficulty regulating their anger because they experience heightened physiological arousal, hostile perceptions of the environment, and antagonistic behavior in response to perceived threats (Chemtob et al. 1997; Novaco and Chemtob 2002).

In a small study of civilians in Northern Ireland (who had been exposed to sectarian violence) comparing people with PTSD vs. cPTSD, those with cPTSD had significantly higher levels of physical aggression and self-harm (Dyer et al. 2009). Alterations of self-perception (e.g., shame) were a significant predictor of aggression toward the self and others.

In looking at people without formal PTSD diagnoses, a study of 10,800 people in Brazil found that people with histories of emotional abuse, neglect, and sexual abuse were more likely to have angry and anxious temperaments (Sudbrack et al. 2015). A study of men who had been sexually abused as children found that they were more likely to be hostile 50 years later, as well as depressed and with physical symptoms (Easton and Kong 2017). Child physical abuse has been found to be linked with aggression, trait anger, and hostility as well as a tendency toward narcissistic traits (Keene and Epps 2016).

Given the relative lack of research on PTSD, cPTSD, and aggression (particularly in civilian populations), we are left to wonder about why some people with cPTSD develop aggression and hostility (externalizing behaviors) and others are prone to turn this anger inward through feelings of self-hatred or develop depression, suicidal ideation, or other internalizing behaviors. In my clinical experience, most people with cPTSD are angry, but this emotion is expressed differently among clients. In the next two sections, I'll describe different ideas for the role of aggression in cPTSD.

Anger as a Result of Feeling Over-Responsible

Veterans witnessing death or being involved in physical harm to others are more likely to develop symptoms of PTSD (Dohrenwend et al. 2006). This data is important as it's been described since the Vietnam War that involvement in harming others is linked with poorer adjustment to trauma. A version of this takes place among civilian populations too, though without the reality of actually physically harming someone (usually), particularly for those who have experienced childhood trauma. As young children our thoughts are our reality. Anger and aggression are important and needed aspects of childhood development, but children need adults around to let them know that angry thoughts won't hurt others. It is vital we learn how to feel anger while maintaining a sense that we are loved and accepted, even when our emotions can feel frightening and destructive. At times we may all wish to rid ourselves of people who frustrate us or present obstacles in our lives, often parents or siblings who keep us from getting something we want, or command us to do something against our wishes. Think of a toddler who sees no reason to wear a coat when it is freezing outside and says to her mother, "I hate you!" A reasonable enough parent likely feels frustrated with this encounter but understands that her daughter is just expressing age-related developmental anger about being controlled. For kids who are being abused or neglected, they have more negative feelings toward people in their lives, and when these feelings can't be expressed or, worse, the child is severely punished for expressing them, the child develops a complicated relationship with anger. In situations where parents are sadistic, a parent is especially envious of her child, wishing on some level that her child was never been born, etc., anger becomes a toxic emotion that terrifies children in response to feeling any kind of danger—as if any aggressive feeling could kill them. And then there are instances when a trusted adult acts so egregious, as to exploit their children for some kind of violent aim, such as child sexual abuse, that children feel that they may die in the face of any intense emotion. Any of these scenarios can lead kids to become adults who can feel more powerful than they actually are, especially in the face of aggressive feelings. Clinically, this can manifest as someone like Darlene, who will act in an aggressive and powerful way as if to prove they will win the "kill or be killed" internal dynamic. Clients like Melanie (whom I've described in previous chapters) are less likely to act overtly aggressive. More often, their aggressive feelings are turned toward themselves. This is likely related to a sense of over-responsibility that we may not learn until later in the therapeutic process.

Melanie had been seeing me for a couple of years when things become stabilized at work. She had been promoted a couple of times, and her panic attacks, which at one point debilitated her, were well under control. It was around this time that she slowly, in measured doses, began to tell me more about her boyfriend, with whom she had moved in with early on in our treatment. I had remained feeling in the dark about this young man, and I knew little about him, other than his occupation. He seemed one-dimensional to me, almost like a cartoon character. Melanie's disclosures about his treatment of her began soon after she started to wonder aloud if they should get married. As soon as she told me about this much stronger commitment, I felt alarmed, though at the time could not articulate (in my own mind) why. Eventually it was clear that there was an ongoing pattern that involved his mistreatment of her. Usually this involved vile and humiliating verbal attacks, but she also felt controlled by him, as he sounded needy and cloying. For example, he required her to let him know where she was nearly all of the time, as he was afraid she would "cheat on him." Although it would be reasonable to assume that her disclosures about her boyfriend might suggest her contemplating getting out of this relationship, it was almost the opposite. The more she told me, the more concerned I became, and the more she talked about marrying him. These aspects of her discussions lasted a long time, and it was the beginning of me really understanding the impact of her trauma background and the degree to which she felt that she deserved to suffer. The more she talked about how badly she was treated, the more she insisted she was bad, damaged, and worthless. And the more she needed to tell me how brilliant and successful he was. At times she compared he and I, although we are not in the same line of work. In this chapter of her therapy, she intimated several times that he was much better at understanding human psychology than myself. The more I knew, the more she protected her boyfriend, and she was incredibly angry with me when I pointed out the aspects of her that felt mistreated and wanted to leave.

Some clinicians might deal with the clinical dilemma posed by Melanie through psychoeducation about emotional abuse and domestic violence, discussing how Melanie's traumatic history mimics her present experience, invoke feminist therapy techniques, or even hope that if Melanie focuses on her own aggression, she could see her way out of this difficult and painful (though in some ways soothing and familiar) situation. Although there might be aspects of therapeutic engagement and change in some of these aforementioned interventions, they are often limited in changing such entrenched patterns involving feelings of aggression and anger in the context of relationships. I have found the most useful way of working in these situations is to think about an old psychoanalytic concept referred to as identification with the aggressor. One way to think about this concept is that it is a variant of Stockholm syndrome. In true Stockholm syndrome, we usually think of feelings involving sympathy, empathy, or admiration that occur in a person who is in a hostage or prisoner situation. In terms of aggression, people with Stockholm syndrome can act toward others as their abuser's act toward them. And of course this does happen, but for people like Melanie, the maltreatment, usually stemming from abusive, exploitive, yet needy caretakers in childhood, leads to aggression, but aggression that is turned inward. It's a kind of self-hatred, and though it can look a lot like masochism or excessive self-destruction, it's not exactly that because there is no real pleasure in suffering. It's more like a self-imposed sadistic trap. Such relationships forge a pseudo sense of agency, as a way to maintain a sense of control over their situation. My preferred conceptualization of these phenomena comes from Ferenczi (1933), who described a process in which the client/victim identifies with the aggressor primarily to know him or her inside and out so that the aggressor's needs can be anticipated. It requires exquisite hypervigilance, an almost preternatural ability to see and identify what goes on inside the minds of others, which provides a sense of cohesion and security. These kinds of connections serve to create the illusion of safety, when the reality is anything but safe. The emotional intimacy from identifying with the aggressor also creates a sense of specialness with a hypervalued other and has themes of vulnerability akin to what we see in people with disorganized attachment styles (Rosbrow 2014). It's like a hypnotic state and involves excessive dissociation.

To deal with identification with the aggressor, we must think about understanding the client's motives for being involved with someone who treats them so negatively, yet offers an intrinsic reward that is difficult for us to understand. In intervening with Melanie, I had to work hard to understand what was great about her boyfriend and to take this in. Eventually, I could offer some of my concerns. But in order to do this, I had to describe this pattern that emerged: she wanted me to know about her boyfriend because on some level, she knew that I would want to protect her. However, this created a triangulation of me vs. him—a relational pattern that was very familiar to her. In terms of therapeutic efficacy, I'm not sure it was interpretations that helped as much as it was her witnessing my struggle to try to help her. At times, I felt as if I bent over backward to try to understand her without judgment. It seemed as if she was mad at me for several months and part of my job was to tolerate feeling bad and useless, which was how she felt. My work with Melanie highlights the benefits of a mentalizing treatment. What I said mattered little; at times it made things worse. It was my thinking and thinking with her about "how to help her" that most likely gave her the courage to leave her boyfriend. Eventually, we could also understand that Melanie, like many people who carry a lot of their own anger, has an investment in finding others who are angry. It allows them to feel that their hostile feelings don't live in *them, they reside in everyone else.* When someone is in this psychic storm, commenting on this latter dynamic may not be useful but can be dealt with later as treatment progresses and people are externally and internally safe enough to think about their own aggressive feelings.

Feeling over-responsible for others has roots in childhood maltreatment because if we believe we have caused a problem, there must be a way to fix it. There is a great deal of psychic value in believing we have caused people to mistreat us. This also weaves in a complementary way of how narcissism has a protective and adaptive value. A key component of trauma, but also narcissistic defense, is control. I personally am very hesitant to pathologize control as I think it is a very normal and adaptive wish. We all want to be in control; we just have to figure out what to do if we don't have it. But the kind of control I am describing with Melanie—that she was responsible for other's mistreatment of her—is as dangerous as it is understandable. By relying on others, we have to relinquish some control. When we allow people into our lives, we risk being injured. We can bypass the idea of being hurt by simply assuming everything is our fault. If we cause our own suffering, it provides a sense of agency. And for people such as Melanie, I think it keeps them from becoming suicidal. It's as if we can simultaneously feel that we are in control, while another part of us feels responsible. This is common in people who dissociate, and it's a kind of "split screen" scenario I described in Chapter 5.

Whether directed at the self or at others, anger is organizing. For people with histories in which many relationships have turned sideways and many people did not have their best interest in mind, feeling angry all of the time can create an internal world in which there are constant adversaries. When things go well or threaten to disrupt that paradigm, clients can become more entrenched in an angry state. It lets us discern the good guys from the bad guys, which is a much clearer narrative—one that's easier than confusion. As Melanie got better and left her boyfriend, confusion was a constant presence in her emotional world, which terrified her and threatened her identity. Her reaction is common among those who let go of a relationship that's organized around them being victimized.

Mind, Body, and Brain: The Neuropsychology of Anger

Chemtob et al. (1997) proposed the Survival Mode theory to explain the strong associations between PTSD and anger/aggression among combat veterans. Perceived threats trigger increased arousal, hostile assessments of external situations, and aggressive behaviors. This makes sense, as anger and aggression are adaptative and prevent helplessness. This is certainly true for people in the military in hostile conflict areas. It also reminds me of a number of cases of men (most often) who told me about being abused as kids by other men and how this abuse usually stopped when they became old enough to start lifting weights. I've also heard this described in situations where someone's mother was being abused by a male partner. Their change in strength allowed them to stop or limit the abuse. However, there is more to PTSD and anger/aggression than just a survival mentality. In adults who have developed PTSD and hostility, evidence suggests that some have preexisting angry traits or an externalizing personality style (Meffert et al. 2008). In several studies looking at veterans, firefighters, and police officers who were involved in combat and first responder roles in response to terrorist attacks, school shootings, and other violent community events, respectively, DiGangi et al. (2013) found that a tendency for hyperarousal *predated* traumatic events. Additionally, DiGangi and colleagues noted that negative emotions, including hostility, anger, as well as behaviors such as avoidance and rumination, represented vulnerability for development of PTSD. The presence of these preexisting factors makes sense, as we know that only a small fraction of the population develops PTSD in response to traumatic events, when such trauma is experienced in adulthood. And, as I've mentioned previously, people who develop PTSD as adults often have histories of child abuse and neglect, which may account for factors that make people more vulnerable to PTSD when they're older and experience trauma.

In addition to these predisposing factors for PTSD, McHugh et al. (2012) offer a novel thesis on the relationship between PTSD and anger involving visual imagery. They emphasize the role of the limbic system (in particular the amygdala) in the experience and rapid processing of visual imagery. As discussed in detail in Chapter 2, the amygdala is thought to be a crucial component of our ability to emotionally process events and is implicated in the physical and psychological effects of trauma. McHugh and colleagues suggest that visual imagery and anger are connected, especially via hypervigilance and a tendency to experience threats particularly when people carry a sense of over-responsibility (Fig. 8.1).

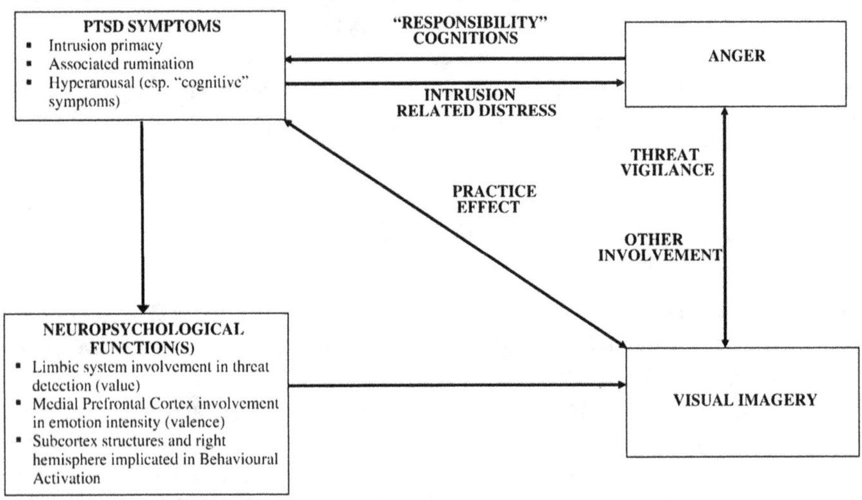

Fig. 8.1 Model of the relationship between PTSD symptoms, neuropsychological function, visual imagery, and anger in PTSD. (McHugh et al. 2012; Elsevier)

This model fits with my description of the weight and importance of feeling overly responsible in reaction to trauma. These authors hypothesize that angry rumination in PTSD may be linked with repetitive, intrusive thoughts as well as visual representations of anger. They note that "visual imaginal processing is more emotionally colored than verbal processing of information and has a more powerful effect than that of verbal representation of equivalent events" (p. 100). I certainly never considered the impact of visual imagery before I read McHugh et al.'s article, but it seems very interesting and relevant. For people with entrenched angry styles who have cPTSD, it's often the case that they cannot talk about their anger. It is acted out. However, I have seen situations where someone with intense acting out anger has also been able to describe the presence of visualizing aggression which is very linked to abuse they themselves endured. Let's return to the situation of Darlene.

When I first met Darlene, I attempted to connect some of her angry states to the presence of cPTSD. This proved helpful as she had an extensive abuse history, including being molested by someone close to her in her family. The abuse went on for years, and evidence indicated that the molestation was known and ignored by others in her family. She said that no one had ever described cPTSD to her before. I then, eventually, tried to suggest that at times in which she felt enraged, maybe there was some sense of fear as well. This proved to be less helpful. In fact, it seemed counterproductive. She continued to note how others were flawed with a reinforced sense of her angry feelings toward them. But there were times when I felt her anger was justified, such as when she recalled the behavior of a bus driver, some of whom used to be infamous for their ill treatment of passengers in our city. But stating that some of her anger might be justified made her more enraged. She then seemed to double down on her aggression, but it was at this point I began to understand her experience of fantasy and visual imagery. She told me that she fantasizes about raping people. I couldn't tell if this was distressing to her. In fact, she seemed to offer this up as justification about why she is so angry. Any attempts to link these fantasies as understandable, given that she was raped, offered little traction. It was as if she couldn't think about the meaning of these fantasies and it seemed as if they were out of her control.

I think what I missed with Darlene was the self-reinforcing nature of her aggression. Darlene felt responsible for her abuse, and her anger toward others provided a sense of organizing cognitions that others were trying to harm her, which were familiar. The component of visualization was not something I routinely ask clients about. Especially since it's hard to deal with anger and I'm often aware how much shame many clients have about it, I think I have erred on the side of assuming that I understand anger and hostility (as if to say something like, *of course you're angry*) which may communicate that I want to deal with issues that *led* to anger, instead of focusing on anger and aggression as important and independent constructs. This does work for many people, but not for people like Darlene who need something more. The article and model presented by McHugh et al. (2012) implies that we may want to consider asking about visual imagery regarding anger and aggression as part of our client's treatment.

Yet, it's the presence of ego-syntonic anger (woven into character structure) and outbursts that may or may not accompany any feeling of aggression that can seem most vexing. In addition, there's often internal (within clients) and external (societal) pressure to avoid talking about aggression. Given its neurobiological substrates, it may be difficult to actually engage in these discussions. Another woman that I spent over two decades treating had an anger problem similar to Darlene, though she was not nearly as conscious of her anger. Her angry outbursts confused her. She also had a very abusive childhood, one that involved severe sadism, such as being tied down and restrained for "punishment." This woman inflicted cruel and verbal abuse on her spouse, children, and anyone who disappointed her, but she rarely remembered these events. She could tell me something happened and others told her that she "got angry," but she could barely remember what she said. Throughout this long-term treatment, I dealt with family members when clinical issues necessitated it (e.g., suicidal crises), and her family also could not recall the extent of her abuse. It was like an explosion. Literally no one in the aftermath could describe what happened, just that something bad had occurred. My client could barely discuss what was on her mind, and attempting to explore any visual aspects of her thoughts was nearly impossible.

Anger and Problems Regarding Ideas of Transference

The discussion about the neurobiology of anger provides additional evidence regarding the difficulty to discuss and treat myriad difficult emotions encompassed under the anger umbrella. It can make us feel helpless as therapists. However, as I've said throughout this book, healing takes place in the context of a supportive therapeutic relationship. In order to develop that relationship, anger and hostility must be under some control toward us, especially in the beginning. Although many seasoned clinicians are aware that certain clients will likely unleash their anger upon them at some point, in the beginning of treatment, in order to feel safe, it's best if anger toward us is somewhat tempered. This does not mean we should shut down all expressions of aggression. In fact, when practicing with the overarching considerations about the therapeutic relationship I have described, no matter which approach is used, we should be curious about our client's complaints about us. Such misgivings can be a useful window into one's psychological life and functioning. In other words, it's often a positive sign if clients complain about us, but more later in therapy. To put an even finer point on it, especially in longer-term treatments, I worry if someone has never complained about me or at the very least been a little aggressive.

For psychodynamic therapists, complaints about us can indicate transference. Whether or not one practices therapy using a psychodynamic model, transference is an important concept. It occurs whether or not we consider it as an aspect of treatment. The rough idea is that transference is when we impose our wishes and feelings toward someone in our adult lives that mirrors feelings we experienced (even unconsciously) toward our primary caretakers when we were young. As therapists, we develop important relationships with our clients, and it is inevitable that transference will be present, possibly in terms of their view of us as therapists but also with others in their lives. What we do with that knowledge, however, depends on the therapeutic approach we're using. To be clear, I don't think we must always *say or do* something about transference. In fact, I think skilled clinicians take note of it without saying anything most of the time. To go back to the concept of mentalizing, what we do with our minds often matters more than what we say.

Transference is thought to occur in virtually all of our relationships. Those aware of older psychoanalytic constructs of transference might be appropriately wary of this discussion. There was a time in analytic treatments in which "working through the transference" was thought to be the main, if not the only, source of therapeutic action, meaning what makes clients better. Transference was thought to be the core window into psychic understanding (Abend and Shaw 1991). Though this may be true in that feelings about important people in client's lives do offer important understandings about trauma specifically, things have shifted in modern psychodynamic approaches. As such, definitions of transference have become more nuanced. Goldberg (2012) notes there are multiple definitions of transference and provides his own definition, which I find extremely useful:

> Transference is a universal mode of human relating in which past experiences with important people and their intrapsychic elaboration, along with archaic modes of thinking and feeling, are preserved, transformed, and brought to interactive life in present day relationships…More unconscious than conscious, transference adds dimensions of depth and intensity to human relationships, while it potentially also constrains and burdens them. Transference is present, dynamic and shifting…. (p. 66)

Goldberg goes on to say that transference becomes a particular focus in analytic treatment. Again, I think this may be shifting, as many psychoanalytic clinicians I know may be mindful of transference, interpreting transference is complicated and risks diminishing the reality the client is experiencing. It is increasingly clear that transference interpretations, when combined with the idea that one's feelings are not matched to the situation, can be difficult for clients to hear because people typically perceive that the issue they discuss in therapy is a complaint or problem that's rooted in "reality," which means that a transference interpretation may question the nature of the complaint. For example, in a treatment focused on uncovering transference, when a woman complains about her husband, the therapist might suggest that the patient's feelings are an echo from the past. In other words, her feelings may not be solely related (or at all related, depending on the therapist) to her husband. The idea is that the emotional weight of the client's complaints is rooted in the past, not the present. She is re-experiencing emotions related to her past as channeled through her current feelings about her husband. I think such comments are genuinely hard for people to hear and I understand why. Especially for people who have survived trauma, understanding the reality of their situation is a vital goal of treatment. People cannot learn to protect themselves if they are constantly questioning their reality. With transference interpretations, the problem is that we risk conveying to clients that they are incapable of realistically appraising their situations. Of course, we are all vulnerable to misperceiving things, particularly involving relationships, and we all have irrational beliefs at times to use the language of CBT. But my approach to dealing with trauma involves a very here-and-now focus, one in which clients are encouraged to take their thoughts seriously. Especially with anger, I start with the idea that the client is reacting to something real. Of course, it's ill-advised to connect with clients around the belief that everyone is awful and everyone else is at fault. But our job is to help people think about and understand their reaction to different situations. Often, people disclose their anger to us bypassing important parts of the story which might help us understand *why* they got angry to begin with. There's always time to think about a client's role in their troubles, but people shouldn't feel crazy when their emotions are intense. This is part of affect regulation.

We need to tread lightly with regard to transference interpretations. This is especially true for clients who seem more vulnerable with a great deal of fear and anger.

Confidence regarding dealing with emotions and relational connecting need to be prioritized before transference interpretations can successfully take place. These characteristics of emotional functioning include a sense of a coherent self, a sense of personal safety, and an experience that others, including the therapist, can provide a caring and stable environment for difficult feelings to emerge without retribution. However, people with cPTSD, which causes them to be oriented in a more practical way, may never achieve a sense of safety. Therefore, we are reliant on some aspects of what Alexander and French (1946) described as the "corrective emotional cure," in which by simply being different from early authority figures, we can help people understand that different kinds of relationships are possible. Again, it all goes back to the therapeutic relationship and our ability to think with clients about their minds and how their psychology works.

When the Therapist Is the Focus of Anger

I describe transference as an introduction to thinking about ways to manage situations in which clients view us as the problem. Again, I often consider complaints about us, when they emerge gradually, as an achievement in long-term therapies for several reasons. First, it's natural that whatever interpersonal problems have occurred outside of treatment will eventually show up in the relationship with the therapist. For people with traumatic histories, they're often waiting (often out of awareness) for the "other shoe to drop," meaning they expect to realize that someone they had hoped to trust could be a "wolf in sheep's clothing." My mixed metaphors aside, what this means is that there is some truth to psychodynamic ideas that when conflict arises between a therapist and client, we get a close-up view of their early, relational experiences. Although I don't point out to clients how they may be treating me like someone in the past who abused them, these enactments, as they are called sometimes, allow us to help clients deal with conflicted feelings about those they care for. This leads to the second benefit of client's complaints about us. If clients have held us in high esteem, it's important that they understand that we can be fallible, but that mistakes can be repaired and relationships can survive. In other words, if we do something that is hurtful or upsetting to our clients, it's important that they can distinguish normal "messed up" behavior from the types of terrifying abuse and exploitation they have been subject to. This is easy to describe in an intellectual sense. But when we are living through these experiences with clients, it can feel frightening, enraging, and overwhelming. Let's return to Melanie's treatment.

Around the time Melanie began to complain about her boyfriend, she started to tell me that her boyfriend did not like me. At first, these were subtle statements, which I took concretely to make a great deal of sense; she had begun to voice concerns about her boyfriend which suggested she was ambivalent about him. If he picked up on this, it would be reasonable for him to view me as a threat. Eventually, she told me that her boyfriend thought she was wasting her money. Practically speaking, this made no sense, as her insurance paid for her treatment, but these comments weren't really about money. It appeared that her boyfriend disagreed with certain ideas about Melanie that we had come up with together during therapy. I noted these remarks and understood the pull she felt between myself and her boyfriend and that this may represent a part of her that really wished for a better life wherein she could feel entitled to be treated well and the part of her that felt destined to be in an unsatisfying relationship. However, it was also the case that Melanie's boyfriend made her feel special and provided her with things that I simply could not. As complaints about me persisted (albeit through the voice of her boyfriend), I started to feel constrained and angry. I felt defensive, as if I needed to justify all of the work we had done. I wanted to remind her where she was when we met and how much things had gotten better. I resisted these pulls and got consultation. Eventually I told Melanie that her boyfriend's complaint might echo some concerns she had about me, but she denied this. A few months went by, and Melanie became convinced that I hated her boyfriend. It was true that I was worried about her relationship and I acknowledged that, yet I was also explicit about the good things she received from him. During the height of this, I showed up 5 minutes late for a session. Though I am occasionally late for that particular hour, I always allow up to, if not more than, 50 minutes, which was our agreed upon appointment time. However, on this occasion, my infraction seemed to burst open the door for generalized anger toward me. She said I was stealing her time, but this was woven into other complaints that sounded vague and confusing to me. She said I had said something harshly in our previous session, which I recalled discussing, but I was not aware of feeling angry. It was easy for me to acknowledge and apologize for my being late, even as I defensively (and not helpfully) pointed out that I make sure to give her all of her time. The other complaints left little for to me address. She said I seemed mad at her in the previous session, that I seemed mad in general. She was so angry she wanted to end therapy.

In the few sessions that followed with Melanie, I needed to tolerate the idea that I had fundamentally failed her. This does not mean a masochistic submission. I did apologize for being late, as was warranted, but for the rest of her general disgust and distrust toward me, I tolerated her thoughts while noting that I thought this was related to her thinking about leaving her boyfriend. In regard to transference, I never once said she was thinking of me like one of the many people who had victimized her. That would have probably ended the treatment and killed off the sense of agency she was desperately trying to find. I use the word killed intentionally, as given Melanie's history of trauma, ideas of death were never far from her mind, given her experience. The line to walk in these situations is not to tolerate abuse or to roll over but at the same time empathize with the part of the client who in that moment, or moments, hates us and needs for us to know it so we can help contain those feelings.

In thinking about it years later, it occurs that a tip off to this coming event was my concrete thinking and my defensiveness. I'd like to imagine that a better version of me could have seen this coming. But as I was caught up in the action of what seemed to be an important and needed expression of Melanie's anger toward me, I could not see it coming, and it was probably better that this was expressed in an authentic and spontaneous way. My consultant, with whom I had a long-term relationship (which is highly helpful in working with traumatized and/or clients dealing with anger), patiently helped me think about the role of anger and helplessness that was felt by both Melanie and myself. One of the greatest vulnerabilities we have as therapists, particularly in long-term therapeutic relationships, is how hard it is to be cast as a villain. But it's a common and necessary development that lead to clients being able to not only express toward us how they may have felt toward others but to realize that relationships are messy, people are fallible, and in all relationships, we will eventually have to tolerate disappointment.

Treating Anger and Aggression

In terms of formal assessment, Sullivan et al. (2019) developed a trauma-related anger scale. It involves questions related to how anger has helped in threatening situations by limiting fear or providing energy, how not being able to avoid distressing thoughts was followed by anger, how vulnerability led to anger, etc. This is the first instrument of its kind and provides a window into the various kinds of anger people with PTSD or cPTSD might experience.

Anger in therapy may not need formal assessment as it presents to us often early in therapy. In dealing with everyone I see, but particularly trauma survivors, I start with the premise that anger is normal and expected. The language I have developed for this with clients is to share that we all have anger and on some level it makes us uncomfortable. This discomfort might be because it bothers others and or it might be because it bothers us, or it could be both. Either way, I emphasize that we all need to develop a healthy relationship with our own aggression. I talk about anger and our aggression as a relationship that needs to be understood and nurtured. That being said, I rarely lead with discussions about aggression unless a client brings it up. But I do intervene when I think doing so can further the discussion. For example, one woman I worked with for over a decade was very hostile and aggressive. She was also paranoid. Although her suspiciousness of me was always on my mind, her anger was directed at others. Early in the therapy, she needed me enough that she had to keep me out of the loop as an object of her attacks on others. Yet, it did seem important that her anger at some point become a focus of clinical attention. In order to facilitate talking about this, I waited for ways in which she had acted aggressively that struck me as funny. One day, she told me about an interaction with an equally aggressive colleague in which she responded with witty and biting sarcasm. I laughed. A lot and for a long time. She was stunned; I imagined she was worried I might judge her. Yet, while I would have tried to avoid acting aggressive in her situation, I thought her wit was quite unmatched. And this person she was describing had been quite hostile to her. I also laughed because I could not personally have imagined having the courage to be as assertive as she was. In a way, I admired it, even though I was not sure how helpful such long-term strategies were. I wait for these moments with clients because it decreases shame about aggression and it allows myself and a client to really connect. Following this, she was much more comfortable telling me about her aggressive actions on social media, over email, and in person. Although I could not summon a part of myself to identify with her aggression in many subsequent situations, she continued to feel safe enough to talk to me about this aspect of her life. She also allowed me to give her suggestions about how to dampen her responses, eventually sending me or bringing into session drafts of emails she needed to send to people she was angry at. Eventually, over a couple of years' time, she stopped these behaviors. She realized with my help that sometimes it was easier to get what she wanted if she was straightforward but also kind (or at least not insulting). It was also around this time she was able to tell me about the constant state of fear she was in from a parent who was hostile all of the time. As her aggressive impulses dimmed, she authentically and spontaneously started to wonder about this parent and how their aggression had shaped her.

Dealing with aggression and anger is difficult, and we have few models about how to do so. I think it's important to walk a balance between breathing life into expressions of aggression and shutting down angry thoughts and feelings because they make us uncomfortable. In terms of aggressive expressions toward us as therapists, I think it's important that we set limits regarding what we allow. One client, when she got angry, felt free to call me all sorts of names. For example, she said I was a "fucking asshole," but that could be the beginning of a diatribe about me. I told her that she needed to find a better way to express herself or the therapy could not continue. Although it's unpleasant to hear these kinds of comments, I don't allow them for another reason. It's simply not helpful for clients to be that aggressive. It's self-reinforcing and does not provide a sense of safety for clients. Clients who are really aggressive are often on some level (even if out of awareness) terrified of actually hurting others. If we allow them to hurt us, we are cohabitating with the aspect of themselves that views themselves as a perpetrator. This is not a situation in which clients can get better, as we are then acting like parents who cannot set limits with a child who has gone too far with their aggression.

Outside of setting limits when needed to keep clients emotionally safe, it's important that we think about anger and aggression as a part of therapy. We need to keep this on our minds so that clients can talk about aggressive and hostile thoughts and ideas and aggressive visualizations. The reality is that the kinds of anger and aggression I am describing can rarely be treated in short-term treatments. Largely, there is no clear evidence to guide mental health professionals in treating angry clients (Saini 2009). This author looked at nine treatments dealing with anger, including cognitive, cognitive behavior therapy, exposure, psychodynamic, psychoeducational, relaxation-based, skills-based, stress inoculation, and multicomponent therapies. All were found to be effective in treating different anger-based therapy concerns. In a 12-session group treatment, using either present-centered therapy or cognitive processing therapy, there were small reductions in anger and hostility among active military members (Miles et al. 2019). The most common short-term treatments for anger, however, are standard cognitive behavioral therapies for anger management. In these treatments, clients are encouraged to notice anger triggers, related physiological arousal and thoughts, and then to develop ways to decrease distress. However, and not surprisingly, a number of different therapies can be helpful to people who present to treatment with anger-related concerns. I often weave in formal anger management when clients are ready to think about different ways of dealing with situations in which they want to not be perceived as aggressive.

Conclusion

Little exists in the way of research to guide us in dealing with anger in people who have cPTSD, and this is a topic that needs more attention. Anger involves our relationship with our own aggressive impulses. Yet, I think therapists who deal with clients with trauma histories understand that anger is a complex topic and that anger has many faces and meanings. It can be primary or a mask for other more vulnerable emotions. It can indicate disappointment. Anger is at once hidden in our culture and also alive via the subcultures on social media and among public figures in some countries who espouse vitriol in an unabandoned way. These facts mirror our own internal relationships with aggression. We know it's there, but we aren't sure how to deal with it. This trickles down to how we act with clients. And while there is no easy answer in how to treat aggression, we need to be open to hear about anger and consider the ways that the culture of mental health has not wanted to deal with some of the more complicated and unpleasant aspects of human nature. Clients can't express their anger if we are not able to tolerate it.

Interventions for Treating Angry and Aggressive Clients

- Start with the idea that aggression and anger are normal.
- If a client is idealizing, know that this may shift but also may be a need aspect or creating safety in the beginning of therapy.
- If you can, use humor to defuse shame about aggression; normalize aggression if this seems reasonable.
- Don't engage in an us vs. them mentality or openly agree with excessive externalization.
- Encourage the development of a relationship with one's aggression; we're all angry and we need to find ways to be compassionate toward our own anger.
- Anger that is turned inward is also an important kind of aggression; it requires patience to understand the nuances and meaning of this.
- Try to identify anger as a clinical issue in people who seem especially angry; if this does not help, shift toward other interventions.
- Adopt an attitude of curiosity if clients complain about the therapist.
- Don't assume you understand what someone is angry about, ask questions; delve into what makes someone angry.
- For people who have anger as part of their personality (trait anger), don't fight with them, but limit insults toward the therapist.

- If it's not too overstimulating and does not create too much physiological arousal, ask about visualizations regarding anger.
- Use anger management strategies if the client is open.
- Consider your own relationship with aggression as a person and a therapist; be mindful of the kind of clients that make you defensive or angry.

References

Abend, S. M., & Shaw, R. R. (1991). Concepts and controversies about the transference neurosis. *Journal of the American Psychoanalytic Association, 39*, 227–239.

Alexander, F., & French, T. M. (1946). *Psychoanalytic therapy: Principals and applications*. New York: Ronald Press.

Burns, J. W., Higdon, L. J., Mullen, J. T., Lansky, D., & Wei, J. M. (1999). Relationships among patient hostility, anger expression, depression, and the working alliance in a work hardening program. *Annals of Behavioral Medicine, 21*(1), 77–82.

Chemtob, C. M., Novaco, R. W., Hamada, R. S., Gross, D. M., & Smith, G. (1997). Anger regulation deficits in combat-related posttraumatic stress disorder. *Journal of Traumatic Stress, 10*, 17–36.

DiGangi, J. A., Gomez, D., Mendoza, L., Jason, L. A., Keys, C. B., & Koenen, K. C. (2013). Pretrauma risk factors for posttraumatic stress disorder: A systematic review of the literature. *Clinical Psychology Review, 33*(6), 728–744.

Dohrenwend, B. P., Turner, J. B., Turse, N. A., Adams, B. G., Koenen, K. C., & Marshall, R. (2006). The psychological risks of Vietnam for U.S. veterans: A revisit with new data and methods. *Science, 313*(5789), 979–982.

Dyer, K. F. W., Dorahy, M. J., Hamilton, G., Corry, M., Shannon, M., MacSherry, A., McRobert, G., Elder, R., & McElhill, B. (2009). Anger, aggression, and self-harm in PTSD and complex PTSD. *Journal of Clinical Psychology, 65*, 1099–1114.

Easton, S. D., & Kong, J. (2017). Mental health indicators fifty years later: A population-based study of men with histories of child sexual abuse. *Child Abuse & Neglect, 63*, 273–283.

Ferenczi, S. (1933). *Confusion of tongues between adults and the child, in final contributions to the problems and methods of psycho-analysis (1955)*. London: Karnac.

Goldberg, S. H. (2012). Transference. In G. O. Gabbard, B. E. Litowitz, & P. Williams (Eds.), *Textbook of psychoanalysis* (2nd ed., pp. 65–77). Arlington: American Psychiatric Publishing.

Gonzalez, O. I., Novaco, R. W., Reger, M. A., & Gahm, G. A. (2016). Anger intensification with combat-related PTSD and depression comorbidity. *Psychological Trauma: Theory, Research, Practice, and Policy, 8*(1), 9–16.

Hoge, C. W., Auchterlonie, J. L., & Milliken, C. S. (2006). Mental health problems, use of mental health services, and attrition from military service after returning from deployment to Iraq or Afghanistan. *Journal of the American Medical Association, 295*(9), 1023–1032.

Keene, A. C., & Epps, J. (2016). Childhood physical abuse and aggression: Shame and narcissistic vulnerability. *Child Abuse & Neglect, 51*, 276–283.

Kohut, H. (1971). *The analysis of the self: A systematic approach to the psychoanalytic treatment of narcissistic personality disorders*. New York: International Universities Press.

Love, A. R., Morland, L. A., Menez, U., Taft, C., MacDonald, A., & Mackintosh, M. A. (2015). "Strength at home" intervention for male veterans perpetrating intimate partner aggression: Perceived needs survey of therapists and pilot effectiveness study. *Journal of Interpersonal Violence, 30*(13), 2344–2362.

Mackintosh, M., Willis, E., & Morland, L. A. (2015, November). Anger reductions in response to evidence-based treatment for PTSD. In M. A. Mackintosh (Chair), *Advances and innovation in treating anger and aggression in trauma exposed populations*. Symposium conducted at the

31st annual meeting of the International Society for Traumatic Stress Studies, New Orleans, LA.

McHugh, T., Forbes, D., Bates, G., Hopwood, M., & Creamer, M. (2012). Anger in PTSD: Is there a need for a concept of PTSD-related posttraumatic anger? *Clinical Psychology Review, 32*(2), 93–104.

Meffert, S. M., Metzler, T. J., Henn-Haase, C., McCaslin, S., Inslicht, S., Chemtob, C., Neylan, T., & Marmar, C. R. (2008). A prospective study of trait anger and PTSD symptoms in police. *Journal of Traumatic Stress, 21*(4), 410–416.

Miles, S. R., Dillon, K. H., Jacoby, V. M., Hale, W. J., Dondanville, K. A., Wachen, J. S., et al. (2019). Changes in anger and aggression after treatment for PTSD in active duty military. *Journal of Clinical Psychology*. Advance online publication. Accessed online on 12th Jan 2020 at https://doi.org/10.1002/jclp.22878.

Mills, J. (2006). *Other banalities*. East Sussex: Routledge.

Novaco, R. W., & Chemtob, C. M. (2002). Anger and combat-related posttraumatic stress disorder. *Journal of Traumatic Stress, 15*, 123–132.

Olatunji, B. O., Ciesielski, B. G., & Tolin, D. F. (2010). Fear and loathing: A meta-analytic review of the specificity of anger in PTSD. *Behavior Therapy, 41*, 93–105.

Rao, S. R., Broome, K. M., & Simpson, D. D. (2004). Depression and hostility as predictors of long-term outcomes among opiate users. *Addiction, 99*(5), 579–589.

Rosbrow, T. (2014). Fear of attachment, ruptured adult relationships, and therapeutic impasse. Attachment: New directions. *Psychotherapy and Relational Psychoanalysis, 8*(3), 227–235.

Russell, J. A., & Fehr, B. (1994). Fuzzy concepts in a fuzzy hierarchy: Varieties of anger. *Journal of Personality and Social Psychology, 67*, 186–205.

Saini, M. (2009). A meta-analysis of the psychological treatment of anger: Developing guidelines for evidence-based practice. *Journal of the American Academy of Psychiatry and the Law, 37*(4), 473–488.

Schell, T. L., Marshall, G. N., & Jaycox, L. H. (2004). All symptoms are not created equal: The prominent role of hyperarousal in the natural course of posttraumatic psychological distress. *Journal of Abnormal Psychology, 113*, 189–197.

Sudbrack, R., Manfro, P. H., Kuhn, I. M., de Carvalho, H. W., & Lara, D. R. (2015). What doesn't kill you makes you stronger and weaker: How childhood trauma relates to temperament traits. *Journal of Psychiatric Research, 62*, 123–129.

Sullivan, C., Jones, R. T., Hauenstein, N., & White, B. (2019). Development of the trauma-related anger scale. *Assessment, 26*(6), 1117–1127.

Wilk, J. E., Quartana, P. J., Clarke-Walper, K., Kok, B. C., & Riviere, L. A. (2015). Aggression in US soldiers post-deployment: Associations with combat exposure and PTSD and the moderating role of trait anger. *Aggressive Behavior, 41*, 556–565.

Chapter 9
Sociocultural Considerations in Trauma Treatment

Culture and the Culture of Avoidance: Thinking About Differences Between Therapist and Client

The trend to avoid race, culture, and class discussions not only mirrors current and historical negations; it's easy to wish that ideas and concepts described in therapeutic work somehow transcend social and racial disparities. We all are just people trying to connect with other people. Right? That is an ideal view, but it's more complicated than that. We are at a puzzling and troubling crossroad in our current history. Some parts of the world are seeing unprecedented levels of hate crimes and overt negative comments by public figures and on social media about certain targeted groups. For example, in the United States, the Federal Bureau of Investigation reported an overall increase in hate crimes directed at people—as opposed to property, which has historically been more common—from 2008 to 2018 (Kaleem 2019). The increases in crimes occurred more among people who were Latino, transgender, or gender nonconforming. Anti-Semitic attacks increased by 13% in 2018 from the previous year, with the highest number of incidents reported in Western countries including the United States, France, Britain, and Germany (Reuters 2019). NAACP reported that 2015 saw increases in hate crimes against African Americans, members of the LGBTQ community, Native Americans, Jews, and Muslims. And while numbers regarding specific hate crimes have fluctuated slightly in recent years, NAACP notes that only 2% of hate crimes are reported to the FBI.

We cannot suppose our clients as being intangible and disentangled from a social context that involves individual experiences and an awareness of discrimination, racism, violence, and the feeling of being "other"—a child or an adult who gets the sense they are different and are constantly stereotyped. These issues become woven into trauma narratives, when there are stories someone can tell. When there are not narratives with language, we can be present and wait to witness and observe the impact of these experiences. If we are really to get to know someone and their

T. M. Greenberg, *Treating Complex Trauma*,
https://doi.org/10.1007/978-3-030-45285-8_9

encounters of adversity related to social contextual issues, tolerating not knowing details of lived experience becomes a part of the therapy as it does with other traumatic events. Let's consider the situation of someone I will refer to as Andrea.

Andrea, a young African American woman, was a successful scientist in her field. She came to therapy because she thought she had "social anxiety." As I got to know her, it seemed that she was depressed. She felt a general sense of hopelessness and unrest, and she also felt a tremendous sense of guilt for having achieved a status of "privilege," even though she worked hard to make ends meet based on her academic salary. I worked with Andrea for several years, and she made it clear that she did not want to discuss race during her first year of therapy, even after she mentioned casually that someone had written a racially offensive slur in the elevator of the building where she lived. It was only after a couple of years that race became a frequent aspect of our conversations, and it was at this point that she was able to tell me about how constant racism and stereotyping impacted her, particularly at work. Once we were able to have these discussions, in which I frequently acknowledged the racism in her workplace as well as how racism impacts people in the United States, she told me stories about how her parents had coached her to be careful when driving or walking because she could be targeted as an African American. She felt confused about these discussions, even as she understood them to reflect the reality of her life in America, particularly where she grew up, which was a geographic area in which systemic racism was widely known. It was important that I labeled these experiences as a kind of trauma, as well as confusing, sad, and enraging. It was equally important that I could acknowledge the unfairness of her situation, including that as a white person, I could not ever really know the constant strain of this kind of discrimination, biased perceptions, and world in which she likely had to work harder than others to achieve the same amount of success. Eventually, she was able to be much more assertive at work, including with people she supervised. She had been allowing her employees to engage in all kinds of behaviors she did not feel comfortable with because she was worried about being seen as "an angry black woman." Interestingly, as I validated that she did not seem assertive enough at work, because of her fears about being stereotyped, she felt safe enough to confront her employees, who welcomed her honesty. I came to learn that her experience of me initially, as a white woman, was that I could not be helpful to her in this regard. She eventually told me that she felt a previous therapist had shied away from race discussions and even minimized her experience as an African American woman.

Although I do think that I helped Andrea with her situation regarding racial discrimination and the sense of hopelessness that stemmed from that, it's important to remember the context of white therapists who help nonwhite clients. In 2015, the clinical psychology workforce was 88% white and 12% racial/ethnic persons (American Psychological Association – APA 2016). Some studies on mental health outcomes research have found that when clients and therapists are ethnically or racially matched, this tends to be related to greater satisfaction and better outcomes

(Meyer et al. 2011; Kim and Kang 2018). This makes sense if we think of the therapist factors we considered in Chapter 1 and the importance of empathy and the therapeutic relationship. This is not to say that we cannot be helpful if we are not ethnically or racially matched with our clients. People we see have all kinds of experiences that we have not lived through, but I'm reminded of the principles of humility emphasized in mentalization-based therapies. We don't know what we don't know. And even if we do think we know, we have to be careful. For example, I have made the mistake of assuming too quickly that I understand some clients who come from lower-class backgrounds. As I come from a lower-class background, I have sometimes not phrased some of my assumptions as questions, which was clearly not helpful for some people. Like all groups, lower-class people are not a monolith. Another mistake I made in this regard was to assume that a nonwhite client who grew up in a predominantly white, rural part of our country may have felt discriminated against. At the time I brought this up, which was early on in therapy, she denied this and said she felt "welcome." It was only after another year of therapy that she recalled experiences of being taunted by white students when she was in junior high school. But even then, it was pretty clear her feelings about social contextual issues were not related to her ethnic identity. Her issues, as she described them, were actually more because of class—her family was wealthy in an area in which few people were. She had many feelings of embarrassment about this, and this stemmed in part from envy of her peers. I should have waited for her to bring up these experiences, but at the same time, I wanted to let her know she could discuss her experiences related to race and ethnicity with me. In another example of how complicated people's reactions to discrimination are and just how hard this can be for well-meaning clinicians, a colleague who grew up in an area of world in which her religious group was a persecuted minority told me that a client of hers who grew up in a similar situation accused her of being prejudiced. Socio-contextual issues are hard to discuss, as there is real desire among many of us to create a space of openness and understanding, but timing and trust in the therapeutic relationship are crucial. Even when we are well meaning, it's hard to get these conversations "just right." And maybe that is how it should be. As therapists, we can't really repair the trauma experienced by people who are discriminated against and unjustly treated. We do have to try to think about the impact of unfair treatment, though, while considering current guidelines of how to talk and think about these issues. By being sensitive to our own biases and assumptions, there may be some healing in our attempts, particularly if we can empower clients and help them not take discrimination personally. I'll discuss more about how to talk and think about these issues with our clients, but we should not assume we understand the specific nuances of what clients experience. In fact, this is a criticism of some of the earlier teaching on working with diverse clients, which I think has unfortunately and unintentionally reinforced stereotypes about some groups.

Trauma, Microaggressions, and Race and Class

Race experiences can have a number of traumatic elements or what Comas-Díaz (2000) refers to as "post-colonization disorder," which involves elements of alienation and identity conflicts from repeated encounters with racism. Racism is defined as prejudice, discrimination, and aggression against a subordinate racial group based on attitudes of superiority by the dominant group (Williams et al. 2018). Given the recent events in our country related to the unfair and violent treatment toward African Americans and others, it seems clear that for many people, simply being a nonwhite person is an experience fraught with fear and elements of trauma. US-born Latino and Mexican-origin persons as well as immigrant groups have more recently experienced increases in fear and anxiety related to immigration enforcement programs in the United States (Martínez et al. 2018). And overall, there have been increases in ethnic prejudice in many Western countries (Thijs et al. 2018).

Bell (1997) has referred to "micro-traumas" due to everyday encounters with racism. A related and more familiar concept is the term "microaggression" which is also linked with experiences of discrimination and often subtle everyday events that denigrate individuals because they are members of particular groups (Pierce et al. 1978). Microaggressions are behaviors and statements, often unconscious or unintentional, that communicate hostile or derogatory messages, particularly to members of targeted social groups (e.g., people of color; lesbian, gay, bisexual, and transgender [LGBT] people; as well as women and stigmatized religious groups) (Sue 2010). Note that in some of the research I will describe, there is a "Q" added to "LGBT." LGBTQ has become a more common phrase in popular culture and in research studies and can mean either "questioning" or "queer." Although some younger groups describe the term "queer" to be a reclaiming of a word that was once a slur, it's not entirely clear that this term is unoffensive to all people in the LGBT community (Gander 2018). Therefore I will limit my use of the term to be respectful while noting the importance of language as a part of a narrative that should be described by people who are included in groups that have been discriminated against.

Several years ago, as the term "microaggressions" became more integrated in the popular culture lexicon, some colleagues mentioned to me that this term seemed to dilute the meaning of the word aggression. However, the value in the concept of microaggressions, as I understand it, is that it accounts for the trend that it's no longer socially acceptable (in many areas, though not all) to make overtly racist, sexist, homophobic, and other derogatory comments. Microaggressions, then, capture the ways people communicate their biases and express discriminatory thoughts. On its face, these comments seem not as overtly aggressive and prejudiced (e.g., no use of racial slurs), but hostile messages are conveyed, nevertheless. Authors have proposed and expanded on beliefs and assumptions that highlight the various ways microaggressions are experienced by people of color (Sue et al. 2007; Sue 2010; Nadal et al. 2014). These themes include *Alien in Own Land* which refers to instances when people assume that nonwhite individuals are foreign born. For example, a bi-racial client living in an almost exclusively white town told me of constant instances in which people asked her, "where she was from." When she answered with the state she was born in and that she was from the United States, they often argued with her regarding her answer, wanting to know where she was *really* from. *Ascription of Intelligence* refers to labeling someone with a certain amount of intelligence based on her or his race. The theme of *Color Blindness* occurs when people deny a person's experiences regarding race, for instance, when people make comments like "There is only one race, the human race," which is denying another's racial reality. The *Criminality/Assumption of Criminal Status* occurs when a person of color is presumed to be deviant. An example of this was expressed to me by an African American client who told me that when she worked in a high-end department store, she was excessively monitored and even followed by security staff. She thought they worried she would steal expensive clothing. Other themes include *Denial of Individual Racism* which is when an individual tries to deny racial biases, and *The Myth of Meritocracy* theme includes statements that emphasize race as having no role in people's life successes. This happens when people say things such as "Everybody can succeed here, if they just work hard enough." The idea with the Myth of Meritocracy is that there is a denial of how much race is an obstacle in the achievement of success. *Pathologizing Cultural Values/Communication Styles* is the idea that the dominant, white cultural values and communication styles are ideal and that anything different is abnormal. A recent example of this involves a young man who was barred from a sport competition because of his hair. The *Second-Class Citizen* theme occurs when a white person is given preferential treatment over a person of color, for example, in customer service situations.

As one can imagine, the term microaggression may just scratch the surface of what is experienced by people of color. One speaker at a recent conference I attended brought up microaggressions and noted that these experiences "Don't seem to be very micro." Research has found that microaggressions do indeed have mental health consequences. Nadal et al. (2014) described that increased racial microaggressions are associated with increases in depression, anxiety, and a negative view of the world. Race-related microaggressions have a negative impact on the self-esteem of Asian Americans, who are often viewed as "perpetual foreigners" (Cheryan and Monin 2005; Wong-Padoongpatt et al. 2017). The burden of microaggressions and perceptions of racial discrimination are associated with suicidal ideation among African Americans (Hollingsworth et al. 2017; Walker et al. 2014). Further in a study of African Americans spanning over two decades, racial discrimination was associated with shortened leukocyte telomere length, which is a marker of accelerated physiologic aging and health decline (Chae et al. 2020). To put this plainly, racism is stressful and acts on the body like other stresses, including abuse and adverse experiences.

Hispanic Americans and African Americans are more likely to report experiencing traumatic events, and they are more likely to describe more experiences of victimization than whites (Andrews et al. 2015; Hatch and Dohrenwend 2007). Another study found increases in PTSD in Hispanic Americans, Native Americans, Pacific Islander Americans, and Southeast Asian refugees (Pole et al. 2008). Additionally,

African Americans also have higher rates of PTSD than white people (Himle et al. 2009). In a nationwide telephone survey, Latinos who perceived their state's immigration policies as unfavorable had worse self-reported mental and physical health. This was particularly true in Latino US citizens who worried about the deportation of a friend or family member (Vargas et al. 2017). Although research is not entirely consistent, overall nonwhite veterans have higher rates of PTSD (Loo 2020).

Regarding immigration experiences, Grinberg and Grinberg (1989) described the immigration process as characterized by cumulative trauma, disorganization, pain, and frustration. Altman (2010), Leary (2006, 2007, 2012), and Tummala-Narra (2007, 2015) have described extensively the ways in which race, histories of colonization, and slavery have influenced perceptions of skin color, unconscious and conscious associations of belonging, ideas of goodness and badness, and the ways these dynamics influence the therapeutic encounter. Particularly for older immigrants raising children in the United States, there are a number of challenges faced in regard to different social and familial roles, and for older adults who have immigrated to the United States, there are a number of stressors related to relative isolation (Akhtar 2011; Tummala-Narra et al. 2013). And as evidenced by relatively recent natural disasters in the United States, people who are both nonwhite and poor are left literally to suffer the consequences of a system that ignores and abandons (Leary 2006; Brown 2008).

Although it is not clear that nonwhites experience more mental health problems than their white counterparts, there is data that nonwhite persons underutilize mental health services and end treatment earlier than white persons (e.g., Leong and Lau 2001). Many of us can imagine the reasons for this. Psychotherapy is an encounter that was developed with a certain type of white upper-middle-class person in mind. Different cultures have different ways of describing emotions. As white upper-middle-class therapists, we risk imposing the "rules" that are unique to our profession to those we treat, and in this way, we are anything but neutral and objective (McWilliams 2003).

Social class is about much more than just the money and material goods somebody possesses. It is also about how one feels, thinks, and acts (Samson and Zaleskiewicz 2020). Diminished resources, uncertainty, and unpredictability are a central part of the lives of lower-class people. The sociocognitive theory of social class suggests that social class constitutes a social environment that individuals inhabit over a prolonged period of time and involves shared experiences, a specific knowledge base, and behaviors that impact relationships with others (Kraus et al. 2012). This involves language and perceptions. Upper-class individuals tend to be more trusting than lower-class individuals (e.g., Chen and Matthews 2001; Pew Research Center 2007). When we are dealing with those from lower-class backgrounds, whether white or nonwhite, we are confronted with a different use of language and perceptions about authority. Sometimes, these differences are pathologized in our field. Regarding perceptions, as someone who has come from a lower-class background, I find that I tend to be more aware of situations of hubris, or at least my perceptions of it. I have noticed in the decades that I have lived in a very high socioeconomic area that I tend to be more sensitive to social situations in which I perceive that someone from a higher class is expecting a level of authority, simply based on their class standing. I have also felt out of place in terms of language. When I first moved to San Francisco, I felt embarrassed by my relatively limited vocabulary given my background as someone from a lower class, even though I was highly educated. As I received a full scholarship toward my graduate school studies, I worried sometimes that I was "faking it," that I was not really as smart as others who had doctorate degrees. I was also known as someone to be very blunt. I was not trying to be aggressive, but I had to learn how to talk about things without being so direct, so as not to alienate colleagues and others from upper-class backgrounds. In a dated book on this topic, *Language and Poverty* (Board of Regents of the University of Wisconsin, 1970, Institute for Research on Poverty, University of Wisconsin, 1970) notes that people from lower-class backgrounds tend to use fewer words to describe the same things as their richer counterparts, what was referred to as "lazy speech." Yet people from impoverished backgrounds are anything but lazy when describing their ideas, and rather, they just tend to be more concise. Lubrano (2004) describes the way that a college education made it difficult to talk with his blue-collar family. It seems for many people that coming from a situation other than that of the white middle to upper middle class can make it hard to adapt to the ways therapy is conducted.

Brown (2008) notes that the contribution of class and classism to individual experience can be used as one means of deepening understanding of the experience of trauma exposure. When I am with clients, I always find it helpful to start with an assumption that something that seems different is cultural or class based. When in doubt, I ask. For example, one person who came from a country in which there was a great deal of oppression and violence against women kept telling me she was "paranoid." Initially I thought perhaps her paranoia had to do with negative assessments in the United States against the particular group she identifies with. I asked her whether she thought her suspiciousness was linked to cultural differences, perceptions of her, etc. She answered me definitively. She said, "No. I'm paranoid. Everyone from my country thinks I am." Indeed this person did have a great deal of clinically important symptoms of paranoia, but even then, I felt it was hard to disassemble her paranoia from adjusting to a new country where there is a great deal of discrimination. I thought of her suspiciousness, in other words, on multiple levels.

Trauma, Microaggressions, and LGBT Persons

In addition to psychotherapy and psychology being a model for white people in the upper classes, it historically has been a heterosexist/heteronormative model. There has been an extensive history of not only pathologizing but criminalizing of homosexual behavior. For example, over two decades ago, I worked with a woman in her 70s who was psychiatrically hospitalized for several months because she was gay. I was able to get her medical records from that time (the late 1950s), and homosexuality was listed as the primary diagnosis. This client had no romantic partner and told me she "tried not to think about being with women" after her hospitalization. In another example, an older client told me about a time in her childhood in which her father was absent for a time, as he was involved in criminal proceedings for having sex with another man.

The first edition of the *Diagnostic and Statistical Manual of Mental Disorders* (APA 1952) classified "homosexuality" as a "sociopathic personality disturbance." In the DSM-II, published in 1968, homosexuality was reclassified as a "sexual deviation." Homosexuality was removed from the DSM in its third edition in 1973. Ironically, even as psychoanalytic theory seemed to pathologize homosexuality in its earlier years, Freud was relatively neutral on the topic. He thought we are all born with bisexual tendencies and said late in his career that he did not think homosexuality should be classified as an illness (Drescher 2015). Many if not most following Freud, however, did pathologize homosexuality, as we see from the first two editions of the DSM. However, in the last few decades, psychoanalytic writing seems to have attempted to correct the extensive pathologizing that took place after Freud. There has been a lot of thoughtful literature regarding work with LGBT populations as well as sex and gender roles. For example, the journals *Gender and Psychoanalysis* and *Studies in Gender and Sexuality* have long covered these topics; Ken Corbett is a very prolific and thoughtful psychoanalyst who has been addressing sexual orientation for the last 25 years; Diane Ehrensaft for almost the same amount of time is a psychoanalytic writer on gender identity and issues impacting trans youth.

Yet, it's hard not to think about the damage done by the mental health field which has labeled homosexuality as an illness. And this mirrors a culture which has struggled to accept aspects of certain rights regarding issues involving LGBT individuals. And though this may be changing in some parts of the world and within the United States, there is still something inherently unique about LGBT issues that are different than race, ethnicity, religion, and class. For most people in these latter situations, there are not the same dilemmas of coming out to family or even with wrestling with identity in the same way—that involves a declarative statement to others who may have opinions on who they are and/or whom they choose to be with. For example, a number of my younger clients who are gay or bisexual enjoy on one level living in an urban area in which they voice few experiences of discrimination or concerns regarding sexual orientation. Yet, when we talk about their families, the story changes to something that is more strained. A common remark might be something like "My mom *says* she's okay with it," with the implication that the reality might be different. Unlike many older clients, the parents of younger clients don't as often seem to just ignore a client's reality about their sexuality. And I hear much less often from younger people that their parents have overtly rejected them, unlike many people in older cohorts. As I discussed regarding microaggressions, there is increased social pressure to be more accepting toward all kinds of differences. Yet, different areas of the United States, our diverse subcultures, and different parts of the world have varying degrees of discrimination and mistreatment of LGBT groups.

LGBT veterans are exposed to higher rates of trauma than their nonveteran LGBT counterparts and non-LGBT veterans. This includes interpersonal and institutional discrimination by fellow service members, citizens, therapy group members, and healthcare providers (Livingston et al. 2019). In medicine, physician biases may result in LGBT clients receiving a lower standard of care or restricted access to services as compared to others not identified as such (Morris et al. 2019). A review of LGBT military personnel and veterans found that they have poorer mental health and well-being; report more stigma and barriers to mental healthcare, which reduces accessing healthcare services; experience more sexual trauma; and have poorer physical health than heterosexual military personnel and veterans (Mark et al. 2019).

Being bullied is more common among LGBT and gender nonconforming adolescents (Camodeca et al. 2019; McBride and Schubotz 2017). Experiences of cyber and in-person social victimization are related to increases in school absences and mental health problems in adulthood, including depression, PTSD, and suicide (Earnshaw et al. 2017; Rivers 2011; Russell et al. 2014). Families that comprise LGBT members experience more microaggressions. A recent study found these aggressions were related to assumptions about (1) family legitimacy; (2) conflicts with family values; and (3) gender role variation within family (Haines et al. 2018).

Stereotypes and Stereotype Threats

Although I have discussed some of the consequences of how certain groups are treated and the impact of this maltreatment, I want to focus on an area of research that has been tremendously helpful to me in thinking about how people are affected by perceptions about them, stereotype threat. The idea of stereotype threat is that stigmatized group members may underperform on diagnostic tests of ability or in other demanding situations through concerns about confirming a negative societal stereotype as belonging to the self. Steele and Aronson's (1995) original article on this topic demonstrated that African Americans underperformed on a verbal reasoning test when participants were told the test was a diagnostic indicator of intellectual ability. Conversely, when the same test was presented as not related to ability, they performed equivalently to their white peers. This was then expanded to include research on females, specifically related to math ability (Steele 1997). In other words, when people are aware of stereotypes that may persist against them, they are more likely to perform poorly in certain situations. For example, women perform worse on a task described as a "mathematical" test as opposed to the same test described as a "problem-solving" task. Framing the task as a mathematical test likely triggers the activation of a negative stereotype in women, as women are stereotypically considered worse in mathematical tasks (Johns et al. 2005). This research has been expanded to include how women perform on simulated driving tests, in the elderly in terms of perceptions on their memory abilities, and even white men when being compared to Asian men regarding math abilities (Aronson et al. 1999; Pavlova et al. 2014; Pennington et al. 2016). It's not clear that people assessed in these studies are even aware of stereotypes (meaning the awareness may be unconscious), but the invocation of stereotypes may increase feelings of anxiety, negative thinking, and mind-wandering (Kiefer and Sekaquaptewa 2007; Pennington et al. 2016).

Stereotype threat is an interesting area of research that offers another way to understand our clients who may be subject to the impact of judgments about who they are. I have incorporated the idea of stereotypes and stereotype threats into therapies for whom these ideas may be helpful. For example, a woman who was struggling considerably with her relatively older age noted that she felt that she was treated differently after she allowed her hair to turn grey and felt that in recent years she began to "look older." As a result she said, she noticed that people started talking loudly to her (as they assumed she may have a hearing impairment; she did not) and questioning her recall of certain events (she had no evidence of cognitive impairment). I talked with her about the idea of stereotype threat and she looked up the research online. She felt "less crazy," as she put it, and did not take as personally the insensitive encounters she experienced with some people, as she understood this in a "scientific way." This did not mean there were not feelings of sadness and anger regarding the culture we live in and the impact of stereotypes; that was something that came later, but the intellectual understanding allowed her to realize that her perceptions of how some people viewed her were inaccurate.

Talking About Differences

How and when to address social context though remains difficult for some therapists and the people we are trying to help. When I look back on my own training, which suggested that we embrace and speak to differences in an active way and right away (e.g., Sue and Sue 1999), I have found that I have alienated people when bringing up racial ideas too soon in treatment. Criticisms of this approach have also noted that it's misleading to lump all diverse groups together, as well as a tendency to ignore intersectionality, the ways that discrimination can occur based on many aspects of not belonging to a white male heterosexual group (Buchanan 2011; Singleton 2013). Cole (2009) described the concept of intersectionality to describe approaches that simultaneously consider the meaning and consequences of multiple categories of identity, difference, and disadvantage. An example of this might be an African American woman who also identifies as a lesbian. It seems impossible to be able to imagine this woman's experiences of discrimination without considering multiple nuances to what she lives through. And she should be the one to describe it. Again, we just don't know what we don't know, but we can be open to learning.

I think there can be a balance between being open to such discussions and rushing in too quickly to assure clients that we "get it." I recall one man I worked many years ago with who was one of only a few African American employees in an organization of over 3000. I brought up the idea that it might be difficult to work in this setting and that perhaps part of his general unrest was being in an organization (that was clearly described by this man) as not being respectful of diversity. He became very anxious and changed the subject. I realized I needed to back off. As I have said,

I tend to consider that immigrant experiences, many "first-generation" experiences, and those involving other people who are among groups prone to discrimination are holding onto a number of difficult emotions that I would place in the category of traumatic or, at the least, very difficult to talk about, particularly with a white therapist. Therefore, I tend to tread cautiously when broaching the subject, just as I would with any person with whom I need to allow time and safety to develop before addressing something painful and traumatic. I hold these kinds of social contextual experiences in my mind until someone feels safe enough with me to address them.

Comas-Díaz (2016) recommends that therapy provide empowerment of clients to "Voice their reality, perceive themselves as a source of authority, and develop critical consciousness to transform themselves and their circumstances. More specifically, the race informed-treatment phases includes (a) assessment and stabilization, (b) desensitization, (c) reprocessing, (d) psychological decolonization, and (e) social action" (pp. 254–255). She also notes that it is generally unhelpful to compare our lives to clients who have experienced racial discrimination or have histories of cultural oppression. She noted an example of a Jewish therapist mentioning to someone who is Native American that both their ancestors had suffered from genocide, implying that the two are interchangeable.

Tummala-Narra (2015) has provided guidelines that implore us to integrate cultural competence into the training of psychotherapy. She, as well as other authors on this topic (e.g., Brown 2008), encourages us to more mindfully integrate race, class, disabilities, immigration, and the experiences of those raised by people who immigrated to this country, sexual orientation, and culture into our work. Tummala-Narra emphasizes increased recognition of indigenous narratives, understanding nuances of language that vary among cultures, as well as an appreciation of social oppression, in addition to self-examination regarding our own cultural narratives and world views.

As I mentioned before, humility and openness seem to be key here. These conversations can be difficult to talk about, and at times it does seem hard to feel that we can get these conversations "just right." Given the heightened awareness of these issues for some, it seems important to realize that we may make mistakes, offer incorrect assumptions, and that some of us may try to quickly assuage client fears that we will not reinjure them or alternatively that some of us could become defensive with an idea that we should not be apologetic. These concerns reflect social discussions on this topic, and I find that I often have to "feel my way through" my individual conversations with clients on topics related to differences. This includes political differences. As a way of concluding this chapter, I'll describe someone who sought me out as a therapist who had very different political views than myself. She knew about these differences because of something I had written online. I am not equating this situation with experiences of discrimination and oppression, but it is a good example of someone I thought I may never be able to help because we were so different.

Amy was in middle age and struggling with iatrogenic injuries from a major surgery she had 5 years before we met. The surgery resulted in her having mild but life-altering paralysis in her legs. At first her situation seemed one I was familiar with, having worked with many people with medical problems, including people who, unfortunately, ended up with the 1% of negative side effects described in the (often not well read) patient consent forms before surgery. Shortly after meeting her, she needed to tell me that she knew we had different political views because of something I had written online that expressed my liberal political ideas. Amy was very vocal about how she felt marginalized in the highly liberal San Francisco Bay Area because she was conservative. In addition to being in the small percentage of people who have a surgical complication, she was also in the 1% in terms of income in the United States. Money never had been and never was going to be an issue for her. Perhaps related to her social class standing, she made it clear to me all of the policies that had been implemented in a previous presidential administration were offensive to her and were designed to help the "poor people" who did not deserve it. She had a number of misconceptions and incorrect facts at her disposal from her favorite news channel and initially espoused these ideas to me, as if to convince me of my ignorance. I thought at times that perhaps I was not the best fit for her treatment, and having come from a lower-class background myself, I experienced some of her comments as gaslighting. Yet, in many ways I genuinely liked Amy. She was smart and clever and I admired her moxie. I thought it was brave on her part to confront me like she did, as it did not seem she wanted to injure me, but more that she was confused. She chose to live in one of the most liberal places in the United States after all. I wondered if this hinted at some ambivalence about her supposedly staunch views. I also did feel some empathy toward her situation. Some people in the area in which I live espouse openness toward all kinds of groups but can be stereotypical and insulting toward people who see political issues differently than they do. I told her that I felt this way and that it seemed unfair to judge anyone based on a mere label. As the therapy progressed, I started to talk with her more openly about her political perspectives. I asked questions about why she thought what she did, and at times, I tuned in to her favorite news channel to see what people were saying. If I saw someone on her channel who had more moderate views, I would note with her that I did not think all people in conservative news were extreme and that having different views should not constitute hatred. Eventually, I found that I could offer ideas about why some of her views might be mistaken, though at first I did this with acknowledgments of problems she had with some very liberal views. Ironically, I found that as someone who is wary of idealization of any person of power (a likely result of my own class background), I could agree that certain mistakes were made by the administration she railed against. This seemed to be especially helpful. At first I worried that she might construe my comments as a merging with her ideas, but actually she seemed to find relief in my words and seemed to respect a different set of ideas. She came from a family and was embedded in a community in which views of all kinds were absolute. Amy had very high ideals of herself, and I think politics was an emotional playground in which we could try on different roles and she could practice not thinking of herself and the world in an all or nothing way. I imagined her views. She imagined mine, and we found a way to not only agree on the terms of our play but to be able to see how someone we cared about could feel so differently about the same issues. There were certain things we could never see eye to eye on, but I was able to genuinely say that I could understand her point of view on some issues. These discussions took place almost in the margins of what became a treatment that dealt with coping with her ongoing disability (which had deeply shaken her foundation of ideas of perfection) and her acceptance of her body. We also discovered the need for her to be more assertive with people in her life who it seemed had always controlled her mind and told her how to think. She was from a family in which there were serious consequences for not seeing everything as others did. The treatment involved some very touching comments, for example, when she very spontaneously complained that some people in her life seemed "way too conservative for her."

To be clear, I don't mean to suggest that being conservative in a liberal area equates to the kind of traumatic events that constant expressions of hostility (racism, homophobia, transphobia, Islamophobia, fears of deportation, etc.) experienced by devalued groups. It is not equivalent, but Amy did teach me a great deal about learning to see someone else's point of view and the importance of humility. To be even more clear, it's important to state that I initially had to work very hard to find empathy toward her experience. At times with Amy, I felt mad, guarded, exposed, and wished I had never written a liberal opinion piece online, as that is something I rarely do. Yet treating Amy was one of the most gratifying clinical experiences I have ever had. I should also mention that despite our differences what seemed to make the treatment gain traction was that we had more similarities than differences. We had a very similar sense of humor; we both loved animals and nature, enjoyed cooking, and both felt worried by how our local communities had changed, to the peril of people who were disadvantaged. I learned much later in her therapy that she had experienced significant childhood abuse, not to mention several adult traumas. This was something she could not mention when we first met; at that time she described an idealized childhood. I think our working out a way to see each other's political views created an environment of mutuality that allowed her to access the reality of both her younger and adult life and the devastating ways her body had failed her. Additionally, although it is cliché to point out, it is important to remember that even with people who seem hard to understand, we are more alike than different.

Conclusion

Discriminated groups suffer mental health consequences from microaggressions and repeated encounters with bias and misunderstanding. Trauma is common in a majority of the population, but people who experience poverty, racism, religious prejudice, homophobia, transphobia, etc. often experience events that can be labeled as traumatic, particularly because of its cumulative nature. Talking about differences with clients is messy but necessary if we are to really get to know them and their experiences. As a therapist I try to let my clients guide these discussions while trying to create a space of openness and willingness to understand and learn.

References

Akhtar, S. (2011). *Immigration and acculturation: Mourning, adaptation, and the next generation*. Jason Aronson.

Altman, N. (2010). *The analyst in the inner city: Race, class and culture though a psychoanalytic lens*. New York: Routledge.

American Psychiatric Association. (1952). *Diagnostic and statistical manual of mental disorders*. Washington, DC: American Psychiatric Association.

American Psychiatric Association. (1968). *Diagnostic and statistical manual of mental disorders* (2nd ed.). Washington, DC: American Psychiatric Press.

American Psychological Association – APA. (2016). *2015 survey of psychology health service providers*. Accessed online on 22nd Jan 2020 at www.apa.org/workforce/publications/15-health-service-providers/index.aspx.

Andrews, A. R., III, Jobe-Shields, L., López, C. M., Metzger, I. W., de Arellano, M. A., Saunders, B., & Kilpatrick, D. G. (2015). Polyvictimization, income, and ethnic differences in trauma-related mental health during adolescence. *Social Psychiatry and Psychiatric Epidemiology, 50*, 1223–1234.

Aronson, J., Lustina, M. J., Good, C., Keough, K., Steele, C. M., & Brown, J. (1999). When White men can't do math: Necessary and sufficient factors in stereotype threat. *Journal of Experimental Social Psychology, 35*(1), 29–46.

Bell, C. (1997). *Public information forum*. Presented at the meetings of the American Psychoanalytic Association, Santa Monica.

Brown, L. S. (2008). *Cultural competence in trauma therapy: Beyond the flashback*. American Psychological Association.

Buchanan, N. T. (2011). Review of microaggressions in everyday life: Race, gender, and sexual orientation [Review of the book microaggressions in everyday life: Race, gender, and sexual orientation, by D. W. Sue]. *Psychology of Women Quarterly, 35*(2), 336–337.

Camodeca, M., Baiocco, R., & Posa, O. (2019). Homophobic bullying and victimization among adolescents: The role of prejudice, moral disengagement, and sexual orientation. *European Journal of Developmental Psychology, 16*(5), 503–521.

Chae, D. H., Wang, Y., Martz, C. D., Slopen, N., Yip, T., Adler, N. E., Fuller-Rowell, T. E., Lin, J., Matthews, K. A., Brody, G. H., Spears, E. C., Puterman, E., & Epel, E. S. (2020). Racial discrimination and telomere shortening among African Americans: The coronary artery risk development in young adults (CARDIA) study. *Health Psychology, 39*(3), 209–219.

Chen, E., & Matthews, K. A. (2001). Cognitive appraisal biases: An approach to understanding the relation between socioeconomic status and cardiovascular reactivity in children. *Annals of Behavioral Medicine, 23*(2), 101–111.

Cheryan, S., & Monin, B. (2005). Where are you really from?: Asian Americans and identity denial. *Journal of Personality and Social Psychology, 89*, 717–730.

Cole, E. R. (2009). Intersectionality and research in psychology. *American Psychologist, 64*(3), 170–180.

Comas-Díaz, L. (2000). An ethnopolitical approach to working with people of color. *American Psychologist, 55*, 1319–1325.

Comas-Díaz, L. (2016). Racial trauma recovery: A race-informed therapeutic approach to racial wounds. In A. N. Alvarez, C. T. H. Liang, & H. A. Neville (Eds.), *Cultural, racial, and ethnic psychology book series. The cost of racism for people of color: Contextualizing experiences of discrimination* (pp. 249–272). Washington, DC: American Psychological Association.

Drescher, J. (2015). Out of DSM: Depathologizing homosexuality. *Behavioral Sciences (Basel, Switzerland), 5*(4), 565–575.

Earnshaw, V. A., Reisner, S. L., Juvonen, J., Hatzenbuehler, M. L., Perrotti, J., & Schuster, M. A. (2017). LGBTQ bullying: Translating research to action in pediatrics. *Pediatrics, 140*(4), 1–10.

Gander, K. (2018 March 21). Is Queer an offensive slur? *Newsweek*. Accessed online on 1st Feb 2020 at https://www.newsweek.com/queer-offensive-slur-855703.

Grinberg, L., & Grinberg, R. (1989). Psychoanalytic perspectives on migration and exile. New Haven: Yale University Press.

Haines, K. M., Reyn Boyer, C., Giovanazzi, C., & Paz Galupo, M. (2018). "Not a real family": Microaggressions directed toward LGBTQ families. *Journal of Homosexuality, 65*(9), 1138–1151.

Hatch, S. L., & Dohrenwend, B. P. (2007). Distribution of traumatic and other stressful life events by race/ethnicity, gender, SES and age: A review of the research. *American Journal of Community Psychology, 40*, 313–332.

Himle, J. A., Baser, R. E., Taylor, R. J., Campbell, R. D., & Jackson, J. S. (2009). Anxiety disorders among African Americans, Blacks of Caribbean descent, and non-Hispanic Whites in the United States. *Journal of Anxiety Disorders, 23*, 578–590.

Hollingsworth, D. W., Cole, A. B., O'Keefe, V. M., Tucker, R. P., Story, C. R., & Wingate, L. R. (2017). Experiencing racial microaggressions influences suicide ideation through perceived burdensomeness in African Americans. *Journal of Counseling Psychology, 64*(1), 104–111.

Johns, M., Schmader, T., & Martens, A. (2005). Knowing is half the battle: Teaching stereotype threat as a means of improving women's math performance. *Psychological Science, 16*, 175–179.

Kaleem, J. (2019 November 12). Latinos and transgender people see big increases in hate crimes, FBI reports. *Los Angeles Times*. Accessed online on 21st Jan 2020 at https://www.latimes.com/world-nation/story/2019-11-12/hate-crimes-fbi-2018.

Kiefer, A. K., & Sekaquaptewa, D. (2007). Implicit stereotypes and women's math performance: How implicit gender-math stereotypes influence women's susceptibility to stereotype threat. *Journal of Experimental Social Psychology, 43*(5), 825–832.

Kim, E., & Kang, M. (2018). The effects of client–counselor racial matching on therapeutic outcome. *Asia Pacific Education Review, 19*(1), 103–110.

Kraus, M. W., Piff, P. K., Mendoza-Denton, R., Rheinschmidt, M. L., & Keltner, D. (2012). Social class, solipsism, and contextualism: How the rich are different from the poor. *Psychological Review, 119*, 546–572.

Leary, K. (2006). In the eye of the storm. *Psychoanalytic Quarterly, 75*, 345–363.

Leary, K. (2007). Racial insult and repair. *Psychoanalytic Dialogues, 17*(4), 539–549.

Leary, K. (2012). Race as an adaptive challenge: Working with diversity in the clinical consulting room. *Psychoanalytic Psychology, 29*, 271–291.

Leong, T. L., & Lau, A. S. L. (2001). Barriers to providing effective mental health services to Asian Americans. *Mental Health Services Research, 3*(4), 201–214.

Livingston, N. A., Berke, D. S., Ruben, M. A., Matza, A. R., & Shipherd, J. C. (2019). Experiences of trauma, discrimination, microaggressions, and minority stress among trauma-exposed LGBT veterans: Unexpected findings and unresolved service gaps. *Psychological Trauma: Theory, Research, Practice, and Policy, 11*(7), 695–703.

Loo, C. M. (2020). *PTSD among ethnic minority veterans*. U.S. Department of Veterans Affairs: PTSD: National Center for PTSD. Accessed online on 25th Jan 2020 at https://www.ptsd.va.gov/professional/treat/type/ethnic_minority_vets.asp.

Lubrano, A. (2004). *Limbo: Blue collar roots, white collar dreams*. Hobeken: Wiley.

Mark, K. M., McNamara, K. A., Gribble, R., Rhead, R., Sharp, M.-L., Stevelink, S. A. M., Schwartz, A., Castro, C., & Fear, N. T. (2019). The health and well-being of LGBTQ serving and ex-serving personnel: A narrative review. *International Review of Psychiatry, 31*(1), 75–94.

Martínez, A. D., Ruelas, L., & Granger, D. A. (2018). Household fear of deportation in relation to chronic stressors and salivary proinflammatory cytokines in Mexican-origin families post-SB 1070. *SSM–Population Health, 5*, 188–200. https://doi.org/10.1016/j.ssmph.2018.06.003.

McBride, R. S., & Schubotz, D. (2017). Living a fairy tale: The educational experiences of transgender and gender non-conforming youth in Northern Ireland. *Child Care in Practice, 23*(3), 292–304.

McWilliams, N. (2003). The educative aspects of psychoanalysis. *Psychoanalytic Psychology, 20*, 245–260.

Meyer, O., Zane, N., & Cho, Y. I. (2011). Understanding the psychological processes of the racial match effect in Asian Americans. *Journal of Counseling Psychology, 58*(3), 335–345.

Morris, M., Cooper, R. L., Ramesh, A., Tabatabai, M., Arcury, T. A., Shinn, M., et al. (2019). Training to reduce LGBTQ-related bias among medical, nursing, and dental students and providers: A systematic review. *BMC Medical Education, 19*, 325. Accessed online on 24th Jan 2020 at https://doi.org/10.1186/s12909-019-1727-3.

NAACP. (2019). *No hate: NAACP tackles hate crimes*. Accessed online on 21st Jan 2020 at https://www.naacp.org/campaigns/no-hate/.

Nadal, K. L., Griffin, K. E., Wong, Y., Hamit, S., & Rasmus, M. (2014). The impact of racial microaggressions on mental health: Counseling implications for clients of color. *Journal of Counseling & Development, 92*(1), 57–66.

Pavlova, M. A., Weber, S., Simoes, E., & Sokolov, A. N. (2014). Gender stereotype susceptibility. *PLoS One, 9*(12), e114802.

Pennington, C. R., Heim, D., Levy, A. R., & Larkin, D. T. (2016). Twenty years of stereotype threat research: A review of psychological mediators. *PLoS One, 11*(1), e0146487. https://doi.org/10.1371/journal.pone.0146487.

Pew Research Center. (2007). *Americans and social trust: Who, where and why*. Accessed online on 25th Jan 2020 at https://www.pewsocialtrends.org/2007/02/22/americans-and-social-trust-who-where-and-why/.

Pierce, C., Carew, J., Pierce-Gonzalez, D., & Willis, D. (1978). An experiment in racism: TV commercials. In C. Pierce (Ed.), *Television and education* (pp. 62–88). Beverly Hills: Sage.

Pole, N., Gone, J., & Kulkarni, M. (2008). Posttraumatic stress disorder among ethnoracial minorities in the United States. *Clinical Psychology: Science and Practice, 15*, 35–61.

Reuters. (2019 May 1). *Anti-Semitic attacks rise worldwide in 2018, led by U.S., West Europe: Study*. Accessed online on 21st Jan 2020 at https://www.reuters.com/article/us-israel-antisemitism/anti-semitic-attacks-rise-worldwide-in-2018-led-by-us-west-europe-stud.

Rivers, I. (2011). *Homophobic bullying: Research and theoretical perspectives*. Oxford: Oxford University Press.

Russell, S. T., Toomey, R. B., Ryan, C., & Diaz, R. M. (2014). Being out at school: The implications for school victimization and young adult adjustment. *American Journal of Orthopsychiatry, 84*(6), 635–643.

Samson, K., & Zaleskiewicz, T. (2020). Social class and interpersonal trust: Partner's warmth, external threats and interpretations of trust betrayal. *European Journal of Social Psychology*. Advance online publication. Accessed online on 25th Jan 2020 at https://doi.org/10.1002/ejsp.2648.

Singleton, K. (2013). Review of microaggressions in everyday life: Race, gender, and sexual orientation [Review of the book microaggressions in everyday life: Race, gender, and sexual orientation, by D. W. Sue]. *Psychoanalytic Psychology, 30*(4), 680–685.

Steele, C. M. (1997). A threat in the air: How stereotypes shape intellectual identity and performance. *American Psychologist, 52*(6), 613–629.

Steele, C. M., & Aronson, J. (1995). Stereotype threat and the intellectual test performance of African Americans. *Journal of Personality and Social Psychology, 69*(5), 797–811.

Sue, D. W. (2010). *Microaggressions in everyday life: Race, gender, and sexual orientation*. Hoboken: Wiley.

Sue, D. W., & Sue, D. (1999). *Counseling the culturally different: Theory and practice* (3rd ed.). New York: Wiley.

Sue, D. W., Bucceri, J., Lin, A. I., Nadal, K. L., & Torino, G. C. (2007). Racial microaggressions and the Asian American experience. *Cultural Diversity and Ethnic Minority Psychology, 13*(1), 72–81.

Thijs, P., Te Grotenhuis, M., & Scheepers, P. (2018). The paradox of rising ethnic prejudice in times of educational expansion and secularization in the Netherlands, 1985–2011. *Social Indicators Research, 139*(2), 653–678.

Tummala-Narra, P. (2007). Skin color and the therapeutic relationship. *Psychoanalytic Psychology, 24*, 255–270.

Tummala-Narra, P. (2015). Cultural competence as a core emphasis of psychoanalytic psychotherapy. *Psychoanalytic Psychology, 32*(2), 275–292.

Tummala-Narra, P., Sathasivam-Rueckery, N., & Sundaram, S. (2013). Voices of Asian Indian immigrants: Mental health implications. *Professional Psychology: Research and Practice, 44*(1), 1–10.

Vargas, E. D., Sanchez, G. R., & Juárez, M. (2017). Fear by association: Perceptions of anti-immigrant policy and health outcomes. *Journal of Health Politics, Policy and Law, 42*(3), 459–483.

Walker, R. L., Salami, T. K., Carter, S. E., & Flowers, K. (2014). Perceived racism and suicide ideation: Mediating role of depression but moderating role of religiosity among African American adults. *Suicide and Life-threatening Behavior, 44*(5), 548–559.

Williams, M. T., Metzger, I. W., Leins, C., & DeLapp, C. (2018). Assessing racial trauma within a DSM–5 framework: The UConn racial/ethnic stress & trauma survey. *Practice Innovations, 3*(4), 242–260.

Wong-Padoongpatt, G., Zane, N., Okazaki, S., & Saw, A. (2017). Decreases in implicit self-esteem explain the racial impact of microaggressions among Asian Americans. *Journal of Counseling Psychology, 64*(5), 574–583.

Chapter 10
Vicarious Trauma and Self-Care for the Trauma Therapist

Compassion Fatigue and the Impact of Vicarious Trauma

The concept of vicarious trauma has often been applied to healthcare and disaster relief workers as well as mental health professionals who work with severely traumatized people. Other labels capturing facets of vicarious trauma have included secondary traumatic stress and compassion fatigue. Lipsky and Burk (2009) encapsulate the burdens and impact of working with traumatized populations under the rubric "traumatic stewardship." For the purpose of this chapter, I will refer to vicarious trauma, secondary traumatic stress, and compassion fatigue somewhat interchangeably and ask for the reader's forgiveness if I leave out subtle differences and distinctions regarding these terms. Although I will describe the aforementioned concepts below, I want to focus this chapter on the emotional strains involved in this work, how there are similarities and differences in terms of how we are impacted, the importance and limitations of our empathy, and ways we can consider how to use our feelings to enhance our work (via countertransference) while taking care of ourselves.

Vicarious trauma has been described as a cumulative transformation in the therapist as a result of empathic engagement with client's traumatic material (Pearlman and Saakvitne 1995). It involves dramatic changes in the way the therapist experiences themselves, others, and the environment (Makadia et al. 2017; McCann and Pearlman 1990). A profound and poignant example of this was when Lipsky, a trauma therapist (Lipsky and Burk 2009), described hiking with her family to the top of a cliff in the Caribbean. While looking over the beautiful scene, Lipsky describes how she began to wonder how many people had jumped from the cliffs. Her thoughts then went to where a helicopter could land in the event someone needed rescuing, if there was a Level 1 trauma center nearby, etc. She realized she had been profoundly changed by the trauma work she had done with clients and how it interfered with her ability to feel enjoyment and pleasure in that otherwise beautiful and serene moment. My first experience with secondary traumatic stress

T. M. Greenberg, *Treating Complex Trauma*,
https://doi.org/10.1007/978-3-030-45285-8_10

was when I was in my early 30s. At that time I was seeing large numbers of hospitalized patients who had hematologic/oncology illnesses, such as leukemia and lymphoma. Many of my patients were young, and I often had extended relationships with them during prolonged hospitalizations for bone marrow transplants. About 40% of people I saw died from their illnesses. Prior to that I had worked with very severely traumatized populations; for many years I worked with families involved with Child Protective Services. Yet, something about the intense exposure to the hospitalized medical patients changed me and my perceptions of health. One example of this was when I was working in the hospital, I could not believe (on some level) that anyone was healthy or not at risk of getting a severe life-threatening cancer! I somehow could compartmentalize my experiences with abused children, though that hardly seems rational, as dealing with people impacted by even severe child maltreatment is much more statistically common than dealing with clients who have severe cancers. In the early years of seeing hospitalized patients, I also was hypochondriacal. A tennis injury drove me to the emergency room; though that was not necessary, but I feared something ominous. As I look back on this now, I think it had something to do with control. When I worked with abused children, I perceived I could have an influence in their lives and outcome. With many of the people I saw in the hospital whose bodies had so severely betrayed them (and this was during a time with fewer treatments available), I felt helpless in a way that was new to me. Additionally, at that age, I had not experienced the death of anyone very close to me. We all have different vulnerabilities, something I will describe later in the chapter.

Secondary traumatic stress involves therapist and other professional caregiver's behaviors and emotions resulting from knowledge about a traumatizing event experienced by significant others, including clients, and resultant symptoms of avoidance, numbing, and hyperarousal, in other words symptoms of PTSD (Figley 1983, 1995). I have also previously linked secondary traumatic stress to witnesses of serious and traumatic life-threatening illness (Greenberg 2012). Figley links secondary traumatic stress to compassion fatigue, which is the emotional residue or strain of exposure of working with those suffering from the consequences of traumatic events. He states that compassion fatigue can occur due to exposure on one case or can be due to a cumulative level of trauma (Figley 1995). Figley notes:

> Compassion Fatigue is a state experienced by those helping people or animals in distress; it is an extreme state of tension and preoccupation with the suffering of those being helped to the degree that it can create a secondary traumatic stress for the helper. We feel the feelings of our clients. We experience their fears. We dream their dreams. Eventually, we lose a certain spark of optimism, humor and hope. We tire. We aren't sick, but we aren't ourselves. (personal communication, 2020)

Trauma has been described as an emotional contagion. When we witness suffering, our experiences can parallel current or anticipated emotions in the person we are with (Miller et al. 1988). I find the idea of how we anticipate emotions especially useful. Psychodynamic clinicians have long known that there is a way that attuned therapists can feel things clients may not have access to. For example, Stern et al. (1998) describe implicit relational knowing, in which behaviors and ideas that have not been symbolically represented allow us to pick up on information about emotions and attitudes that we respond to out of conscious awareness. Consider the example of Jed:

Jed was asleep when a firefighter burst into his apartment and told him he had to leave. Flames were engulfing his multistory building. He came in with a clear narrative about what happened, told me about his trip to the emergency room (for smoke inhalation) and what his plan was to meet with his insurance agent, find a new apartment, etc. There was little emotion involved in his telling of his harrowing experience. I, on the other hand, could not think. In the first couple of sessions after the fire, we were having seemingly rational conversations, but in the split screen scenario I have described in other parts of this book, I was silently panicked. I was worried about him but not in any way I could describe. Physically, he was fine. Emotionally, he seemed well-organized and composed, perhaps too much so. In subsequent sessions, I braced myself for what I thought would be or should be intense emotion. That interfered with my ability to listen to him. And even more disturbing to me, I wondered what I would do in the same situation. I feel especially embarrassed about this part of my reaction. I wondered if I should call my insurance agent and check on how much coverage I have. Granted, I've known friends and acquaintances in this situation. In California thousands of people have lost their homes due to increases in wildfires all over the state and faulty wiring in very old buildings in the city in which I live. If I consider it rationally, thinking about fire insurance coverage is a good idea, but it was my preoccupation with my own safety, my sense of disorganization and panic which bothered me. Clearly this man was dissociative (something that was already an issue in his treatment), and as is often true with dissociative people, I filled my mind with what I thought emotions should be in Jed. This is what is sometimes perceived as an unconscious communication by a client. My panic and disorganization possibly mirrored his state of mind, but only I was aware of it. Yet, even though it has been several years, I wonder if my initial excessive attunement, if that is what it was, disrupted his ability to find me containing and helpful in the beginning of his crisis.

Figley (2002) suggests that empathy plays a key role in the development of compassion fatigue. Through empathic responding, therapists experience the emotional distress of a client, and this contributes directly to the development of compassion fatigue. Cerney (1995) goes a step further and suggests that therapists can take over the "pathology" of their clients. I am hesitant to embrace the term pathology when thinking about normal and understandable responses to trauma, but the idea is that we can absorb the suffering of the people we see. Waugaman (2009) speculates that overidentification with clients can lead to vicarious trauma. Overidentification is thought to involve an excessive involvement in the lives of others. When we do this with clients, it's difficult to think because we are excessively involved and thinking too much about our own experience. This is one way of thinking about how I felt with Jed. The line between overidentification and empathy can be murky, however.

Most of us are wired with the capacity for empathic responses. Neuroscientists have described the multiple brain activities involved in literally feeling the physical and emotional pain of others. For example, observing another person's action, pain, or affect can trigger parts of the same neural networks responsible for executing those same actions and experiencing those same feelings firsthand (Armstrong 2017). Extreme empathy that results in compassion fatigue can have both costs and benefits. Some note that compassion fatigue is characterized by physical and emotional exhaustion and a pronounced reduction in the ability to feel empathy and compassion for others (Elwood et al. 2011). Alternatively, a beautiful paper by Boulanger (2018) describes that vicarious trauma and the kind of empathy therapists are engaged in can be a therapeutic tool that allows us to connect with aspects of client's lives that we may find too difficult to think about. She described the ways she was able to overcome feelings of horror and the inability to think (which parallel those of her client) when treating a veteran who had been involved in violence against civilians while in Vietnam. Boulanger suggests this kind of immersion in another's experience may be useful or even necessary in order to be optimally helpful in working with people who have been subject to extreme trauma.

Too Much Empathy? The Risk of Burnout and Potential Consequences

As therapists we often come into the field with a predisposition for feeling empathy and an ability to understand and identify with others. As we age in this profession, many of us get better at mentalizing being able to pick up on nuances of feelings in others. I sometimes joke with my own consultant, who has been practicing for almost 40 years that he and some people in his cohort almost seem like mind-readers! For example, I'll describe a case in a few sentences, and he seems to hit exactly on what is going on and what my struggles might be. Granted, I've known him a long time, and we have a good collaborative relationship; he knows my strengths and vulnerabilities. I have wondered, though, if after seeing hundreds of clients if we develop unconscious algorithms based on subtle verbal and nonverbal cues. Or perhaps some of us simply get better at thinking because we are less rattled. On the value of growing older, psychoanalyst Joyce Slochower (2019) stated about her work as an older therapist, "I've never felt better about my work. I trust my analytic intuition; I can work deeply with far more ease than in earlier years. I have a sense of clinical wisdom that I certainly lacked as a young analyst. When I don't know what's going on, I can stay in the process without the kind of anxiety that plagues my younger supervisees" (p. 552).

Note that psychoanalysts are required to undergo several years of their own treatment; many therapists in the field have more than one extended therapy or analysis. It is often the case that many therapists who work on themselves professionally and personally get better with age. It takes less time to figure out what might be going on with a client, we feel more confident, and hopefully we have a clearer sense of the limitations of our abilities. However, particularly if we work with very traumatized people, there is a threshold to what we can endure. In thinking about colleagues who are emotionally healthy and who continue to enjoy the work well into their 70s and 80s, one commonality I've noticed is their ability to set limits. They say no to referrals that don't seem like a good fit, and they realize the limits of their emotional capacity. I recently asked one senior colleague to take on a lovely but very traumatized person in his practice, and after he politely declined he said, "I have to limit the number of clients I take, even if I am intrigued and I can maybe help them. If I don't do this, I'll feel compelled to retire." This seems like a good model.

If we are not careful, compassion fatigue, secondary traumatic stress, and vicarious trauma can take their toll. I think of burnout as the endpoint of these latter states. To put it succulently, I consider burnout as a state of mind in a therapist or clinician that makes me hesitant in referring to them, as I worry they may be too cynical or exhausted to treat someone with complex trauma. In some cases, burned out clinicians can pose a danger to the people they treat. I can't say this with certainty in all or even the majority of cases of burned out clinicians. As I'll discuss, there is limited research on this topic. We all have our struggles as trauma therapists, and many of us have complicated and difficult histories. Our backgrounds can certainly be assets when seeing people with cPTSD. But let me provide an example which will illustrate burnout and my hesitancy in providing referrals to those I imagine might be suffering too much to help others.

Dr. Johnson was a late middle-aged psychiatrist who had a reputation for treating people with trauma histories. I met Dr. Johnson when I was in training and had known him for over two decades. I always had a positive view of him, and I found him to be both psychologically astute and patient with clients, as well as very good regarding medications. I referred people to him for almost as long as I had been in practice, until several years ago. I began to notice he seemed not to take seriously some of the issues clients presented to him. For example, in one situation when a client needed a lot of attention in getting off an antidepressant (one that is notorious for complicated side effects in trying to decrease the dosage), he told the client "he did not want to deal with it." He suggested this client stay on the medication, though it was causing her unpleasant side effects and she really wanted to taper her dosage. Following that, with another client of mine, whom he and I had seen for several years and whom I'll refer to as Mary, Dr. Johnson began to talk with Mary about his personal struggles. He disclosed things to Mary that I can't repeat here, as they would provide too much identifying detail, but these were personal and family-related facts I could never imagine discussing with a client under any circumstance. Eventually, Mary's psychiatric sessions became therapy sessions for Dr. Johnson. For the most part, Mary was not actually (or consciously) disturbed about this; she loved having access to a "doctor's mind" and problems. Mary and I eventually understood it as "evening the playing field for her." Indeed, Mary had often complained that she did not know enough about me. She wanted personal details of my life, and I would not provide them in enough detail to satisfy her. I'm not opposed to self-disclosure, but Mary wanted information about me that I did not feel comfortable sharing. For example, after my mother died (and I had been away from work for a couple of weeks), she was enraged that I did not tell her the details of how she died. She looked this information up online and wanted me to talk about it with her.

Mary seemed to have no access to empathy about what it might be like for me to discuss the details of my mother's death, who had died relatively young, not to mention suddenly. As Mary had been in mental healthcare her entire life, it seemed a triumph for her that Dr. Johnson was so open, as other clinicians had been more austere and judicious regarding self-disclosure. At the same time, Mary often presented to me after sessions with Dr. Johnson seeming guilty and conflicted. She knew on some level something was wrong, and it was both exciting and overstimulating for her. In the sessions with Dr. Johnson, they were not dealing with issues she needed to be addressed which she did voice was frustrating, but Mary was more focused on the victory she felt in regard to her "getting" Dr. Johnson to talk about himself. Related to what she imagined my response might be (which in reality was a mixture of shock, horror, disgust, curiosity, and disbelief), she recited every confession and aspect of the TMI—too much information—that was inflicted and spilled out by Dr. Johnson. It appeared to be reenactment for Mary, but not one that would warrant the outrage or even concern I expected. Chronic abuse and exploitation was in Mary's background. She felt special in the relationship with Dr. Johnson in which she had become (in her mind) an important person with whom he could spill his secrets. She imagined she was the only one he talked to this way. When Dr. Johnson lost his license for reasons related to competency and a number of patient complaints which included the use of substances during sessions, Mary kept in contact with him, well after he retired. They became friends on social media. They traded emails about how they were doing. Any comments I made regarding how this relationship did not seem to be designed to suit Mary were met with ideas that I did not understand how special Dr. Johnson was. In terms of my ability to help Mary think about the actual intrusion and exploitive aspects of this psychiatric relationship, their ongoing contact rendered me helpless and useless for a long time regarding this specific issue.

Dr. Johnson and Mary's relationship illustrates the complicated trail of damage that can result from a clinician who may be suffering from burnout. In the multiple versions of Dr. Johnson I have known, with the exception of one clinician, they all started out as sought-out experts in their fields. They were highly regarded and they really seemed to help people. In fact, I have seen a number of people after a previous clinician either lost their license and/or died by suicide following boundary violations. I heard in most cases how helpful and empathic the clinician was. This is hard to explain; it may be that something tragic happened to these doctors later in their careers. It may be that certain maladaptive coping behaviors (i.e., substance abuse) worsened. We don't really know in detail what happens for many clinicians who cross the line.

Freudenberger (1974) used the term "burnout" to conceptualize a type of stress associated with feelings of exhaustion, disconnection, and self-doubt derived from emotionally involved work in helping professions. Burnout is associated with physical and emotional fatigue, depersonalization, negative feelings or attitudes toward clients and job tasks, cynicism, and decreased professional efficacy (Maslach 1986; Maslach and Jackson 1981; Schutte et al. 2000). Although it may seem to be the case, it's not clear that burnout is linked with clinician boundary violations. Much of the data is anecdotal. In fact, I looked at several articles which stated that both burnout and vicarious trauma are linked with boundary violations (e.g., Everall and Paulson 2004; Neumann and Gamble 1995), but there were no studies listed. Even experts who have written extensively on boundary violations find it hard to categorize exactly what leads to serious missteps, but burnout is not at the top of the list. Gabbard (2006) notes that therapist factors such as divorce, death of a parent or spouse, or death of a client by suicide have been associated with therapists who have committed serious boundary violations. Sexual misconduct with a client was associated with factors related to therapist dissatisfaction with their personal life such as loneliness, divorce or a relationship crisis, a parent's death, personal illness, and financial concerns (Lamb et al. 2003; Norris et al. 2003). Guy et al. (1993) reported that therapists who were substantially impacted by divorce were more likely to maintain social contact with clients after termination of the therapy.

To be clear, burnout should not be equated with impairment (Norcross and VandenBos 2018). There is not enough data to make this leap, as intuitive as it may seem. I think it's reasonable to assume that we can't be as good at our jobs if we are overwhelmed and preoccupied with our work or personal lives, however. Kahill (1988) described five core areas that impact the burnout professional, involving (1) physical symptoms, including a variety of physical complaints such as headaches, exhaustion, and gastrointestinal distress; (2) emotional symptoms involving irritability, depression, anxiety, and sense of helplessness; (3) behavioral symptoms such as aggression, callousness, cynicism, defensiveness, and substance abuse; (4) work-related symptoms such as frequent absenteeism; and (5) interpersonal problems including withdrawing from clients and overintellectualizing or dehumanizing clients. In addition, authors note that client acuity and intensity of problems that seem beyond the scope of practice for the clinician are related to burnout (Maslach and Jackson 1981). Regarding the latter, in a medical school I worked for, we used to temper expectations among medical students when working with highly traumatized clients, who were often marginally housed, with many adverse events in their recent and past histories by reminding the students that they could not provide their patients with a "life transplant." These young professionals wanted to do just that, but there was only so much that could be offered. It's difficult for anyone—though I think especially when clinicians are young—to confront injustice and tragedy. For the empathically attuned person, it can seem that just a few wrong turns and a lack of privilege can lead to disastrous life circumstance that many of us may imagine being in. Seeing trauma is terrifying as well as contagious.

Interestingly, a higher sense of trust in work settings is associated with a reduction in compassion fatigue and related symptoms (Johnson et al. 2016). One study found that bilingual Latina or Latino clinicians endorsed lower degrees of burnout relative to their monolingual, English colleagues (Teran et al. 2017). These authors described that the "lower levels of burnout among this [therapist] sample could be explained by significant pride, satisfaction, and connection to their ethnic and cultural identities" (p. 27). This study is illuminating in a number of ways but I think illustrates that we need to feel connected to professional communities as well as our clients, even in hard times, and to have a sense of overall meaning and purpose.

A measured sense of optimism and hopefulness is required in order to take care of some of the people that need our help. It seems that in order to do this work effectively in the long term, we need to hold onto aspects of hope in the resiliency of the human spirit. How to do this without being naïve, overly empathic, or overly identifying is complicated, however. Empathy is predictive of the development of vicarious trauma and compassion fatigue as are past traumas in clinicians, exposure to trauma, and distress of clients, including treating a high number of traumatized individuals (Turgoose and Maddox 2017). Some studies have not found that therapist trauma history is correlated with secondary traumatic stress, but this may have to do with the nature of the clients treated. It is possible that therapists experience more symptoms of vicarious trauma among people who have similar backgrounds. For example, in one study among mental health disaster workers following the terrorist attacks of September 11, 2001, past trauma history was not related with secondary traumatic stress (Creamer and Liddle 2005). However, heavier prior trauma caseload, less professional experience, youth, and therapist's discussion of trauma work (meaning about client's) in his or her own therapy were connected with symptoms of secondary traumatic stress, measured by reported distress, and symptoms of intrusion and avoidance. In one review of the literature, over half of therapists reported moderate symptoms of burnout (Simionato and Simpson 2018). Psychotherapist factors connected with burnout included neuroticism (defined as anxiety, depressive tendencies, negativity, hypochondriacal concerns, or, as Lahey [2009] describes it, relatively stable tendencies to respond with negative emotions to threat, frustration, or loss), rigid thinking style, excessive conscientiousness, perfectionism, overinvolvement in client problems, as well as younger age and having less work experience. Interestingly, "disagreeable" traits, such as egocentrism, less compassion, competitiveness, and high introverted traits (e.g., shyness), were also associated with increased job stress due to less interpersonal connection with clients (Simionato and Simpson 2018).

The interpersonal connection we have with clients can be a protective factor against burnout. Although I have a reputation for and a genuine comfort level with being someone who can work with those who are more challenging (which I suppose is code for angry) clients, I have found that I need to be thoughtful about whom I see. As I have gotten older, I have learned that I need to balance my practice with those who may present as challenging right at the start of therapy and with those clients who initially expect and desire more warmth and collaboration.

It's always somewhat fraught when I say (partly in jest) to younger colleagues that it took me 10 years to have a basic sense of what I was doing as a psychologist and another 20 to feel competent. At almost 30 years of treating clients, I am still learning. This is a field in which there can be a great benefit to growing older, as long as we remember we need others to help us in the challenging work that we do. I have noticed at times when I am supervising people new to the field, I sometimes can't tell if they are describing something that is really happening with the client or if this is some dynamic or issue present in themselves, or both. I think when we are new to the field, there is a risk of overidentifying with the clients that we treat. Yet, as we saw with Dr. Johnson, clinicians who are highly experienced can be subject to difficulties. Our younger colleagues may have an advantage of not succumbing to some of the pitfalls associated with being an "expert" and the potential grandiosity that can be associated with that. However, no matter our age and experience level, we can all be vulnerable to the impact of our work. This may have something to do with our own personal histories.

Therapist Vulnerabilities

Understanding what is on the minds of our clients is the key to doing this work well, and there is evidence that as therapists we are especially likely to be able to relate to our clients and their suffering. For example, one study found that almost 70% of female psychologists and 33% of male psychologists surveyed acknowledged a history of physical or sexual abuse as children and more than one-third acknowledged experiencing some form of abuse as adults (Pope and Feldman-Summers 1992). Compared with women from other professions, female mental health professionals acknowledged far greater histories of childhood abuse, parental alcoholism, and dysfunction in their family of origin and were more likely to have experienced the death of a family member or the psychiatric hospitalization of a parent (Elliott and Guy 1993). Such experiences result in therapists having served in a caregiving or parenting role as children (Racusin et al. 1981). However, having experienced the same issues as clients can be thought of as an advantage. In substance abuse treatment settings, 60–70% of treatment providers are former substance users themselves (Fialk 2019). It can be helpful for people with eating disorders to see a therapist that has struggled in a similar way but is "in recovery" (Verbeek 2018). If we think back to Chapter 1 and what makes us good clinicians, the therapeutic relationship and empathy are vital, and I do think there can be some advantage when we have experienced some of the same things as our clients. However, it seems important that we have a conscious idea of similarities, that we don't overidentify with them and risk a merging of identities and hopefully have a bit more practice working through our own difficulties. In other words, if we want to help our patients, it's important to *be a patient ourselves*, many times throughout our careers.

There is a less flattering side to some of us who enter the field. Although there can be aspects of altruism and a desire to help people, therapists have often been referred to with the mocking label as "wounded healers." Norcross and VandenBos (2018) note that sometimes therapists have been drawn into the field so that they can exercise influence or live vicariously through their clients, or more disquietingly to seek power and control. These authors state further that some therapists tend to be people with histories of being loners and of being lonely. Pope and Tabachnick (1994) found that psychologist survey respondents acknowledged depression, relationship difficulties, anxiety, and self-esteem/self-confidence problems. Of these clinicians, 60% acknowledged being significantly depressed at some time during their careers, 29% reported having felt suicidal, and nearly 4% had attempted suicide. In another study, more than 50% of psychologists reported that fears about clients negatively impacted their personal functioning, including sleep, diet, concentration, and focus (Pope and Tabachnick 1993). These worries were focused on the lack of available clinical resources to meet a client's needs, the possibility that a client would file a complaint, and on possible criticism by colleagues. Psychologists reporting work or personal distress acknowledged that their distress adversely impacted the quality of service provided to clients, with 5% reporting that the care they provided was inadequate, and in another sample almost 60% of the practicing psychologists surveyed acknowledged working when too distressed to be effective (Guy et al. 1989; Pope et al. 1987).

I realize that some of this research may be daunting. We all have complicated reasons we chose this career. I think it's important that we consider our assets and limitations and how these contributed to our choice in becoming psychotherapists. I wonder how much this happens, however. Thinking about my own therapies in which I have been a patient, I have noticed a pregnant silence when bringing up this topic. I have felt that my therapists and some colleagues don't want to describe or think about the fact that we might have mixed motives for our career choice. More worrisome to me has been an attitude of colleagues who idealize being a therapist, as if we have some special knowledge or power. This just does not seem helpful. Surely we learn certain skills and if we get good at them, we can help people. But this does not mean we can help everyone, and it definitely does not mean we necessarily have special advantages in our private lives. Although we are in a field in which people can and do idealize us, it's important to hold in mind the reality that we are far from perfect.

It's helpful to focus on the ways our own experiences can be useful to clients, as long as we can provide good boundaries and avoid becoming merged with them. Whenever I have a client in which I fear the latter could happen, I seek out consultation with a trusted colleague and with whom I can be open about my own vulnerabilities as a therapist. And of course our own personal therapies help. In order to be effective, we need to have dealt with our own personal issues, including the number of different reasons we chose this profession.

It also goes without saying that for those of us in private practice and even some community settings, there is a financial investment in keeping people in therapy. Whether it's what we get paid per hour or even RVU systems which is an example of rewarding clinician productivity, we may be incentivized to keep people in treatment when we are not a good fit for them. Once I became more comfortable with this inherent and complicated risk of being in private practice, I became much more assertive in my own thinking and even talking with clients about the importance of us both feeling that I am the right person to treat them. There is also an ethical obligation to protect clients if we do not feel we are the right fit. This is something I discuss in the first month or so of seeing someone in which the therapy has not gained a comfort level or traction that I would expect. I'm not talking here about someone who is guarded because of cPTSD, as that is something I can usually speak to early on. Clients in this situation can often acknowledge they are hesitant, but have a sense of being connected to me, nevertheless. They might be guarded with me about some topics but not all aspects of conversation. For people who are not the right fit, I am thinking about clients where it is clear that my personality does not seem to be a good match. For example, I use humor a lot with the people I see and sometimes clients find this annoying. Of course I can back this off if I sense I am bothering someone or they tell me about it. Whatever the reason, not everyone likes me and that is perfectly fine. Clients deserve therapy with someone they can like and connect with. It's a protective factor when things get difficult in treatment. Empathy is more than an intellectual exercise; it means getting to really know someone's internal experience if they allow that. If it seems I might have difficulty with being a match for someone, there are many talented people I can refer to. My point here is that we all have limitations and vulnerabilities and it's important we can learn what these are so we can help clients find people with whom they might match better.

Dealing with difficult emotions is crucial to doing this work, but this starts with us knowing ourselves and being open to the ways we can't help everyone. Once we decide we can help people with complex trauma histories, when we think we can be the right fit, we need to be prepared to deal with countertransference and related emotions that can guide us in helping them.

Countertransference and the Importance of Therapist's Emotions

Our emotions and our ability to acknowledge them to ourselves, within our own consultation/supervision, and to use our feelings as information with our clients are crucial to being effective in our work with people who have survived trauma. Countertransference applies to the feelings we have as therapists in response to the dynamics present in our clients. A definition of countertransference is that it refers to feelings in our clients, which get stirred up in the therapist. These feelings are thought to be an identification with the client's unconscious material or wishes or with a client's internal self-representation that takes place in a relational context (Carnochan 2001; Kernberg 1988). Our reactions when we are with people we are treating matter because our thoughts and feelings not only lie at the heart of a relational and meaningful encounter but can also provide important clues as to what our clients are experiencing emotionally. In other words, our emotional responses to them help identify what they are experiencing, consciously and unconsciously. As a simple example of this, I might find myself feeling angry with a client while listening to her. One hypothesis regarding this feeling of anger is that, in fact, the client is angry but is unable to be aware of it. The notion of projective identification is one way to explain this. Klein (1975) postulated that unconscious anger gets located in the therapist as an early form of communication. Far from being a magical process in which emotions "get put into" the other, Gabbard (2000) has described this process as a "nudge," in which clients unconsciously urge the therapist to be cast in a role of some important person from their past. In the case of my client, my anger may not only be reflective of her anger toward myself but also an expression that she expects that others will be angry with her. I also think that as we get more experienced in doing this work, therapists just get incredibly good at anticipating the feelings clients will have as I described previously in this chapter. In fact, as I have gotten older, I don't really find the aforementioned ideas of Klein or Gabbard to be as compelling as I once did. While I do think it's true that some clients are perhaps better communicators of thoughts and feelings that are out of awareness, I think more experienced clinicians develop unconscious, complex algorithms based on hundreds of people seen and these experienced therapists can just surmise things more quickly than some younger colleagues.

The value in contemporary ideas on countertransference is an increased appreciation of the multiple forms of communication that we are all capable of. Countertransference feelings are particularly useful in working with clients who have difficulty symbolizing. Especially in more vulnerable populations, which include clients with complex PTSD, our emotional responses can help us to acknowledge the extent of vulnerability and fear often present in our clients but which cannot always be verbalized. A large part of the work is the holding and containing of these feelings. I emphasize this because I feel strongly that the majority of things we feel in terms of complicated emotions should be worked through in our own minds (and with the help of colleagues) and rarely spoken when we are with clients. I use my feelings or even dreams about my clients all the time in my own supervision and in my own thinking about clients, but this is to get a sense of what may be going on, not something I need to say to them. To be clear, I am extremely talkative as a therapist, and I voice thoughts and associations, but regarding feelings, I tend to keep those private. It's always a huge risk when we discuss our personal feelings with clients, and I think ill-advised with most people who have cPTSD, especially when we are getting to know someone.

Working with people with cPTSD causes us to face our own vulnerability. In order to not merge with our clients or defensively distance ourselves, we need a heightened awareness of our emotional responses to our clients, as well as an awareness of our feelings about our own histories, including our own traumas. This is not easy to do. And in order to help our traumatized clients, we need to be able to handle all of the complicated feelings our clients bring up, especially the negative feelings we need to bear.

Winnicott (1949) provided acknowledgment of the fact that we can sometimes feel hatred or anger toward our clients. He stated that therapists should not deny that hatred or other intense feelings exist and that denying hatred in particular can lead to "therapy that is adapted to the needs of the therapist rather than to the needs of the patient" (Winnicott 1949, p. 74). Of course, it's difficult to acknowledge intense negative feelings toward a client. But if we do not deal with them, we and our clients pay the price. This involves managing our feelings toward individual clients as well as the work in general. Thorne (1989) suggested that therapists who do not acknowledge the difficult and at times grueling nature of our work are mendacious, deluded, or incompetent.

Our negative feelings can inform our work and need to be felt in order to help mentalize what our clients are going through. At the same time, if we are too overwhelmed with negative feelings, we lose our ability to be truly empathic. I've noticed that instead of wading through difficult feelings, sometimes therapists can become super caretakers, which has its own set of costs.

Over-responsibility and the Trappings of the Super Therapist

Becoming compulsive about caretaking is likely a way therapists try to avoid overwhelming feelings such as anger, grief, sadness, and loss. Some therapists may suffer from the avoidance symptoms observed in PTSD: they cut off their feelings and become focused on survival—the survival of the people they are caring for and their own survival through the attempt to eliminate difficult feelings. Norcross and VandenBos (2018) suggest that some individuals are drawn to the work of being a therapist guided by a belief that their caring has special or curative powers. This is indeed problematic. However, in many cases, I tend to think of the super therapist as someone who also may have evolved into this role as a way to protect themselves from the intense feelings involved in this work. Paradoxically, it can start through what is often required to become really good at clinical work. Conscientious clinicians get a lot of training; they seek out supervision, their own therapy, consultation groups and classes, read articles to stay abreast of the literature, etc. This is all in addition to seeing clients. Such motivated clinicians do tend to work a lot, as all of the aforementioned activities are non-billable time and/or we pay for them. Most of us do need to work in order to pay our bills, and the extensive hours of professional development and clinical hours add up quickly.

Additionally, being with clients involves a lot of isolation, particularly when we are in private practice. We don't have people to regularly check in with unless we work to make that happen. Confidentiality can be an ongoing burden. In addition to all of the emotions we hold, we also steal away secrets that we can't just talk to anyone about. A common example of how this strain can manifest is when someone posts too much information about a client situation on listservs. I am on a number of these lists, and even though we are frequently reminded to keep identifying details out of clinical descriptions when asking for referrals, for example, there seem to be inevitable lapses. It's as if our secrets spill out and way too much identifying detail can be revealed. Spiegel (1990) described the tendency of therapists to split off the emotional impact of their work from the rest of their life. This seems reasonable; we can't really come home and unload our day onto our family members without risking confidentiality, not to mention burdening them with a host of intense emotions that are hard to understand out of context. Interestingly, there is a body of research within experimental psychology that suggests that holding secrets carries a literal physical burden. For example, one study found that the more burdensome the secret and the more thought devoted to it, people perceived literal distances to be farther, felt physical tasks would require more effort, and were less likely to help others with physical activities. In other words, secret-keepers experience certain ideas similar to carrying physical weight (Slepian et al. 2012). As far as

I know, this line of research has not looked at the burdens of secrets therapists hold, but confidentiality and the related isolation add further demands on us. The "one-way intimacy" (Norcross and VandenBos 2018) required of our work involves a number of losses. If we stop and think about it, it is a lot to deal with. When a therapist lapses into super therapist mode, they are often preventing themselves from feeling.

I think that therapists who work all of the time, avoid vacations, see too many clients in one day, and don't allow realistic breaks between sessions (such as going back to back, which negates biological needs for snacks, water, and using the bathroom) are avoiding thinking about their own needs. They can get caught up in a cycle of caretaking in which the only thing they want to think about is what is on the minds of others. I think that these therapists have a wish that once they are not working, they can fold back into a gratifying emotional life, but I wonder how much this happens. Particularly these days, we all have phones and devices that can alert us to any kind of contact related to our work. How realistic is it that some of us really take time away?

Halevi and Idisis (2018) found that therapists with a better differentiated sense of self were less likely to develop symptoms of secondary traumatic stress. MacKay (2017) notes that over-responsibility is linked with therapist burnout and secondary traumatic stress. As professional caretakers, we might believe that we can offer better support than anyone else. As some therapists become well known or develop a good reputation for dealing with certain kinds of clients, a kind of compulsive need to work seems to take over for some. Certainly in private practice, there are worries if referrals will keep coming. I've sometimes wondered if people who work excessively are worried that if they slow down, their referrals might as well. Further it may be that the more experienced we become, the more complicated and traumatized clients come our way. This is a compliment and a marker of success. But how much work is too much? Just because we are good at something does not mean we should not allow ourselves to say no to referrals or to stop and think what we want our professional lives to look like. For trauma therapists who become compulsive around the work, they can lose their identity as a person and become only a caretaker. In my experience with a number of health professionals, nothing good seems to come from that.

Therapist Self-Care

Norcross (2000) noted the lack of research and writing on therapist self-care and described it as "unsettling." I will describe some of the ways that I have thought about self-care while realizing that this issue is both personal and individualized. I imagine most clinicians have thought about this a lot, and I do not want to suggest my ideas are superior. They are not. I'll describe what has worked for me, often through modeling what I have observed in senior colleagues who seem to fare well in doing this work long term. However, an excellent book on this topic is one I have referenced several times throughout this chapter. *Leaving It at the Office* (2nd Ed. Norcross and VandenBos 2018) is a stellar resource. And while its parroted things I have gleaned along the way in my career and will describe below, the book provides longer discussions of many things that I described more briefly in this chapter.

The ways we can feel helpless with our clients are a normal part of what witnesses to suffering experience. Compassion fatigue and the development of secondary traumatic stress symptoms may be unavoidable. However, therapists can help themselves by monitoring the tendency toward avoidance of feelings and keeping an eye on a sense of over-responsibility. We bear a great deal of trauma in our work, but by managing our emotions and staying aware of our own symptoms, we can ultimately gain more control. Trauma can remind us not only of how much we need other people to treat us well but also of our own vulnerabilities and the times in our lives in which others put their needs before ours. For some of us, thoughts of our own vulnerability can be terrifying. This seems normal and is a risk inherent in our work and the injured parts of us we bring into our careers.

What I have found most helpful for me in treating traumatized clients is allowing myself to feel the intense emotionality and grief that I encounter in the work. I don't do this with clients. Although I may feel intense emotions when I am with them and I allow myself to look sad or even slightly tearful at times, a full expression of emotion is something I keep out of the room. It took me a long time to learn how to modulate my emotions with traumatized persons; I used to shut off and overintellectualize in order to move away from intense feelings. I get consultation once a week, and I've seen the same consultant for several years, and with him I can express the full extent of my emotions about my clients. I think when I was younger I used to feel that if I had strong emotions about a client, then I must be doing something wrong. I don't feel this way anymore. In fact, one colleague I really admire mentioned she thinks in some ways we become more emotional as the years go on because we can handle the intensity of emotions brought on in the course of our work. When I deal with my feelings about my clients and the trauma they have been or are being subjected to, I make sure I have safe outlets. For example, I cry sometimes when I talk with my consultant about a particularly sad, tragic, and unfair clinical set of circumstances involving a client. These are sometimes cases when I may be identifying with someone too much and I want to think through my vulnerabilities as well as the reality of a tragic situation. I also talk with my consultant when I feel angry at a client and I can't quite make sense of it. Choi (2011) found that supportive supervision can lower vicarious traumatization levels. For those working in institutions, a high amount of empowerment within the organization, defined by a sense of meaning, self-efficacy, and self-determination and a sense of agency regarding being able to influence outcomes within their organization, leads to lower levels of traumatic stress (Choi 2017). I can feel alone sometimes regarding the intensity of feelings I need to hold, and so my own supervision and access to a professional community, including people I can refer to, are vital to my sense of professional well-being.

In addition to acknowledging how we feel and developing a caring professional community, it is important to manage vicarious trauma and compassion fatigue by setting boundaries. Limits and boundaries allow us to stay involved without having to experience the same thing as our clients. When we care for our clients and our work, it can be easy to feel the same things they do. This is the true root of empathic communication. However, it is important to avoid empathic merging. Boundaries are protective. In my practice, I allow myself time between sessions to reset after therapeutic hours that involve a lot of strong emotions. I allow 10–15 minutes between clients. I will up the time between sessions with people who require a lot of me emotionally. For example, I may see someone who is very complicated before lunch. With clients who are especially dissociative, I make sure they are spaced out during all days of the week, and I never see two clients in a row who experience a lot of dissociative processes. Others may be heartier, but I personally need more time to emotionally digest after seeing people who manifest these kinds of cPTSD symptoms. I have found this increases my ability to think and be more present with all of the clients I see in a day.

I use ideas regarding boundaries to inform how I spend my time away from work. I tend to take a couple vacations a year, at least. And if I find I am thinking too much about work, I try to sort this out myself (by thinking about what emotions are being brought up by the client or clients I am preoccupied with), or I bring it up in consultation. When that has not helped, I get back into therapy.

Regarding out of session contacts, I explain in writing in my consent form and verbally what the limits of emails and texting are and what constitutes an emergency. I personally do not mind emails that might go into some detail about something that is going on as long as clients understand the inherent confidentiality limitations associated with electronic communications. But I explain there may be a delay in how quickly I get back to them. I also let clients know that if I am busy, they may not get a detailed response from me but that I will be able to think about their email. I realize some colleagues have more stringent limits regarding emails, but I do find that sometimes there can be useful information that can be expressed in writing in between sessions. I explain to clients that texting should be reserved for practice-related details, like appointment changes. If something acute is going on that needs to be addressed, I let people know they can contact me to set up a phone appointment if contact is needed before the next session. In an emergency, I will do this on the same day, but I find it containing for both myself and clients to maintain this level of control regarding contact outside of in-person meetings.

Other than dealing with my emotions, the other simple practice that has helped me more than anything is to not have my phone with me all of the time. I explain to my clients that when I am covering my practice (which is most of the time if I am not on vacation), I will be unavailable from my phone for a few hours at a time. I will check it, but not every minute. I don't look at my phone (meaning email, texts, or calls) when I am exercising, when I am running errands, when I am in nature (which is mostly at the beach with my dogs), or when I am with friends or family for meals. For me, I can get too distracted by my phone, and this interferes when I am trying to connect with people outside of work. My phone keeps me from being in the present moment, and so I had to develop boundaries around it. Others may need something different, but this is what works for me.

Not surprisingly, mindfulness is found to be protective of compassion fatigue (Turgoose and Maddox 2017). Mindfulness integrates several self-care strategies that impact the body, provides boundaries between our clients and ourselves, and helps to quiet our own anxious and unquiet minds (Norcross and VandenBos 2018). Formal mindfulness can be a struggle, but it starts with trying to be present in moments both inside and outside of work. It should be noted that modern mindfulness apps have meditations as short as 3 minutes, so the truly mindfully motivated among us could even practice this between clients. I have a ways to go in terms of this admirable goal, but I try to do an informal body scan at least once a day to notice what is going on in my body and where I am tense. Other helpful mindfulness strategies involve paying attention to our breathing when we are with clients and grounding ourselves in our bodies.

In order to survive the trauma in our work, we need good relationships outside of the office. As gratifying as our work can be, we need others where we can have more than one-way intimacy. I think an important aspect of close interpersonal relationships outside of work is that we can be involved with people who don't idealize us or see us as an expert and who hold us to account as normal people who have good and negative aspects. Our relationships are not only grounding, they feed us, which is extremely important when we spend our professional lives taking care of others.

Conclusion

As gratifying as it is, there is a price we pay for doing this work. It is stressful and demanding, and if we are not careful, we can become too traumatized to think with people who desperately need our help. Although it is a lot of work to become skilled in our fields, it's important that we avoid the trappings of being a super therapist. Our vulnerabilities are as important as our strengths, and we should recognize both, including how our own backgrounds may make us especially empathic but also at risk in certain clinical situations. We teach assertiveness and self-care to our clients, but this can feel empty and unrewarding if we fail to set limits ourselves. Thinking seriously about our self-care, including engaging in our own therapy and supervision, is crucial to aging well when working with traumatized populations. Our work can be lonely and isolating. We need to develop a professional community with people who can remind us of the challenges and rewards of this work and personal relationships with people with whom we can be ourselves, with the reality of imperfect selves exposed. We need safety as much as our clients do and we have to work hard to achieve that. And though I will say this again in my suggested interventions below, perhaps the best thing we can do to preserve ourselves in our line of work is this: When things are going well at work, when you really can tell you have helped someone, stop and allow yourself to recognize how amazing it is that you've probably overcome something difficult in order for you to help someone else in need.

Self-Care Interventions

- Be thoughtful about caseload. For example, if certain clients pose challenges, limit the numbers of these kinds of clients if possible.
- Really take time to think about the structure of your day if you have the luxury of controlling it.
- If certain clients are triggering, space them throughout the week and/or allow longer breaks after challenging clients.
- Take real breaks from work. Not just vacations but times when clients are not being thought about.
- If you suddenly become "famous" in your community and everyone wants to refer to you, take it with a grain of salt. There are many talented clinicians around.
- It's nice to be successful, but long-term success involves a measured pace, not a hurried one.
- Good therapists will always have referrals. Saying no to referrals won't close your practice.
- Engage in activities that don't have to do with client care.
- Develop creative pursuits. Therapists often are very talented at many kinds of artistic endeavors.
- Exercise. It's the most powerful treatment for depression and very helpful for anxiety and stress.
- Consider spending time in nature, even if it's just having lunch in a park on a nice day.
- Consider frequent consultation, either individually or in a group.
- Consider seeking a therapist, even if you've had therapy before.
- If you start to feel overly responsible, can't stop thinking about work, then really consider getting back into therapy.
- Nurture relationships, whether with a partner or other family and friends.
- Animals are amazing healers. If you like animals, consider getting a pet if you don't already have one. Or find ways to see them in nature or volunteer in organizations that care for animals.
- Spend time thinking about the kinds of people who can take care of you when you need it.
- Many of us in the field often have one-sided relationships. Find people who need you but whom you can need.
- If meditation works for you, do it often.
- Think about your relationship with electronic devices and social media. Both can lead to compulsive behaviors and lower quality of life.
- Communicate to clients right away what your limits are regarding out of office contact. It's more than important for risk management and clinical reasons; it relates to thinking about the realities of your availability and what you are comfortable with.
- When things are going well at work, when you really can tell you have helped someone, stop and allow yourself to recognize how amazing it is that you've probably overcome something difficult in order for you to help someone else in need.

References

Armstrong, K. (2017, December 29). 'I feel your pain:' The neuroscience of empathy. *Association of Psychological Science.* Accessed online on 3rd Feb 2020 at https://www.psychologicalscience.org/observer/i-feel-your-pain-the-neuroscience-of-empathy.

Boulanger, G. (2018). When is vicarious trauma a necessary therapeutic tool? *Psychoanalytic Psychology, 35*(1), 60–69.

Carnochan, P. G. M. (2001). *Looking for ground: Countertransference and the problem of value in psychoanalysis* (Relational perspectives book series). Hillsdale: The Analytic Press.

Cerney, M. S. (1995). Treating the "heroic treaters". In C. R. Figley (Ed.), *Brunner/Mazel psychological stress series, no. 23. Compassion fatigue: Coping with secondary traumatic stress disorder in those who treat the traumatized* (pp. 131–149). New York: Brunner/Mazel.

Choi, G.-Y. (2011). Organizational impacts on the secondary traumatic stress of social workers assisting family violence or sexual assault survivors. *Administration in Social Work, 35*(3), 225–242.

Choi, G.-Y. (2017). Secondary traumatic stress and empowerment among social workers working with family violence or sexual assault survivors. *Journal of Social Work, 17*(3), 358–378. https://doi.org/10.1177/1468017316640194.

Creamer, T. L., & Liddle, B. J. (2005). Secondary traumatic stress among disaster mental health workers responding to the September 11 attacks. *Journal of Traumatic Stress, 18*, 89–96.

Elliott, D. M., & Guy, J. D. (1993). Mental health professionals versus non-mental health professionals: Childhood trauma and adult functioning. *Professional Psychology: Research and Practice, 24*, 83–90.

Elwood, L. S., Mott, J., Lohr, J. M., & Galovski, T. E. (2011). Secondary trauma symptoms in clinicians: A critical review of the construct, specificity, and implications for trauma-focused treatment. *Clinical Psychology Review, 31*, 25–36.

Everall, R. D., & Paulson, B. L. (2004). Burnout and secondary traumatic stress: Impact on ethical behaviour. *Canadian Journal of Counselling, 38*(1), 25–35.

Fialk, A. (2019). *Wounded versus non-wounded healers and substance abuse treatment: Countertransference considerations.* Dissertation Abstracts International Section A: Humanities and Social Sciences, 80(1–A(E)).

Figley, C. R. (1983). Catastrophe: An overview of family reactions. In C. R. Figley & H. I. McHubblin (Eds.), *Stress and the family* (Coping with catastrophe) (Vol. 2, pp. 3–20). New York: Brunner/Mazel.

Figley, C. R. (Ed.). (1995). *Brunner/Mazel psychological stress series, no. 23. Compassion fatigue: Coping with secondary traumatic stress disorder in those who treat the traumatized.* New York: Brunner/Mazel.

Figley, C. R. (2002). Compassion fatigue: Psychotherapists' chronic lack of self-care. *Journal of Clinical Psychology, 58*, 1433–1441.

Freudenberger, H. J. (1974). Staff burnout-out. *Journal of Social Issues, 30*, 156–165.

Gabbard, G. (2000). The integration of psychoanalytic and neuroscientific thought in the realm of personality. In J. Sandler, R. Michels, & P. Fonagy (Eds.), *Changing ideas in a changing world: The revolution in psychoanalysis* (pp. 155–162). London: Karnac.

Gabbard, G. (2006). Sexual and nonsexual boundary violations in psychoanalysis and psychotherapy. In S. Akhtar (Ed.), *Interpersonal boundaries: Variations and violations* (pp. 39–48). Oxford: Jason Aronson.

Greenberg, T. M. (2012). *When someone you love has a chronic illness.* Springville Utah: Cedar Fort/Plain Sight Publishing.

Guy, J. D., Poelstra, P. L., & Stark, M. J. (1989). Personal distress and therapeutic effectiveness: National survey of psychologists practicing psychotherapy. *Professional Psychology: Research and Practice, 20*(1), 48–50.

Guy, J. D., French, R. J., Poelstra, P. L., & Brown, C. K. (1993). Therapeutic terminations: How psychotherapists say good-bye. *Psychotherapy in Private Practice, 12*(2), 73–82.

Halevi, E., & Idisis, Y. (2018). Who helps the helper? Differentiation of self as an indicator for resisting vicarious traumatization. *Psychological Trauma: Theory, Research, Practice, and Policy, 10*(6), 698–705.

Johnson, H., Worthington, R., Gredecki, N., & Wilks-Riley, F. R. (2016). The relationship between trust in work colleagues, impact of boundary violations and burnout among staff within a forensic psychiatric service. *Journal of Forensic Practice, 18*(1), 64–75.

Kahill, S. (1988). Interventions for burnout in the helping professions: A review of the empirical evidence. *Canadian Journal of Counselling, 22*(3), 162–169.

Kernberg, O. F. (1988). Object relations theory in clinical practice. *Psychoanalytic Quarterly, 57*, 481–504.

Klein, M. (1975). In M. Masud & R. Khan (Eds.), *Envy and gratitude and other works 1946–1963*. London: The Hogarth.

Lahey, B. B. (2009). Public health significance of neuroticism. *American Psychologist, 64*(4), 241–256.

Lamb, D. H., Catanzaro, S. J., & Moorman, A. S. (2003). Psychologists reflect on their sexual relationships with clients, supervisees, and students: Occurrence, impact, rationales and collegial intervention. *Professional Psychology: Research and Practice, 34*(1), 102–107.

Lipsky, L. V. D., & Burk, C. (2009). *Trauma stewardship*. San Francisco: Berrett-Koehler Publishers.

MacKay, L. M. (2017). Differentiation of self: Enhancing therapist resilience when working with relational trauma. *Australian and New Zealand Journal of Family Therapy, 38*(4), 637–656.

Makadia, R., Sabin-Farrell, R., & Turpin, G. (2017). Indirect exposure to client trauma and the impact on trainee clinical psychologists: Secondary traumatic stress or vicarious traumatization? *Clinical Psychology & Psychotherapy, 24*(5), 1059–1068.

Maslach, C. (1986). *Maslach burnout inventory manual* (3rd ed.). Palo Alto: Consulting Psychologists Press.

Maslach, C., & Jackson, S. E. (1981). The measurement of experienced burnout. *Journal of Organizational Behavior, 2*, 99–113.

McCann, I. L., & Pearlman, L. A. (1990). Vicarious traumatization: A framework for understanding the psychological effects of working with victims. *Journal of Traumatic Stress, 3*(1), 131–149.

Miller, K. I., Stiff, J. B., & Ellis, B. H. (1988). Communication and empathy as precursors to burnout among human service workers. *Communication Monographs, 55*(3), 250–265.

Neumann, D. A., & Gamble, S. J. (1995). Issues in the professional development of psychotherapists: Countertransference and vicarious traumatization in the new trauma therapist. *Psychotherapy: Theory, Research, Practice, Training, 32*(2), 341–347.

Norcross, J. C. (2000). Psychotherapist self-care: Practitioner-tested, research-informed strategies. *Professional Psychology: Research and Practice, 31*(6), 710–713.

Norcross, J. C., & VandenBos, G. R. (2018). *Leaving it at the office: A guide to psychotherapist self-care* (2nd ed.). New York: Guilford Press.

Norris, D. M., Gutheil, T. G., & Strasburger, L. H. (2003). This couldn't happen to me: Boundary problems and sexual misconduct in the psychotherapy relationship. *Psychiatric Services, 54*, 517–522.

Pearlman, L. A., & Saakvitne, K. W. (1995). *Trauma and the therapist: Countertransference and vicarious traumatization in psychotherapy with incest survivors*. New York: Norton.

Pope, K. S., & Feldman-Summers, S. (1992). National survey of psychologists' sexual and physical abuse history and their evaluation of training and competence in these areas. *Professional Psychology: Research and Practice, 23*, 353–361.

Pope, K. S., & Tabachnick, B. G. (1993). Therapists' anger, hate, fear, and sexual feelings: National survey of therapist responses, client characteristics, critical events, formal complaints, and training. *Professional Psychology: Research and Practice, 24*, 142–152.

Pope, K. S., & Tabachnick, B. G. (1994). Therapists as patients: A national survey of psychologists' experiences, problems, and beliefs. *Professional Psychology: Research and Practice, 25*, 247–258.

Pope, K. S., Tabachnick, B. G., & Keith-Spiegel, P. (1987). Ethics of practice: The beliefs and behaviors of psychologists as therapists. *American Psychologist, 42*, 993–1006.

Racusin, G. R., Abramowitz, S. I., & Winter, W. D. (1981). Becoming a therapist: Family dynamics and career choice. *Professional Psychology, 12*(2), 271–279. https://doi.org/10.1037/0735-7028.12.2.271.

Schutte, N., Toppinen, S., Kalimo, R., & Schaufeli, W. (2000). The factorial validity of the Maslach Burnout Inventory-General Survey (MBI-GS) across occupational groups and nations. *Journal of Occupational and Organizational Psychology, 73*, 53–66.

Simionato, G. K., & Simpson, S. (2018). Personal risk factors associated with burnout among psychotherapists: A systematic review of the literature. *Journal of Clinical Psychology, 74*(9), 1431–1456.

Slepian, M. L., Masicampo, E. J., Toosi, N. R., & Ambady, N. (2012). The physical burdens of secrecy. *Journal of Experimental Psychology: General, 141*(4), 619–624.

Slochower, J. (2019). Getting better all the time? *Psychoanalytic Dialogues, 29*(5), 548–559.

Spiegel, P. B. (1990). Confidentiality endangered under some circumstances without special management. *Psychotherapy: Theory, Research, Practice, Training, 27*(4), 636–643.

Stern, D. N., Sander, L. W., Nahum, J. P., Harrison, A. M., Lyons-Ruth, K., Morgan, A. C., The Process of Change Study Group, et al. (1998). Non-interpretive mechanisms in psychoanalytic therapy. The 'something more' than interpretation. *The International Journal of Psychoanalysis, 79*, 903–921.

Teran, V. G., Fuentes, M. A., Atallah, D. G., & Yang, Y. (2017). Risk and protective factors impacting burnout in bilingual, Latina/o clinicians: An exploratory study. *Professional Psychology: Research and Practice, 48*(1), 22–29.

Thorne, B. (1989). The blessing and curse of empathy. In W. Dryden & L. Spurling (Eds.), *On becoming a psychotherapist* (pp. 53–68). London: Routledge.

Turgoose, D., & Maddox, L. (2017). Predictors of compassion fatigue in mental health professionals: A narrative review. *Traumatology, 23*(2), 172–185.

Verbeek, L. (2018). 'The recovered therapist': Working with body image disturbance and eating disorders—Researching the countertransference. In P. Valerio (Ed.), *Introduction to countertransference in therapeutic practice: A myriad of mirrors* (pp. 185–199). Routledge/Taylor & Francis Group.

Winnicott, D. W. (1949). Hate in the counter-transference. *International Journal of Psychoanalysis, 30*, 69–74.

Waugaman, R. M. (2009). Book review: Coasting in the countertransference: Conflicts of self interest between analyst and patient. By Irwin Hirsch. *Journal of the American Psychoanalytic Association, 57*, 507–511.

Index

T. M. Greenberg, *Treating Complex Trauma*,
https://doi.org/10.1007/978-3-030-45285-8

S

T

V

GPSR Compliance
The European Union's (EU) General Product Safety Regulation (GPSR) is a set of rules that requires consumer products to be safe and our obligations to ensure this.

If you have any concerns about our products, you can contact us on

ProductSafety@springernature.com

In case Publisher is established outside the EU, the EU authorized representative is:

Springer Nature Customer Service Center GmbH
Europaplatz 3
69115 Heidelberg, Germany

www.ingramcontent.com/pod-product-compliance
Lightning Source LLC
Chambersburg PA
CBHW071732061025
33644CB00003B/130
* 9 7 8 3 0 3 0 4 5 2 8 4 1 *